# Take Control of Your Tinnitus

## Here's How

Seventh Edition

Neil G. Bauman, Ph.D.

Integrity First Publications

Lynden, WA

http://www.IntegrityFirstPublications.com

*Take Control of Your Tinnitus*
*—Here's How*

*Seventh Edition*

Another **Integrity First** book in the series:

*Everything You Wanted to Know About Your Hearing Loss But Were Afraid to Ask*
*(Because You Knew You Wouldn't Hear the Answers Anyway!)*



ISBN 978-1-935939-21-4



Integrity First Publications
1013 Ridgeway Drive,
Lynden, WA 98264-1057
Phone: (360) 778-1266
FAX: (360) 389-5226
Email: info@IntegrityFirstPublications.com
Website: http://IntegrityFirstPublications.com

*Printed in the United States of America*

# Warning—Disclaimer

This book is for your education and reference. It is neither a medical manual nor a guide to self-treatment for medical problems. Do not construe this book as giving personal medical advice or instruction. The author is not a medical doctor and neither prescribes treatment nor treats medical problems and does not intend that you attempt to do so either. If you suspect that you have a medical problem related to your ears, seek competent professional medical help. Use the information in this book to help you make informed decisions, not as a substitute for any treatment that your doctor may have prescribed for you.

The information and opinions expressed in this book are the result of careful research. They are believed to be accurate and sound, based on the best judgment available to the author. If you fail to consult appropriate health professionals, you assume the risk of any injuries. Neither Integrity First Publications, the Center for Hearing Loss Help, nor the author assumes any responsibility for damages or losses incurred as a result of using the information in this book, nor for any errors or omissions. It is the responsibility of each reader to exercise good judgment in using any information contained in this book.

# Contents

# About the Author

Neil G. Bauman, Ph.D., (Dr. Neil), is the Director and CEO of The Center for Hearing Loss Help. He is a hearing loss coping skills specialist, researcher, author and speaker on issues pertaining to ears and hearing loss. No stranger to hearing loss himself, he has lived with a life-long, severe, hereditary hearing loss, not to mention life-long tinnitus.

Dr. Neil did not let his hearing loss stop him from achieving what he wanted to do. He earned several degrees in fields ranging from forestry to ancient astronomy (Ph.D.) and theology (Th.D.) in addition to his extensive studies in fields related to ears and hearing loss.

Over the years, Dr. Neil has helped thousands of hard of hearing people understand and successfully live with their hearing losses and other ear conditions, including tinnitus. To this end, he provides education, support and counsel to hard of hearing people through personal contact, as well as through his books, articles and presentations.

A prolific writer, Dr. Neil is the author of eleven books and more than 900 articles on hearing-loss-related topics (http://hearinglosshelp.com/blog/). (See the back of this book for a list of his books or go to http://hearinglosshelp.com/shop/category/books/.) In addition, he is a dynamic speaker. His presentations are in demand throughout the USA and Canada.

You can reach him at:

Neil Bauman, Ph.D.
Center for Hearing Loss Help
1013 Ridgeway Drive
Lynden, WA 98264-1057
Phone: (360) 778-1266
FAX: (260) 389-5226
Email: neil@hearinglosshelp.com
Web site: http://hearinglosshelp.com

# Preface

Tinnitus is a stranger that one day suddenly invaded your life—unwanted and unbidden to be sure—but there nevertheless. How you cope with this stranger is up to you. There are a number of things you can do to either eliminate your tinnitus, or at least help bring it under your control, so that it no longer interferes with your life.

Tinnitus is not one disease—in fact, it is not a disease at all—but rather, a group of diverse disorders with different physiology, different causes and consequently, different treatments. Unlike most books on tinnitus that focus on one pet way of relieving tinnitus, this comprehensive tinnitus book explains a number of the different "kinds" of tinnitus people may have, and then gives you numerous therapies and remedies you can try in order to eliminate or alleviate your tinnitus.

No one remedy has proven to work for every person with tinnitus. Some things work for some people, and other things work for others. You have to find what specific treatments work for you with your own particular kind of tinnitus. Some remedies only work for very specific kinds of tinnitus. Thus, the closer you match the remedy to the kind of tinnitus you have, the better your chances of success.

I do not specifically recommend any of the remedies I mention in this book. I have sought out the most promising and effective remedies, and am simply bringing them to your attention for your consideration. What you do with this information is up to you.

All the products and treatments in this book are reputable (I believe), and have helped a number of the people that have tried them. However, there are no guarantees of success. I am not making any claims as to the efficacy of any of these tinnitus treatments. I have simply reported the results that have come to my attention. Try any of them that "tickle your fancy". Ignore those that don't. The choice is yours.

I have had constant tinnitus for many decades now. I've used some of the remedies and treatments explained in these pages myself. The good news is that I have kept my tinnitus under control so that it does not bother me, even though my ears ring constantly day and night. However, you can rest assured that if my tinnitus begins to bother me, these are the various remedies I will turn to in order to bring it under control again. I believe they will work for you too.

I wish you well in your quest to bring your tinnitus under control.

Neil Bauman, Ph.D.
Lynden, WA

# Part I

# What Is Tinnitus?

Chapter 1

# Introduction to Tinnitus

## My Ears Are Ringing

Tinnitus (pronounced either TIN-ih-tus or ti-NIGH-tus) is the word we use to describe hearing certain phantom sounds. A simple dictionary definition of tinnitus is "the sensation of noise, often ringing or roaring in your ears that comes from inside your head in the absence of any external sound".

A more complete definition of tinnitus is "any noise produced in either your ears and/or the subconscious portions of your brain that is experienced, in large part, from the conscious portion of your mind spending time in a feedback loop that is constantly moving from hearing noise to experiencing negative emotions, ad infinitum".[1]

Note: There are two basic kinds of tinnitus—subjective tinnitus and objective tinnitus. The above and other generalized statements are true only of the common subjective kind of tinnitus, but are not true of the less common objective form of tinnitus. (See the section "Subjective vs. Objective Tinnitus" in Chapter 2 for an explanation of the difference between subjective and objective tinnitus.)

One person wrote tinnitus expert Dr. Jonathan Hazell (now retired), "Doctor, please confirm that this noise is not all in my head, and that I am not going mad". Dr. Hazell wrote back, "With pleasure! You are not going mad! And yes, it is all in your head, but then, so are your ears!" If you have tinnitus, you are hearing noises that no one else can hear, but they are very real to you. And no, you are not going crazy, although you may feel like it sometimes.

…ere are no external sounds corresponding to the sounds you are …itus is really a phantom sound. Even so, your brain actually … in your auditory system that you perceive and "hear" as real … no mistake about it; to you tinnitus sounds are just as real as any external sounds.

According to tinnitus researcher, Fatima Husain, Ph.D., "everyone has some low level of noise (one can say neural noise) in the brain, but in the case of tinnitus, for some reason, the neural noise is not suppressed and rises to the level of consciousness. In short, tinnitus is a perception of noise the brain is generating within itself. By the time you hear tinnitus, your ears are no longer involved."[2]

**The Sound of Silence**

I've probably had tinnitus all my life. When I was a boy, I didn't know there was such a thing as tinnitus. All I knew was that when it was totally quiet (and that's easy to experience when you have a severe hearing loss) I could still hear a "background" sound—what I now know was tinnitus. I called this sound (my tinnitus) by the oxymoronic term, the "sound of silence".

Interestingly enough, although children may experience tinnitus, they rarely mention it unless directly asked about it.[3] This is probably especially true in respect to those of us born with significant hearing losses. To us, the presence of tinnitus is normal. Thus it never crosses our minds that others do not "hear" these same phantom sounds.

Some people say their ears are ringing (mine are ringing right now as I write this) while others call it head noise. Appropriately enough, tinnitus is actually a Latin word meaning "a ringing or jingling". It is derived from "tinnire" "to tinkle" or "to ring like a bell".

Tinnitus may be a symptom of something gone wrong in your auditory system;[4] but then again, there may be nothing wrong with your ears at all. In some people, tinnitus may be the only "physical" symptom of emotional problems such as anxiety, depression or severe stress.[5]

In truth, tinnitus may not be a problem when it occurs alone as a single factor, but when other factors also become involved, (for example, progressive hearing loss, depression or allergies) then these two or more factors may synergistically lead to tinnitus becoming a problem.[6]

Tinnitus is noise that, in some cases, begins as the result of a middle or inner ear disorder. Later, it may become thoroughly enmeshed in the neurology of your brain and, in fact, may literally become a very loud, persistent and emotionally distressing "memory loop".[7]

Sometimes your inner ears generate tinnitus. Other times your ears and your brain team up, and together generate your tinnitus. However, the latest research reveals that most forms of tinnitus are the result of abnormalities in your central nervous system (brain) caused by neural plasticity—a fancy way of saying that changes in your brain are responsible for your tinnitus.[8] Thus, in the final analysis, your tinnitus always has something to do with your brain.[9]

Since tinnitus is often the result of neural plasticity, effectively treating tinnitus requires an understanding of neural plasticity and how it relates to tinnitus.[10] (See the section on "Neural Plasticity" in Chapter 3 for more on this subject.)

Furthermore, tinnitus does not just arise from the auditory parts of our brains. Using Functional Magnetic Resonance Imaging (fMRI) techniques, researchers have detected tinnitus-related activity in various other parts of our brains. Interestingly enough, tinnitus-related activity doesn't always occur in the same brain regions in all people.[11] This is because there are a number of different types of tinnitus.

**MRI Scans, Tinnitus and Hearing Loss**

Normal Magnetic Resonance Imaging (MRI) scans can be extremely noisy—ranging from 82 to 131 dB[12]—noisy enough to damage hearing, or trigger or aggravate tinnitus and hyperacusis.

Numbers of people have reported tinnitus after having an MRI. Others have reported their existing tinnitus got worse. Therefore, be sure to wear proper ear protection if you are having an MRI.[13] Good foam earplugs with a protection factor of about 30 dB should prevent ear damage or tinnitus.

One researcher reported temporary hearing loss in 43% of the patients scanned without ear protection or with improperly fitted earplugs. Hearing normally returns to normal in a few minutes to a few hours, but can take several weeks. In some cases, permanent hearing loss has occurred.[14]

In the future, doctors using fMRI scans may be able to identify the presence or absence of tinnitus, detect different types of tinnitus and even show the effectiveness of various tinnitus treatments. However, up to now, researchers have been able to distinguish between unilateral and bilateral tinnitus using fMRI techniques.[15]

Researchers are busily working on the three areas related to tinnitus—the somatic (physical) component of tinnitus, how this relates to the tinnitus sounds we hear (auditory component) and to the distress tinnitus causes us (psychological component).[16] This research supports the theory that tinnitus arises in the brain and is due to altered neural pathways.[17]

### Hearing Loss and Tinnitus

It is not necessary to even have a hearing loss to have tinnitus. Many people who have no hearing loss at all experience tinnitus and may find it hard to tolerate. In fact, researchers have found that up to 27% of those with normal hearing suffer from tinnitus.[18] Of all the people that have tinnitus, roughly one-third of them have normal hearing, at least in the commonly tested frequencies below 8,000 Hz. (They may, however, prove to have significant hearing loss in the high frequencies between 8,000 and 20,000 Hz that are seldom tested.) Perhaps just as surprising, one-third of those who have profound hearing losses do not have any tinnitus whatsoever.[19] Interestingly enough, tinnitus is almost unknown in those born totally deaf.[20]

Tinnitus itself does not cause hearing loss; nor does hearing loss as such cause tinnitus. Hearing loss and tinnitus can, and very often do, go together.[21] In fact, the odds of having tinnitus increases with the degree of hearing loss when measured at 4 kHz.[22] Tinnitus is most commonly associated with inner ear hearing losses. That is why it often accompanies age-related hearing loss. However, tinnitus can accompany any kind of hearing loss whether conductive or sensorineural.

Note that more than half of the people that are really bothered by their tinnitus have accompanying psychological injuries or illnesses such as post-traumatic stress disorder, depression, anxiety, obsessive-compulsive disorder, stress, etc.[23]

In one survey of people with tinnitus, 70% reported they also had hearing loss, 31% had problems sleeping, 24% suffered from depression/anxiety or other mental health issues, 21% had hyperacusis, 16% had hypertension (high blood pressure), 11% had temporomandibular joint problems (TMJ) and 6% had Meniere's disease.[24]

### "Exploding Head" Syndrome

A lady explained, "A horrible, loud explosion woke me up last night and made me scream out a bit. It was really scary! What's happening?"

What this lady experienced goes by the ghastly-sounding name of "Exploding Head" syndrome. In spite of its grisly name, your head doesn't really explode—you just hear a loud exploding sound.

"Exploding Head" syndrome is relatively rare. You may experience a very loud and sudden noise such as a loud bang similar to a bomb exploding,[25] a gun going off, a clash of cymbals, a door slamming, a roaring sound, waves crashing against rocks, loud voices or screams, a ringing noise, a terrific bang on a tin tray, the sound of electrical arcing (buzzing)[26] or any other form of loud, indecipherable noise that seems to originate from inside your head. It most often occurs just before deep sleep (and sometimes upon coming out of deep sleep) and wakes you up.[27] It can certainly scare you and set your heart to pounding.

## Super-Sensitivity to Sound

Severe tinnitus is often accompanied by conditions such as hyperacusis, hypersensitivity to sounds,[28] distortion of sounds, phonophobia, depression,[29] misophonia and even "exploding head syndrome".

### Sound Sensitivity (Hyperacusis)

Almost half of the people who seek help for their tinnitus also have sound sensitivity.[31] Although hyperacusis occurs in 9 - 15% of the population at large, it is even more common among tinnitus sufferers.[32] This is likely because sound sensitivity is linked with various conditions also common to tinnitus such as: noise exposure, hearing loss, various ear conditions, head or neck injury, dental or jaw problems, a side effect of ototoxic drugs, surgery, etc.[33]

If you have hyperacusis, you may worry that it indicates you will have bothersome tinnitus in the future. You can set your mind at rest. "A study of 309 tinnitus patients found that 18.4% of them also struggled with hyperacusis. However, there appeared to be no correlation between hyperacusis and the degree of annoyance caused by their tinnitus. In other words, hyperacusis did not measurably make their tinnitus worse."[34]

### Hyperacusis

Note that hyperacusis results from increased **gain** within your auditory pathways and is determined solely by the physical characteristics of sound such as its intensity and frequency.[30]

As professor Richard Salvi at the State University of New York at Buffalo explained, "Damage to the inner ear can lead to a drastic reduction in neural output from the cochlea. Unfortunately, the brain's auditory cortex may sometimes overcompensate for this decreased neural output—magnifying the brain sensation of (and sensitivity to) sound. Hyperacusis is the product of this overstimulation."[35]

### Kinds of Hyperacusis

Since hyperacusis is a general term referring to all kinds of supersensitivity to sound, think of their being three types of hyperacusis.

First, there is loudness hyperacusis where you have a lowered loudness discomfort level. That is, you have a reduced tolerance to sound such that you now perceive normal sounds as being too loud. This is the kind of hyperacusis most people think of when they talk about hyperacusis. Typically, it is just called **hyperacusis**.

Second, there is annoyance hyperacusis. This is where a person is particularly annoyed by certain sounds, i.e. has a dislike of specific sounds. This kind of hyperacusis is often referred to as **misophonia**.

Third, there is fear hyperacusis where you have a fear or phobia of certain sounds, or all sounds in general. This kind of hyperacusis is often referred to as **phonophobia**.[36]

If you have hyperacusis in addition to your

tinnitus, you need to be treated for it at the same time as you are being treated for your tinnitus.[37]

## Misophonia

Misophonia results from enhanced functional connections between your auditory system, limbic (emotional) system and autonomic nervous system. This means you will react to specific **patterns** of sound, with the loudness of the sound being either secondary or irrelevant. In misophonia, the meaning of a given sound and your past history of encountering it is crucial. The auditory characteristics of the sound only play a secondary role.[38]

Misophonia is a learned response. You weren't born with it. This means that if you have misophonia, you might report that a particular sound is a problem in some situations, but not in others.[39]

The simple way to understand the difference between hyperacusis and misophonia is that with hyperacusis, your brain has turned up its internal volume so you hear all sounds louder than normal. These sounds are now so loud they bother you. However, if you have misophonia, it's not the volume of the sound that bothers you, but your association with a particular sound. For example, the sound of cars crashing may unduly bother you because you lost a family member in an auto accident.

## Phonophobia

Misophonia can cause any kind of negative emotional response, but phonophobia specifically causes a **fear** reaction due to sound. Phonophobia is a subcategory of misophonia. A defining feature of phonophobia is the anticipation that sound will be uncomfortably loud. Thus, phonophobia refers to a person's state of mind with respect to sounds.[40]

## Recruitment

Many people confuse recruitment with hyperacusis. Recruitment refers to abnormally rapid growth in the **perception** of loudness, and is associated with sensorineural hearing loss and normal loudness discomfort levels. This means your dynamic range is compressed, but you have normal tolerance to louder sounds. (Note: Your dynamic range is the range in decibels [dB] between the softest sound you can hear and the loudest sound you can stand.)

If you have reduced tolerance to sounds, you need to be aware of the **sensitizing** effects of using hearing protection and the **desensitizing** effects of using therapeutic sound.[41] In other words, wearing ear protectors when you do not really need to makes your sound sensitivity worse. Conversely, exposing your ears to the proper level of sounds slowly expands your dynamic range, and thus your sound sensitivity gradually disappears.

## The Impact of Tinnitus

Many people worry about their tinnitus. To them tinnitus is quite threatening. They are sure that something is wrong with their hearing or with their brain. They fear that hearing tinnitus means they have some kind of serious illness. They are convinced that they have permanently damaged their ears. Usually it is the other way around—a hearing loss may trigger tinnitus. Still, tinnitus is only twice as common in those with hearing losses compared to those with normal hearing. Some people even mistakenly believe that their tinnitus heralds the onset of some serious disease such as a brain tumor, stroke, or some serious mental disorder.[42] Set your mind at ease. This is almost never true.

Then, too, many people fear their tinnitus will get louder and continue forever. Some feel threatened because their tinnitus is invading their "right to

### Interesting Facts About Tinnitus

Here are some cool facts about tinnitus gleaned from the Tinnitus Data Archive compiled from patient records at the Oregon Health and Science University's Tinnitus Clinic. These data only relate to people who seek help for their tinnitus, not to all people that have tinnitus.

- About 2½ times more men than women seek help for their tinnitus. (This is likely because more men than women work in loud environments and thus get tinnitus, rather than because men are more likely to seek help than women. Probably the opposite is true.)

- 80% of all people seeking help for their tinnitus are at least 40 years old. (This may reflect that it takes time to cause tinnitus to become permanent from repeatedly exposing your ears to loud sounds. Initially, tinnitus often tends to be temporary. Thus, younger people are more likely to have temporary tinnitus and consequently not seek help.)

- Tinnitus comes on gradually or suddenly about equally.

- Left-sided tinnitus is reported more often than right-sided tinnitus.[43] (This could reflect that when you drive with your window open, your left ear gets the brunt of traffic noise. It also reflects that more people are right-handed and thus shoot right-handed, thus exposing their left ear to the brunt of the rifle blast. In contrast, the right ear is turned away and tucked down thus partially protecting it.)

silence". They fear that tinnitus will spoil their peace and quiet, interfere with their concentration at work and play, and ruin their ability to sleep at night.

The impact tinnitus has on a person's life can vary enormously. Some people can completely ignore their tinnitus. For many others, tinnitus is only a mild irritation. However, for the unfortunate few, tinnitus is totally debilitating.

In one survey of people with tinnitus, 33% reported that their tinnitus, while annoying, did not significantly impact their lives; 18% reported trouble sleeping; 16% had trouble concentrating; 13% regularly experienced anxiety; 7% felt socially isolated; 7% were unable to work and another 7% had ongoing depression. Only 4% reported they barely noticed their tinnitus.[44]

Note that since this survey was of American Tinnitus Association members only, and since ATA members are much more likely to be bothered by their tinnitus than the typical person with tinnitus, this latter figure is probably drastically low.

These same people reported on a scale of 1 to 10 the impact their tinnitus had on their daily lives. (See box below.)

| Scale of 1 – 10 | % at this Level |
|---|---|
| 1 | 4 |
| 2 | 12 |
| 3 | 19 |
| 4 | 11 |
| 5 | 12 |
| 6 | 10 |
| 7 | 12 |
| 8 | 11 |
| 9 | 4 |
| 10 | 5[45] |

You might think the people that are most distressed by their tinnitus have the loudest tinnitus, but this is not necessarily the case. For example, one person can have loud tinnitus and yet not feel distressed by it, while another person can experience soft tinnitus and yet feel greatly distressed by it. In fact, two people can experience the same loudness and pitch of tinnitus, yet one person basically ignores their tinnitus and the other person is greatly bothered by theirs.[46]

People with severe tinnitus often have problems sleeping. One study revealed that more than 50% of the people who seek help for their tinnitus report problems sleeping because of their tinnitus.[47] In addition, people with tinnitus may be irritable, frustrated and tense. They cannot concentrate on anything other than their tinnitus. For example, in one small study of people with moderate to severe tinnitus, those with tinnitus performed less well on tests that required working memory and attention.[48]

Furthermore, people with severe tinnitus may experience frequent mood swings and feel anxious and/or depressed. As a result, they are constantly under stress, perform poorly, and lose their joy of living. In extreme cases, some even entertain thoughts of suicide. Many go to great lengths to find help and relentlessly pursue a cure for their tinnitus.

---

**Chapter 1 Endnotes**

1 Hogan, 1998. p. 30.
2 Forstag, 2014. p. 17.
3 Moller, 2011. p. 39.
4 Sauer, 1992. p. 22.
5 Hogan, 1998. p. 41.
6 Levine, 2004. p. 108.
7 Hogan, 1998. pp. 49-50.
8 Moller, 2011. p. xi.
9 Hogan, 1998. pp. 48-49.
10 Moller, 2011. p. xii.
11 Functional Magnetic Resonance Imaging, 2000. p. 1.
12 Shellock, Frank. Acoustic Noise and MRI Procedures. 2015. p. 1.
13 Functional Magnetic Resonance Imaging, 2000. p. 2.
14 Shellock, Frank. Acoustic Noise and MRI Procedures. 2015. p. 1.
15 Functional Magnetic Resonance Imaging, 2000. p. 1.
16 Functional Magnetic Resonance Imaging, 2000. p. 2.
17 Lockwood, 1999. p. 1.
18 Noise, Its Effects on Hearing and Tinnitus. 1988.
19 Hazell, p. 41.
20 McCall, 1991. p. 163.
21 Information About Tinnitus, 1988.
22 Moller, 2011. pp. 29-37.
23 Beck, 2014. p. 29.
24 Results from ATA's Membership Survey, 2014. p. 8.
25 Moller, 2011. pp. 25-27.
26 Exploding Head Syndrome, 2011. p. 1.
27 American Sleep Association, 2007. p. 1.
28 Moller, 2011. pp. 9-12.
29 Moller, 2011. p. xi.
30 Moller, 2011. pp. 575-596.
31 Mayes, 2010. p. 134.
32 Moller, 2011. p. 455.
33 Mayes, 2010. p. 37.
34 Guimaraes, 2014. p. 28.
35 Kurian, 2014. p. 22.
36 Kurian, 2014. p. 22.
37 Moller, 2011. pp. 575-596.

38 Moller, 2011. pp. 575-596.
39 Henry, 2010a. p. 9.
40 Henry, 2010a. p. 9.
41 Henry, 2010a. pp. 9-10.
42 Hazell, p. 41.
43 Henry, 2010a. p. 8.
44 Results from ATA's Membership Survey, 2014. p. 8.
45 Results from ATA's Membership Survey, 2014. p. 8.
46 Mayes, 2010. p. 16.
47 Mayes, 2010. p. 109.
48 Craggs-Hinton, 2007. p. 2.

## Chapter 2

# More About Tinnitus

## How Common Is Tinnitus?

Tinnitus is relatively common. Approximately 17% of the general population **have** tinnitus. This means that 17 out of every 100 people around the world have some degree of tinnitus. "Some studies have reported that as many as 80% of the adult population experience tinnitus at some point" in their lives. Six large population studies of adults revealed that between 4% and 15% experienced **prolonged** tinnitus.[1]

Tinnitus is about twice as common in hard of hearing people as it is in hearing people. About two-thirds of hard of hearing people suffer from some degree of tinnitus.[2] Other authorities put this figure as high as 95%.

In studies in the United States, tinnitus that lasted more than 3 months was present in 1.6% of adults aged 18 - 44 years; 4.6% of adults aged 45 – 64 years; and 9.0% of adults 60 years old and older. In adults between the ages of 21 and 84 years, 10.6% reported tinnitus of at least moderate severity.[3]

Furthermore, the estimated prevalence in the USA of people experiencing tinnitus at any time is 25.3%. The incidence of experiencing frequent (almost always or at least once a day) tinnitus is 7.9%. These figures may be low because only 10% to 15% of people with persistent tinnitus seek medical evaluation.

In the USA, the prevalence of experiencing any tinnitus in a given year increases with age, peaking at 31.4% in the 60 to 69 year age group.

Interestingly enough, the prevalence of tinnitus is higher among males, non-Hispanic whites, people who are overweight or those with a diagnosis of hypertension, diabetes mellitus, anxiety disorder or dyslipidemia (an abnormal amount of cholesterol or triglycerides in their blood). In addition, people with a history of loud noise exposure from using firearms or occupational or leisure activities, as would be expected, also have a higher incidence of tinnitus.[4]

The American Tinnitus Association estimates that about 45 million Americans have tinnitus to some degree. However, there is a big difference between just **having** tinnitus and **suffering** from tinnitus. About 12 million have tinnitus severely enough that they seek medical advice.[5]

In Canada, about 6 million people have varying degrees of tinnitus. About 1.3 million Canadians **suffer** from tinnitus severely enough that they seek help. Of these, about 200,000 suffer from tinnitus so severely that they cannot function normally.[6]

Suffering from severe tinnitus is no laughing matter. Tinnitus causes significant suffering in about 4% of the general population.[7] In another study, 2.4% of the population responded "yes" to the statement, "tinnitus plagues me all day".[8]

In the USA, about 2 million people have such severe tinnitus that they cannot function normally.[9] To them, tinnitus is totally debilitating and disrupts their entire lives. They are constantly under stress, perform poorly, and lose their joy of living.

**Intractable Tinnitus**

Did you know that extreme tinnitus is considered the third most difficult malady with which to live? Only intractable pain and intractable vertigo are ahead of it.[10]

Actors William Shatner (Captain Kirk) and Leonard Nimoy (Mr. Spock) of Star Trek fame both got severe tinnitus as a result of an explosion on the Star Trek set. Shatner's tinnitus almost drove him to suicide.

Incidentally, tinnitus disproportionately affects the people most likely to least understand it: older adults and people with low incomes.[11]

The good news, if you can see good news in having tinnitus, is that about 75% of the people who have tinnitus do **not** suffer from it. For them, it is just simply there.

Tinnitus gets more common as we age. For example, about 8% of those under 50 have tinnitus all or most of the time. After age 50, about 20% of the population report constant tinnitus, a jump of 250%. About 33% of the elderly have tinnitus.[12]

A study in England found that 17.5% of the participants between 40 and 60 years of age reported tinnitus. This figure rose to 22.2% in those above the age of 60.[13] A Brazilian study of 498 patients found that nearly 43% of all elderly subjects had tinnitus, with almost 59% of all cases having tinnitus in both ears.[14] Severe tinnitus affects less than 1% of those under 50, but about 4% of those over 50.[15]

**Tinnitus Has Been Around for a Long Time**

Tinnitus is not a modern problem. It has been around for thousands of years. In fact, it is mentioned as early as 400 BC in the writings of Hippocrates, often called the "Father of Medicine".[16]

Unfortunately, more and more young adults are flirting with tinnitus by exposing their ears to excessively loud sounds. According to the November 2009 issue of the Journal of Clinical Nursing, "75% of 18 to 30 year-olds that go to nightclubs and concerts may experience tinnitus". If this continues, it is only a matter of time until we see an epidemic of tinnitus among younger people.

One often-asked question is, "Will my tinnitus get worse as I get older?" I have good news for you. The results of a recent study indicate that tinnitus in elderly people is no more severe or distracting than it is in younger people, even though it is much more common.[17]

## What Is Tinnitus Like?

Tinnitus can manifest itself as a wide variety of sounds, volumes and patterns. Tinnitus sounds are **single**, **unmodulated** (simple) and generally **unformed** sounds. Basically, tinnitus is a single, meaningless sound, repeated endlessly. Tinnitus can be intermittent or constant. You may hear a single tone or multiple sounds. Furthermore, you may perceive its volume as ranging from subtle to shattering![18]

If you have tinnitus, you know what it sounds like—at least to you. For those of you who do not have tinnitus, our tinnitus may be a ringing, roaring, rushing, rumbling, blowing, beating, banging, buzzing, clicking, chirping, clanging, drumming, fluttering, hissing, humming, pulsating, sizzling, whooshing, whistling or dreadful shrieking noise in our ears. To some people, tinnitus sounds like crickets chirping, birds twittering, bees humming, clocks ticking, water rushing, machines clanking, bells ringing, owls hooting, jet engines roaring, glass breaking, radio static or chain saws running.[19, 20]

**Hear What Tinnitus Sounds Like for Yourself**

If you don't have tinnitus and would like to hear what some people with tinnitus put up with day in and day out, here are some simulated tinnitus sounds that give you an idea of just how mind-rending tinnitus can be. Of course there are many other tinnitus sounds, but these sounds at least give you a clue as to their variety and to the degree of annoyance of some tinnitus sounds. The American Tinnitus Association has kindly provided eight simulated tinnitus sound samples on their website at https://www.ata.org/understanding-facts/symptoms. The National Health Service in the United Kingdom has 11 tinnitus sounds on their website that you may listen to. You can hear these sounds at http://www.hearing.nihr.ac.uk/public/auditory-examples-sounds-of-tinnitus.

Interestingly enough, tinnitus is always a simple sound although it may have a tonal quality to it. In contrast, if you are "hearing" more complex phantom sounds such as music, singing or what sounds like a TV, radio or stereo playing from another room, you are very likely experiencing Musical Ear syndrome (non-psychiatric auditory hallucinations) instead of, or in addition to, your tinnitus.[21]

**Predominant Tinnitus Sounds**

| Tinnitus Sound | % |
|---|---|
| Ringing | 57 |
| Hissing | 20 |
| Clear tone | 17 |
| High tension wire | 14 |
| Buzzing | 12 |
| Sizzling | 8 |
| Transformer noise | 7 |
| Crickets chirping | 6 |
| Humming | 6 |
| Pulsating | 6 |
| Whistling | 6 |
| Ocean roar | 5 |
| Clicking | 1 |
| Pounding | 1[22] |

Another study listed the results as: Ringing - 34%, Hissing – 25%, Buzzing/Humming – 11%, Screeching/Whistling - 9%, Roaring – 2%, Clicking/Pulsing – 1% and Other – 8%.[23]

Musical Ear syndrome is a "sister" condition to tinnitus. You can learn about these non-tinnitus phantom sounds (sometimes, but erroneously, called "musical tinnitus") and how to control them in my companion book *Phantom Voices, Ethereal Music & Other Spooky Sounds*. (See inside the back cover for information on obtaining your copy of this most helpful book, or go to http://hearinglosshelp.com/shop/category/books/ and scroll down to the book on Musical Ear Syndrome.)

In contrast to the figures in the "Predominant Tinnitus Sounds" sidebar, one author wrote that about 30% of those with tinnitus hear a pure tone, while about 10% hear white noise. Also, about 30% hear a high-pitched whistle; the rest hear the various noises described in the sidebar.[24] Much of this is due to the fact that people describe the same tinnitus sound using different descriptors. For example, what I call a high-pitched ringing

> **White Noise**
>
> White noise is a sound containing a blend of all audible frequencies distributed over the various audible frequencies with equal energy per frequency. Most people hear white noise as a hissing sound or much like the static you heard in years gone by when an FM radio was not tuned to any station. (For more information on white noise see the sidebar in the section "White Noise vs. Pink Noise" and the sidebar in the section "Which Tinnitus Therapy Sound Is Right for Me?", both in Chapter 21.)

or whining sound, others may describe as a hissing sound or as white noise. One person's buzzing sound may be another person's humming sound.

What frequency do most people hear their tinnitus at? Typically people hear tinnitus as a high-frequency sound (55%), rather than a low frequency sound (9%). The rest fall in between these frequencies, but still tend to bunch more towards the higher end of the mid-frequencies (Fig. 2-1). This should not be surprising since people typically hear their tinnitus near the frequency of their greatest hearing loss, and most people have high-frequency hearing loss.

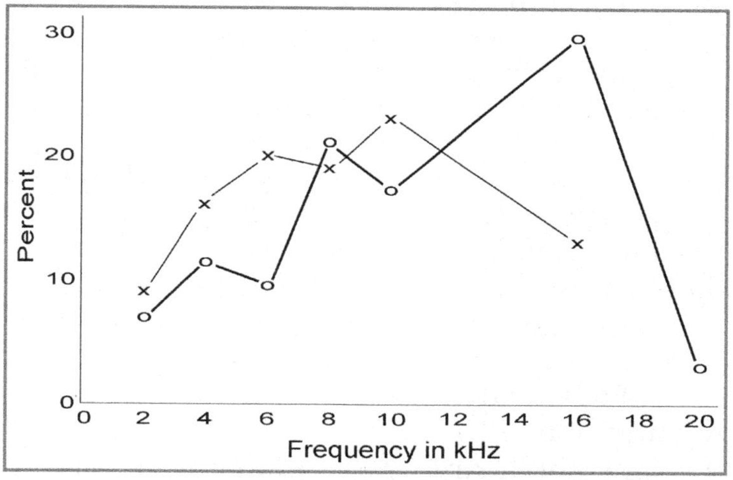

Fig. 2-1. Graph showing the frequency distribution of tinnitus.

A study of 1,514 people with tinnitus revealed that most people heard their tinnitus in the higher frequencies—the "X" line in Fig. 2-1.[25] Another study of approximately 1,337 people revealed a slightly different distribution of tinnitus frequencies—the "O" line in Fig. 2-1.[26] Note that the average of both lines is more or less a normal curve, but it is somewhat skewed towards the higher frequencies.

In a study of more than 1,500 people with tinnitus, about 80% reported that their tinnitus had a tonal quality. The rest said it was just plain noise.[27] Most people find that the noise-type of tinnitus is less severe (and less disturbing) than the tonal type of tinnitus.[28]

In which ear do most people hear their tinnitus? Interestingly enough, 56% hear their tinnitus in both ears at the same time, 10% in their left ear, 10% in their right ear, and 24% just hear it inside their head somewhere and not specifically associated with either ear.[29] In another study, 63% heard their tinnitus in both ears, 11% in their right ear,14% in their left ear, and 12% heard it just in their heads.[30]

Your tinnitus may be constant. It may come and go. It may pulsate. It may even change over a period of hours or days. In one survey, 72% experienced their tinnitus all the time, 18% heard their tinnitus frequently and only 10% had occasional tinnitus.[31] In another study, 30% described their tinnitus as constant—always the same volume and sound, 61% described it as constant, but the volume and/or sound changed from time to time, while 9% said their tinnitus came and went.[32]

Fifty-one percent of people reported their tinnitus came on gradually (taking more than one month to reach full volume), while for others tinnitus just suddenly "appeared". Seven percent reported their tinnitus took between a week and a month to reach full volume, while 39% noticed their tinnitus appeared within a week.[33]

There are varying degrees of tinnitus. For some, it is a mild background sound. For others, it is a serious handicap. For example, after taking certain anti-cancer drugs, Ruby heard what sounded like the roar of Niagara Falls in one ear and a broken washing machine in her other ear.

To me tinnitus is usually a high-pitched ringing or whine (much like a high-speed turbine running), and less often a soft shhh sound or a low rumbling noise like an 18-wheeler idling outside the house. Sometimes I hear birds twittering in my right ear. Occasionally I hear a loud roaring sound like a freight train bearing down right on top of me.

Pam hears what sounds like birds chirping and occasionally an owl hooting. When Una shakes her head, she hears the pure tone "F". The rest of the time she hears what sounds like a piece of sheet metal being hammered or a constant high-pitched tone.

One lady explained, "I have a constant ringing in my ears. Occasionally I hear beautiful chimes playing an unknown melody or scale in my left ear. The chimes are almost a welcome sound over that constant and irritating ringing in both ears." Another lady explained, "I've had ringing for years now, since I was about 30 years old. Lately, I've been hearing chimes in my right ear!"

If you have tinnitus, you don't necessarily just hear one constant tinnitus sound. Many people do, to be sure, but many others hear multiple tinnitus sounds. They may hear these multiple sounds at the same time, or their tinnitus may vary in volume, pitch and sound depending on a variety of factors as they go about their daily lives. For example, Mrs. Parker, who had a severe case of tinnitus, used to hear what sounded like a cow bell, a door bell, a tune, a noise like rushing water and a roaring like traffic in a tunnel—all at once.[34] One unfortunate person heard seven different tinnitus sounds at the same time.[35]

**Number of Tinnitus Sounds Heard**

In one study of 1,627 people with tinnitus, 53% only heard one tinnitus sound, 26% heard two tinnitus sounds while 16% heard three or more tinnitus sounds at the same time. (The remaining 5% were unsure just how many tinnitus sounds they actually hear.)[36]

The constant racket that tinnitus produces may make it seem difficult to hear or understand others. In actual fact, tinnitus does not "mask" your hearing, although it often seems that way if you have loud tinnitus and a hearing loss at the same time. But tinnitus can certainly cause so much distraction and distress that you may find it impossible to concentrate on what people are saying. Fortunately, my tinnitus normally remains at a constant, relatively low volume. Occasionally it becomes so loud I don't like to talk to others because it seems hard to hear them through all the racket. Even the great musician, Beethoven, complained, "My ears whistle and buzz continually day and night. I can say I am living a wretched life."[37] His tinnitus bothered him so much that in 1801, he actually contemplated suicide.[38]

Composer Robert Schumann also suffered from tinnitus. During his last years he heard a constant A-flat tone.[39]

There is an enormous difference between mild or short lasting tinnitus and loud, severe, constant tinnitus day in and day out. The mild tinnitus some have does not bother them much. However, in extreme cases, tinnitus is debilitating and can disrupt your entire life.

**Smetana Composed a String Quartet for His Tinnitus**

Bedrich Smetana (1824-1884), the Czech composer, later in life had hearing loss accompanied by severe tinnitus. He once remarked despairingly about the pounding and intense hissing in his head, as if he were standing under a big waterfall.[40]

His tinnitus had been a constant "high E" sound, which he memorialized in his autobiographical 1876 E-minor composition for string quartets, entitled *From My Life*. In the finale, *Vivace*, of his String Quartet No. 1, he had the first violin play a persistent high E to mimic his high-pitched "piercing, whistling" tinnitus that rang almost continually in his ears.[41]

The loudness you "hear" your tinnitus at may remain constant or it may vary throughout a day, throughout an hour, or even more frequently.[42] Researchers have found that no matter how loud we perceive our tinnitus, its actual volume is always under 20 dB and for many people it is only 5 dB to 10 dB.[43] In fact, about two thirds of tinnitus

**How Tinnitus Affects Your Life**

Tinnitus can have a great impact on your life. The following table reveals that some people have great difficulty coping with their tinnitus, while other people don't seem to have much of a problem with their tinnitus. The results are shown as percentages. The first part of the table includes data from about 1,600 people with tinnitus, while the second part of the table includes data from about 1,100 people.[44]

| My tinnitus: | None | Some | Often* | |
|---|---|---|---|---|
| Interferes with my sleep | 29 | 45 | 25 | |
| Makes me feel irritable or nervous | 18 | 43 | 38 | |
| Makes me feel tired or ill | 47 | 28 | 25 | |
| Makes it difficult to relax | 18 | 35 | 45 | |
| Makes me uncomfortable in quiet | 26 | 24 | 45 | |
| Makes it difficult to concentrate | 22 | 33 | 38 | |
| Makes it harder to interact pleasantly | 31 | 32 | 30 | |
| | None | Slight | Mod. | Lots* |
| Amount of effort to ignore tinnitus | 7 | 29 | 32 | 32 |
| Amount of discomfort from tinnitus | 9 | 21 | 26 | 33 |
| Interference with work activities | 24 | 24 | 30 | 22 |
| Interference with social activities | 15 | 21 | 26 | 27 |
| Interference with overall enjoyment | 8 | 19 | 39 | 34 |

* Row totals do not always add up to 100%

sufferers can have their tinnitus masked by other sounds only 14 dB or less above their hearing threshold.[45]

## Subjective vs. Objective Tinnitus

There are two basic kinds or forms of tinnitus, subjective tinnitus and objective tinnitus.

### Subjective Tinnitus

Subjective tinnitus is the common (neurophysiologic) type of tinnitus that the vast majority of people with tinnitus have. It is often associated with hearing loss. It is subjective, because only you can hear (perceive) the noises in your head because they are produced in your auditory system and heard only in your brain. Subjective tinnitus sounds include the common ringing, roaring, hissing and kindred sounds. There are a number of forms of subjective tinnitus. Thus, it really is a group of disorders rather than a single disorder.[46] The majority of this book deals with this kind of tinnitus.

### Objective Tinnitus

Objective tinnitus consists of real sounds produced in your body that other people can hear if they listen closely. (A doctor may have to listen with a stethoscope in order to hear them.) Fewer than 5% of the people with tinnitus have this type of tinnitus.[47]

The sounds of objective tinnitus come from your head and neck—but not from your auditory system. What you are really hearing is body sounds such as blood flowing in the blood vessels close to your ears, which can produce a throbbing sound that pulses in step with your heart beat. This may be from an aneurysm or other vascular malformation, a tumor near your ears or narrowed blood vessels in your head or neck that causes turbulent blood flow in blood vessels near your ears. Doctors call these forms of tinnitus "pulsatile tinnitus" because they all vary in unison to your pulse (heart beat).

Muscle spasms or rhythmic muscular contractions of your soft palate and facial muscles (palatal myoclonus) can also produce objective tinnitus. In these cases, you may hear clicks or cracklings.[48] You can even get objective tinnitus by hearing the spontaneous otoacoustic emissions from your outer hair cells.[49]

The good news is that your doctor can often correct objective tinnitus through medical or surgical means.

## Somatic vs. Neurophysiologic Tinnitus

Whenever you consciously perceive your tinnitus, the **perception** of your tinnitus results from active processing by your auditory nervous system (auditory cortex). Although the final destination of your tinnitus always is your auditory cortex, the origin of your tinnitus can be from either outside or within your auditory nervous system.

If your tinnitus is triggered in your inner ears or brain we refer to it by the fancy technical term "neurophysiologic tinnitus". Sometimes doctors call it sensorineural tinnitus, or more rarely, otological tinnitus. However, the vast majority of the time we simply refer to it as tinnitus[50] because this is the kind of tinnitus most people experience.

However, if your tinnitus is triggered elsewhere in your body, we refer to it as somatic tinnitus—from the Greek word "soma"—body. Sometimes people refer to this kind of tinnitus as somatosensory tinnitus or even body tinnitus.

## How Bad Is My Tinnitus?—Standardized Tinnitus Evaluation

For some people, tinnitus seriously affects the quality of their lives. For other people, tinnitus is more of an annoyance. And for numbers of people, tinnitus isn't a problem. It is just "there".

In order for health care professionals to categorize the degree to which tinnitus affects a person's quality of life, and to be able to compare the effects of tinnitus between people, they came up with the Tinnitus Handicap Inventory (THI).

### Tinnitus Handicap Inventory

The Tinnitus Handicap Inventory is just a standardized means of determining how much your tinnitus bothers you. It consists of 25 questions to which you answer "yes", "sometimes" or "no".

To take this tinnitus evaluation, grab a piece of paper and number the lines from 1 to 25. Beside each number answer "yes", "sometimes" or "no" to each of the following THI questions.

**Tinnitus Handicap Inventory Questions**

1. Because of your tinnitus, is it difficult for you to concentrate?
2. Does the loudness of your tinnitus make it difficult for you to hear people?
3. Does your tinnitus make you angry?
4. Does your tinnitus make you feel confused?
5. Because of your tinnitus, do you feel desperate?
6. Do you complain a great deal about your tinnitus?
7. Because of your tinnitus, do you have trouble falling asleep at night?
8. Do you feel as though you cannot escape your tinnitus?
9. Does your tinnitus interfere with your ability to enjoy your social activities (such as going out to dinner or to the movies)?
10. Because of your tinnitus, do you feel frustrated?

11. Because of your tinnitus, do you feel that you have a terrible disease?
12. Does your tinnitus make it difficult for you to enjoy life?
13. Does your tinnitus interfere with your job or household responsibilities?
14. Because of your tinnitus, do you find that you are often irritable?
15. Because of your tinnitus, is a difficult for you to read?
16. Does your tinnitus make you upset?
17. Do you feel that your tinnitus problem has placed stress on your relationships with members of your family and friends?
18. Do you find it difficult to focus your attention away from your tinnitus and on other things?
19. Do you feel that you have no control over your tinnitus?
20. Because of your tinnitus, do you often feel tired?
21. Because of your tinnitus, do you feel depressed?
22. Does your tinnitus make you feel anxious?
23. Do you feel that you can no longer cope with your tinnitus?
24. Does your tinnitus get worse when you are under stress?
25. Does your tinnitus make you feel insecure?[51]

Here is how to score your Tinnitus Handicap Inventory. Each "yes" answer gets 4 points, each "sometimes" answer gets 2 points and each "no" answer gets 0 points. Add up all the points to get your total Tinnitus Handicap Inventory.

Here's how to interpret your Tinnitus Handicap Inventory score.

| Score | Degree of Handicap | Grade |
|---|---|---|
| 0-16 | Slight or no handicap | 1 |
| 18-36 | Mild handicap | 2 |
| 38-56 | Moderate handicap | 3 |
| 58-76 | Severe handicap | 4 |
| 78-100 | Catastrophic handicap | 5[52] |

Many people don't seek help for their tinnitus until their Tinnitus Handicap Inventory reaches the severe level. Dr. Jastreboff found that the initial average THI score of his patients was 64[53] by the time they finally contacted him.

Your THI not only helps health care professionals know how much your tinnitus affects your quality of life, you can also use it yourself.

For example, you can compare how well any tinnitus treatment is working by periodically taking the Tinnitus Handicap Inventory again. Don't do this too often, perhaps every three months or so. You need to allow enough time to see if a given tinnitus treatment is working for you. If your score drops, good things are happening. In that case, this treatment is one you probably want to continue. If the treatment doesn't make any difference to your THI score, it's ineffective and you might want to stop that treatment and try one of the many other tinnitus treatments explained in this book.

Furthermore, you can use the THI to let you know when you can stop tinnitus treatments because you now have your tinnitus under control.

A good goal is to stop treatment when your tinnitus is no longer a factor in your life. Typically that would mean you Tinnitus Handicap Inventory score has dropped to 20 or less. Of course, the lower the score, the better.

## Tinnitus Functional Index

A newer, more accurate **Tinnitus Functional Index** (TFI) was developed in 2012. You can see a copy of the Tinnitus Functional Index at http://www.ncrar.research.va.gov/Education/Documents/TinnitusDocuments/TFI.pdf.

Like the Tinnitus Handicap Inventory, the Tinnitus Functional Index also consists of 25 questions. You answer each question by choosing a number ranging between 0 and 10. When finished, you add up your total score and interpret it as follows:

| Score | Degree of Tinnitus Problem |
|---|---|
| 0-17 | not a problem |
| 18-31 | small problem |
| 32-53 | moderate problem |
| 54-72 | big problem |
| 73-100 | very big problem |

Note that when using the Tinnitus, Functional Index, a "meaningful change" occurs whenever TFI scores are reduced by 13 points or more.[54]

**Chapter 2 Endnotes**


1 Moller, 2011. pp. 29-37.
2 McCall, 1991. p. 163.
3 Tunkel, 2014. p. S2.
4 Tunkel, 2014. pp. S3-S4.
5 Information About Tinnitus, 1988.
6 Info-Tinnitus, Causes and Factors in the Hearing System, 1990.
7 Jastreboff, 1997a. p. 1.
8 Moller, 2011. pp. 29-37.
9 American Tinnitus Association, 2002. p. 1.
10 Hogan, 1998. p. 61.
11 Henry, 2010b. p. 26.
12 Dobie, p. 45.
13 Moller, 2011. pp. 29-37.
14 Gibrin, 2013. p. 19.
15 Dobie, p. 45.
16 Connor, 2003. p. 1.
17 Press, 1997. p. 14.
18 American Tinnitus Association, 2002. p. 1.
19 Discovering and Understanding Tinnitus, 1997. p. 2.
20 Craggs-Hinton, 2007. p. 1.
21 Bauman, 2011b. p. 26.
22 Tinnitus Archive, 2004. p. 3.
23 Results from ATA's Membership Survey, 2014. p. 7.
24 Hickish, p. 47.
25 Tinnitus Archive, 2004. p. 1.
26 Phua, Peter. 2015. p. 1.
27 Discovering and Understanding Tinnitus, 1997. p. 2.
28 Press, 1997. p. 13.
29 Discovering and Understanding Tinnitus, 1997. p. 2.
30 Results from ATA's Membership Survey, 2014. p. 7.
31 McCall, 1991. p. 163.
32 Results from ATA's Membership Survey, 2014. p. 7.
33 Tinnitus Archive, 2004. p. 2.
34 Trauma of Sensory Loss, p. 203.
35 Sauer, 1992. p. 22.
36 Tinnitus Attributes, 1996. p. 2.
37 Hickish, p. 48.
38 Conner, 2003. p. 1.
39 Lean, 2004. p. 1.
40 Cohn, 2004. p. 1.
41 Bedrich Smetana, 2004. p. 2.
42 Sauer, 1992. p. 22.
43 Hickish, p. 48.
44 Tinnitus Archive, 2004. p. 4.
45 Discovering and Understanding Tinnitus, 1997. p. 2.
46 Moller, 2011. p. 9.

47 Sweetow, 1998. p. 1.
48 Tinnitus & Your Hearing, 1998. p. 1.
49 Lockwood, 2001b. p. 472.
50 Henry, 2010a. p. 2.
51 Newman, 1996. pp. 143-148.
52 McCombe, 1999. pp. 388-393.
53 Robb, 2015. p. 19.
54 Tinnitus Functional Index, 2015. p. 1.

## Chapter 3

# Tinnitus Is More Complex Than You Think

Tinnitus is a surprisingly complex subject—not a simple subject like people used to think. In the past, conventional wisdom assumed that tinnitus resulted from damage to the hair cells in the cochlea. They thought that these damaged hair cells then sent abnormal signals to our brains, which we heard as tinnitus. (Incidentally, many people still hold this belief today.)

Researchers figured this was why tinnitus was so closely associated with sensorineural hearing loss. They further reasoned that cutting the auditory nerve or destroying the cochlea should provide immediate and total relief from tinnitus.

Does this happen? No, it does not! The reality is quite different. First, about 10% of people suffering from tinnitus have normal hearing, so their tinnitus can't be caused from damaged hair cells. Second, attempts to cure tinnitus by cutting the auditory nerve are successful less than 25% of the time.

Unfortunately, people who have had their auditory nerves cut find their tinnitus frequently stays the same or gets worse, even though they are now completely deaf. Furthermore, get this—more than 50% of the people who have had their auditory nerves cut (for example, as a result of surgery for acoustic neuromas) **develop** tinnitus where they didn't have any before. Thus, it became obvious that there had to be another explanation for the cause of tinnitus. They now know that tinnitus largely develops within the brain, not just in the cochlea or auditory nerve.

The previous way of understanding tinnitus also did not explain why more than 75% of the people with tinnitus were not disturbed by it. In fact, about two-thirds of all the people who experience moderate tinnitus do not suffer from the noise. These people seek no medical or mental health attention. Furthermore, they have no significant negative emotional responses to the noises they hear.[1]

We, (people who are not bothered by their tinnitus), myself included, can easily hear our tinnitus whenever we focus our attention on it, but we are not unduly bothered by it. In the past, doctors assumed that we just had very soft, or mild, tinnitus that was easily masked by other sounds. They thought the other 25% suffered from severe tinnitus. Again, reality is totally different.

Guess what! There is absolutely no correlation between how severe our tinnitus is and how much it bothers us. For example, mild tinnitus totally debilitates some people, while loud tinnitus does not bother others. In fact, as I mentioned in Chapter 1, it is possible to find two people with identical hearing and identical tinnitus in terms of loudness, yet one person ignores it while the other suffers profoundly. Why?

It seems likely that the brains of people that suffer from tinnitus are particularly susceptible to focus on the perception of tinnitus. At the same time, they ascribe a negative emotional component to their tinnitus.[2]

Fortunately, in the past few years tinnitus research has accelerated. Much of this impetus to find a tinnitus cure stems from the thousands of military personnel returning from overseas service now suffering from severe tinnitus.

As researchers probe more and more into our brains in order to find the cause of tinnitus, they are finding that the more they look, the more complex the problem becomes. Even so, they are beginning to understand what goes on in our brains that makes tinnitus a life-shattering condition for some people, yet only a minor annoyance for others.

Although our current state of understanding tinnitus is still far from complete, this chapter will give you some insight into the complexities of tinnitus, and thus why no one single remedy works for all people.

We now know that tinnitus may or may not have something to do with our ears. However, tinnitus **always** has something to do with our brains. In fact, it has **lots** to do with the various parts of our brains.

It appears that in many cases, both our ears and our brains work together in generating the sounds we call tinnitus. You see, bothersome tinnitus is really a psychosomatic condition. It has both a physical component and a significant mental or emotional component. To put it another way, tinnitus is always both a medical and a psychological phenomenon.[3]

Thus, tinnitus is really a complex intermingling of neural plasticity, deficient brain chemistry, phantom auditory perception, hair cell damage, and negative emotional experiences such as fear, stress, anxiety and depression, among other variables.[4]

Read this next statement carefully. It is very important.

**Certain things can trigger your tinnitus, but whether your tinnitus bothers you or not has nothing to do with what triggered it in the first place.**

This is because how loud and intrusive you perceive your tinnitus to be is affected by many factors such as your actual circumstances, your expectations, any stress you are under and your emotional state.[5]

It is now obvious that there are several different mechanisms that generate a number of different kinds of tinnitus in the general population, not just one. In fact, there may be several different mechanisms that may generate tinnitus in any given person![6] Studies have shown that not only do changes occur in our brain's auditory circuits, but changes also occur in non-auditory areas of our brains that are involved in such things as integrating information from our other senses, decision-making and evaluating our emotions.[7]

Furthermore, our brains have filters that determine which sensory perceptions they will bring to our conscious attention. If we are bothered by our tinnitus, these filters determine that our brains need to pay close attention to our tinnitus sounds (something we don't want our brains to do). In addition, our autonomic nervous systems and the amygdala (part of our limbic [emotional] systems) further increases the sensitivity of our auditory systems. Thus, we perceive our tinnitus as louder and more intrusive. And this, in turn, increases our level of stress. The "emotional" parts of our brains define how we will **react** to hearing our tinnitus, as opposed to the fact of just perceiving (hearing) our tinnitus.[8]

In one study, researchers explained, "Perhaps the most remarkable finding was that activity directly linked to tinnitus was very extensive, and spanned a large proportion of the parts of the brain." In fact, "Tinnitus–linked brain activity extended far beyond circumscribed auditory cortical regions, encompassing almost all of the auditory cortex, along with other parts of the brain." "In contrast, the brain responses to a sound we played that mimicked tinnitus were localized to just a tiny area."

What this means is that, "Tinnitus is represented very differently in the brain to normal sounds, even ones that sound the same, and therefore, these cannot necessarily be used as a basis for understanding tinnitus or targeting treatment".[9]

Such discoveries add to our understanding of tinnitus. They also show why treating tinnitus is so complex and challenging, and why treating tinnitus does not have just one simple solution.

## Neural Plasticity

Some of the complex issues involving tinnitus result from neural plasticity. Neural plasticity is just a fancy way of saying that our brains are not necessarily organized in just one way and then set in stone, but that they can change, given the right conditions. Neural plasticity can be good—for example, rebuilding parts of our brains damaged by a stroke.

On the other hand, doctors are now beginning to understand how neural plasticity can also reprogram our brains in ways that are not to our benefit. When this happens, neural plasticity can be bad—causing changes leading to tinnitus or hyperacusis, for example.

Normally, after our auditory systems are fully developed, they work the way God designed them to work. As a result, there is no need for major changes, although minor changes are always taking place.

However, hearing loss can throw a monkey wrench into the gear-works and thus activate neural plasticity. You can also invoke neural plasticity by doing things such as exposing your ears to loud noise, accidentally injuring your ears or deliberately creating change though behavioral training such as Cognitive Behavior Therapy (see Chapter 18), for example.

Neural plasticity can result in a number of changes in our brains. It can cause changes in the way sounds are processed; changes in how active certain auditory neurons are; and changes in how auditory and related information is routed along new pathways. This means that when neural plasticity kicks in, changes in one part of our auditory systems ultimately produce changes in a number of other parts of our brains.[10] Furthermore, neural plasticity can cause more neurons to become excited while inhibition (suppression of unwanted neuronal activity) is reduced.

## Neuronal Activity—The Balance Between Being Excited or Inhibited

Normally the neurons in the auditory circuits in our brains are kept in balance—neither being too active (excited), nor being too inactive (inhibited). When no sounds are present, neuronal activity in our auditory circuits is low. However, when our ears hear something, neuronal activity increases. Our brains interpret this increased activity as sound.

When hair cells in our inner ears sustain damage or die, the corresponding parts of the auditory circuits in our brains become more active (excited) than they would otherwise be. Although this seems exactly backwards, we'll see why in a moment. When this happens, neuronal activity resembles the same level of activity that is normally seen when sound is present.

As we age, or when the hair cells are damaged, there are now fewer inhibitory (gamma-Aminobutyric acid [GABA]) neurotransmitter receptors, whose job is to dampen (inhibit) this extraneous activity in our auditory pathways. At the same time, the number of excitatory (glutamate) neurotransmitter receptors increases resulting in even higher levels of neuronal activity.

Currently, researchers believe that if something can be done to restore the normal balance between neurons being excited and neurons being inhibited, tinnitus will cease to be a problem.

In a similar way, exposing your ears to loud noise can result in tinnitus because of neuronal excitability. Exposure to loud sound triggers some of the nerve cells (neurons) in the dorsal cochlear nucleus in the brain to fire erratically. This uncontrolled activity eventually leads to tinnitus.

Here's how it works. There are five different KCNQ potassium channels in our bodies, but only two are important in tinnitus—KCNQ2 and KCNQ3.[11] These potassium channels affect neuronal activity. Under normal conditions, these cells fire regularly and then return to their resting states. It's these potassium channels that help to drag down the cellular electrical activity to its resting state. This allows the cells to function with a regular pattern.

However, after exposure to loud sound, the KCNQ2 and KCNQ3 potassium channels that help regulate the neuron's electrical activity do not function properly. The result is that the cells remain constantly active, being unable to reach their resting states. This, in turn, results is continuous, random, irregular bursts of activity creating the sensation of constant noise when none exists.[12]

Putting this in simple terms—when everything is functioning properly, if some auditory neurons in your brain get too excited and "talk" out of turn so to speak, other surrounding neurons tell them to "shut up". This maintains order in the auditory cortex and prevents tinnitus.

However, when you have a hearing loss, a good number of neurons in your auditory cortex are deprived of normal sound signals. This is because for each frequency of sound you hear there are neurons dedicated to processing that sound frequency. Damage to your inner ear (typically death of hair cells) deprives the corresponding neurons in the auditory circuits in your brain of "hearing" real sound signals.

The result is that these neurons have nothing to do. Since neurons are not happy when they are not doing anything, they find a "new job". It seems they "rewire" themselves so that they are no longer excited by the frequencies they were originally tuned to. Instead, they tune in to (are excited by) the frequency of their neighboring neurons. When too many neurons begin to "talk out of turn" like this, and not enough other neurons tell them to "shut up", things get a bit wild.

What you are now seeing is neural plasticity at work. This shifts the normal balance between excitation and inhibition more to the side of excitation. Thus, overall activity in your auditory system increases. We call this increased activity tinnitus. The good news is that studies have shown that if these neurons are stimulated with sounds at their original frequencies, then neural plasticity does not develop.[13] That is why people with hearing loss typically experience improvement in their tinnitus when hearing aids restore the missing sounds to levels the hard of hearing ear can still hear. This is one good reason to wear hearing aids if you have bothersome tinnitus resulting from hearing loss.

Another change in neuronal activity resulting from damage to, or the death of, inner ear hair cells is an increase in synchrony. Synchrony just means that a bunch of nearby neurons fire at the same time. (Incidentally, damage from loud noise or ototoxic drugs can cause an increase in synchronous firing. We "hear" this resulting synchronized, spontaneous neural activity as tinnitus.)[14]

If this situation is allowed to continue, it becomes the new norm and you end up with constant, permanent tinnitus. These brain neurons don't know that you don't want to hear this aggravating new sound. They are simply "doing their jobs".[15]

The good news is that this "rowdy", synchronized behavior can be modified by behavioral training such that the neurons that aren't directly stimulated are now inhibited when enough of the surrounding neurons tell the "tinnitus neurons" to "shut up". Thus, the volume of your tinnitus goes down, and things become more normal again.[16]

## Tonotopic Organization

Another change caused by neural plasticity is remodeling of the frequency (tonotopic) organization in your auditory pathways.[17]

The hair cells in your cochleas are arranged in order by frequency. Those hair cells sensitive to high-frequency sounds are situated at the base of the cochlea. Those hair cells that are sensitive to low-frequency sounds lie at the apex (tip) of the cochlea. This ordering of the hair cells according to frequency (much like the notes on a piano keyboard) is referred to as tonotopic organization.

It should come as no surprise then that the various parts of our brains involved in processing sound also exhibit this same tonotopic organization. As a result of this tonotopic organization, each neuron in these areas of our brains is only capable of responding to a limited range of frequencies and responds most sensitively to a single frequency.[18]

With neural plasticity, this tonotopic map can be somewhat reorganized to give inordinate representation to frequencies of sound near the edge of our normal hearing at the expense of frequencies in the regions of our greatest hearing loss.[19, 20] Using the analogy of a piano keyboard, in people with hearing loss, these "brain keyboards" are missing "keys" corresponding to their hearing loss, and have extra "keys" corresponding to frequencies of sound close to their hearing loss.

In people with tinnitus, these extra keys often match the pitch of their tinnitus.[21] That is why we typically hear our tinnitus at a pitch near the frequency of our greatest hearing loss.[22]

However, not everyone hears their tinnitus at the frequency of their greatest loss. For example, my greatest loss is between 500 and 2,000 Hz, yet I hear my typical tinnitus as a very high-frequency sound, the very frequencies at which I have my **best** hearing. My hearing loss is genetic.

Because of such conflicting examples, researchers have sought to determine whether tinnitus resulting from different causes such as noise exposure, head trauma, stroke, etc. result in unique tinnitus pitches. In a study of 509 ears, they found the tinnitus pitch was generally highest in people who had acute acoustic trauma and lowest in tinnitus caused by use of estrogen and progesterone.[23]

Certain drugs also cause different pitches of tinnitus. (See Chapter 7 for more on this.)

Thus, it appears that the pitch of your tinnitus is dependent on the exact cause of your tinnitus. This is important because it may lead to unique treatment options depending on the specific cause of your tinnitus.[24]

For reasons as yet unknown, once something activates neural plasticity, sometimes this activity does not stop. The resulting changes may become permanent.[25] The good news is that reversing these neural-plasticity changes is often possible by means of special treatments. For example, neural plasticity changes can result from using tinnitus retraining therapy, Neuromonics, Cognitive Behavior Therapy, and other therapies. (I explain these various treatments in Part III.)

## Our Current Understanding of Tinnitus

People that suffer from tinnitus, as opposed to those whose tinnitus does not cause them distress, need to learn the connection between their auditory (hearing) systems, limbic (emotional) systems and their tinnitus. Briefly, here is how this is thought to tie together.

Sound signals are sent up our auditory nerves to the subconscious parts of our brains. Besides the auditory system where sound is processed, there are a number of other brain structures that have input into how sounds are processed, or whether certain sounds are even processed at all. Once the sound signals reach the subconscious parts of our brains, they are split and processed by at least two (and probably more) separate, but interconnected, systems—namely the auditory system and the limbic system. The interactions between these two systems are complex.

Although the limbic system is the seat of our emotions, various parts of it also have other functions. For example, recent research has shown that particular parts of the limbic system are involved in deciding the value of our thoughts, perceptions and behaviors.[26]

One part of the limbic system, the ventromedial prefrontal cortex, is thought to act as a "gatekeeper". Typically, we ignore the majority of the auditory signals passing through our auditory systems because these are unimportant background sounds that we do not want to be bothered hearing. (For example, how many people raptly listen to the sounds their refrigerators make? More likely you are not even aware your fridge is making any sounds.)

The "gatekeeper's" job is to filter out and reject such sounds. However, the "gatekeeper" must recognize and pass on those sounds that it perceives as threatening or a warning of some kind. For example, when the "gatekeeper" receives a tinnitus signal, it has to decide whether this sound should be considered valuable information and passed on, or worthless information that needs to be suppressed.[27]

When the "gatekeeper" system isn't working well, you are not able to suppress your unimportant thoughts, behaviors and perceptions—including phantom perceptions such as your tinnitus. Thus, it appears that people with bothersome tinnitus are not able to regulate the hyperactivity in their auditory systems that may originally be triggered by loss of hearing.[28] This is in stark contrast to people with no tinnitus, or people with tinnitus that does not bother them. For these latter people, tinnitus signals are largely suppressed. However, this apparently does not happen to people with bothersome tinnitus.

Researchers have been puzzling over this question, "Why doesn't the "gatekeeper" block the tinnitus signals from these people too?" Now they think they have discovered the answer.

In recent studies, researchers have discovered that a part of the limbic system of people with tinnitus is structurally different and significantly smaller in size than it is in people without bothersome tinnitus. They think that the loss in volume in this area reflects fewer neurons there. Thus, the "gatekeeper" doesn't have enough "horsepower" to do its job effectively. As a result, it is less successful at suppressing unwanted signals. Consequently, these people begin to hear their tinnitus.[29]

**Depression, Chronic Pain and Tinnitus**

Interestingly enough, the same differences in the "gatekeeper" (ventromedial prefrontal cortex) are found in people with depression and chronic pain as they are in people with chronic tinnitus.[30] In the future, this may lead to similar treatments for tinnitus as is used for people with chronic pain, for example.

If your limbic system does not sufficiently inhibit your tinnitus, here's what happens. You first experience tinnitus either in your ears or in the temporal lobe of your brain. This strange new tinnitus sound can trigger a pathway of fear, phonophobia, hyperacusis, depression[31], disgust, frustration, annoyance, anxiety or panic.[32] Thus, as a tinnitus sufferer, you are someone whose brain detects this noise, and then your limbic system interprets this new sound as **dangerous or threatening to your well-being** in some manner.

Your hippocampus (part of your limbic system) quickly decides how important this new sound is. If your brain is emotionally stimulated (fear, anxiety, panic, depression, stress, etc.) by the noise, your brain's emotional center pulls its internal "fire alarm".[33]

When this happens, norepinephrine (nor-epp-ih-NEFF-rin) is released and suffuses your brain. Norepinephrine essentially heightens the sensitivity of the brain areas that receive it, making your sensory circuits more sensitive Essentially, it sets your brain on edge.[34] Another way of saying this is that it sets your internal auditory volume control to high—and guess what—your tinnitus now sounds much louder too!

The hippocampus part of your brain directs the release of dopamine that leads to your riveting your attention on the source of your fear—the strange tinnitus sounds. It also puts your muscles at readiness to react accordingly (fight or flight mode).[35] At this point, your whole body is focused on your tinnitus.

This is exactly opposite to what you want to happen. As a tinnitus sufferer, you need to understand that hearing tinnitus is completely acceptable and unworthy of any special attention. Furthermore; you need to understand that it is just an auditory perception—neither good nor bad—but simply something that you perceive.[36] It is not something to fear.

In addition, you must learn that tinnitus can be eliminated **only** if the sound becomes irrelevant, meaningless and unimportant to you. When sounds become unimportant, your brain begins to ignore them. The result is that these sounds then begin to fade into the background much the same as do traffic noises or the sounds from your fridge or furnace after you become used to them.

## A Neurophysiological Model of Tinnitus

Much of our current understanding of tinnitus has come through the dedicated research of Dr. Pawel Jastreboff. Dr. Jastreboff, a world-famous neuro-scientist, developed the neurophysiological model of tinnitus. This model takes into account the complex relationships between other systems in our brains in addition to our auditory systems.

In Dr. Jastreboff's model of tinnitus, the two major players are the limbic system and the autonomic nervous system (Fig. 3-1). The limbic system within our brains generates our emotions. It is here that we feel such negative emotions as fear, anxiety, thirst and hunger.

Our autonomic nervous systems work closely with our limbic systems. They control many of the functions of our bodies, especially all the stress-related actions such as the "fight or flight" reaction whenever danger presents itself.

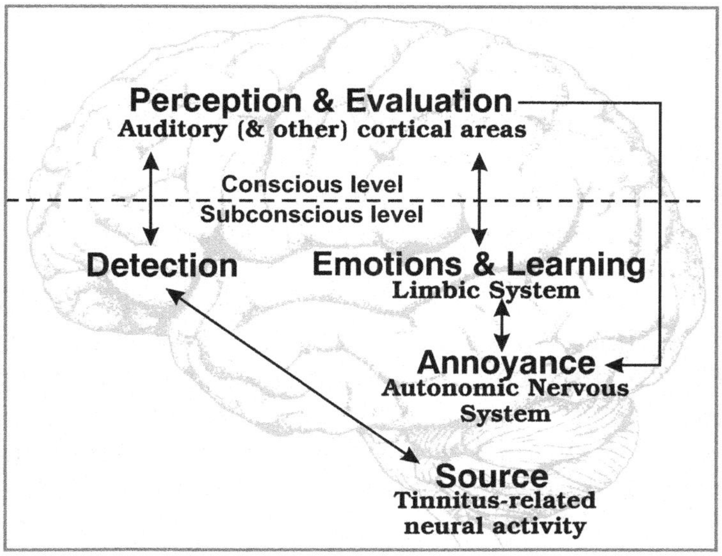


Fig. 3-1. This is a diagrammatic representation of Dr. Jastreboff's neuro-physiological model of tinnitus. The source of tinnitus may be the electrical signals from any active neurons in our auditory systems. At the subconscious level several things happen. Detection filters (clusters of neurons) tune in to this signal. If it does not have any negative significance it is largely ignored and not brought to the conscious level. If it is persistent or has negative significance this signal is sent to our limbic and autonomic nervous systems where a conditioned response is learned and set up—still at the subconscious level. A response is then sent to the conscious level of our brains where we hear it as tinnitus. Note that the unpleasant "sounds" of tinnitus result solely from the negative stimulation of our limbic and autonomic nervous systems. Both of these systems lie outside of our auditory systems. Thus tinnitus is not connected directly to our ears.

At this point, we need to review what happens to any sound signals from the time they leave our ears until we hear them in the conscious parts of our brains. Our ears send all the sound signals they generate to our brains. These sounds are not separated—they are just one big mass of signals—some meaningful, some insignificant, some just random neuronal activity. There, in our brainstems at the bottom of our brains, millions and millions of neurons (nerve cells) in numerous neuronal networks begin sorting and filtering these signals (Fig. 3-2). Our brains initially sort and filter these sound signals without our even being aware of it since this is done in the subconscious parts of our brains.

The subconscious parts of our brains enhance (make louder) certain signals and reduce or suppress others. This happens whenever we consciously focus our attention on or away from certain sounds. When we focus on people talking, for example, our lower brain separates out and inhibits non-speech-like sounds. It does this by sending down neural messages to reduce the activity of the nerves bringing up unwanted noise. When we want to hear just one person when many are speaking at once, we pinpoint in space the voice we want to hear. We do this by focusing our attention on the person we want to hear and ignoring others speaking

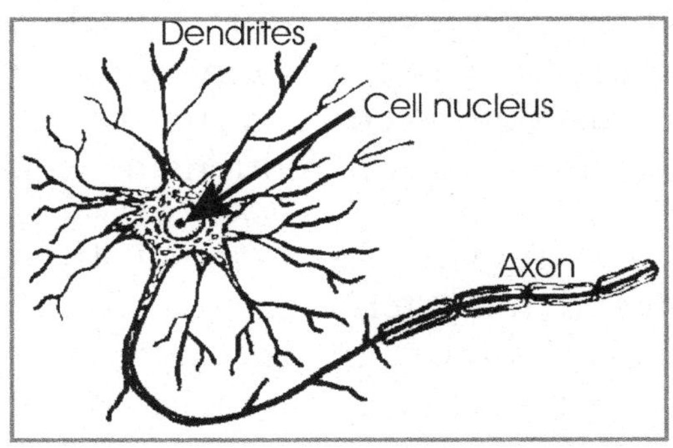


Fig. 3-2. A neuron or nerve cell. Our bodies have several billion nerve cells in them. The dendrites receive stimulation from other nerve cells. The axon carries nerve impulses to other nerve cells or their dendrites. This vast interconnected array of nerve cells is called a neuronal network.

around us. Our brains then attempt to neurologically suppress any sounds coming from other locations.

We also need to understand that in the absence of sound—that is, in total silence—our auditory pathways still have considerable neuronal activity going on. However, this activity is random. Normally, our nervous systems filter out all this random activity before it reaches our conscious level. Therefore, we do not perceive it as sound.

Whenever there is sound around us, the neuronal activity within our auditory systems increases. The big difference is that this activity is more regular and synchronized. When the patterns of electrical activity within our auditory nerves closely reflect the sounds that reach our ears, these signals undergo further extensive processing in several centers within our auditory pathways.

Only after these auditory signals have been extensively processed and filtered by our neuronal networks are they sent to the auditory processing centers in the conscious parts of our brains. Up to this point we have not heard a thing. All processing has been done in our subconscious. Speech sounds have not yet been identified as words. Now, our temporal lobes organize these sounds into words and we "hear" them. At the same time, this information is routed to other centers of thought, action, sight, and so on.[37]

These sound signals get further processed as they pass through our limbic systems. Here is where we react to many sounds. For example, the sound of a loved one's voice may bring us feelings of joy. Some sounds may evoke fear, such as a gunshot nearby in the middle of the night. Other sounds do not draw any response from us at all—like the sounds our refrigerators make. It is obvious that some sounds induce strong positive emotions in us. Others give rise to negative emotions. And some do not affect our emotions at all. Dr. Jastreboff discovered that people who are bothered by tinnitus typically have strong negative emotions associated with their tinnitus.

As you might expect, these negative emotions bring on strong negative reactions. Often these reactions involve such things as having trouble sleeping, being unable to pay attention to anything other than our tinnitus, and suppressing our positive emotions.

The reason for this is because the neuronal networks in our brains sort all sounds according to their significance. The important sounds get high priority and are brought to our attention. Insignificant sounds are filtered out (inhibited or suppressed). The rules controlling this sorting are not fixed, but change throughout our lives (neural plasticity). Therefore, with proper training, we can enhance our perception of certain sounds we always want to hear. At the same time, we can train our brains to filter out other less significant sounds.

When we "hear" a certain signal over and over, and as long as we do not associate any emotion with it, our neuronal networks begin to filter it out. This means that less and less often are such signals passed on to our limbic (emotional) and cortical (auditory) centers for further processing. In contrast, any sounds associated with something significant, particularly sounds related to danger, are immediately enhanced and strongly activate those areas responsible for our emotions and conscious response.

It takes time to become conditioned to a given sound. In the beginning, new sounds have no meaning to us. We have to learn to associate a sound with its meaning. Then we learn to associate certain emotions with it. In time, we become conditioned to certain sounds. For example, if we are going to cross a road and a car horn sounds, we instinctively jump back. Why? It is simply because we have learned to associate the sound of a car horn with danger. Now, because of the strong negative emotions associated with danger, it has become a conditioned reflex. We cannot easily change this by our conscious will. This is why I just cannot say, "My tinnitus will not bother me anymore", and have it immediately come true. However, any type of conditioned reflex that we learn, we can also unlearn and/or relearn differently. It will take time and effort, but we can do it.

For example, I originally learned to type using the standard keyboard (QWERTY) layout. After 35 years of typing this way, I decided one day a number of years ago to change the layout of the keys to the Dvorak layout in order to type more efficiently. Now I had to unlearn everything I knew about typing and start all over again. (It's quite a pain to go from typing over 100 words per minute to 0!) It was also totally frustrating. My fingers wanted to go back to their old habits. I made numerous mistakes. However, slowly I retrained my brain. The mistakes became fewer and fewer, and my speed slowly increased.

Now I type using the Dvorak layout just like I used to do with the QWERTY layout. My fingers have learned a new reflex action. When my eyes see a certain letter, I do not have to consciously think which finger to press—it is now automatic. In fact, I can no longer touch-type using a standard (QWERTY) keyboard layout any more—I have to look at the keys. I have totally unlearned one way and learned another way.

In the same manner, we can teach our brains to unlearn their conditioned reflexes to tinnitus and relearn another conditioned reflex—ignore tinnitus.

Research has shown that people with normal hearing are aware of only a small portion of the sounds reaching their ears. As I have previously explained, our brains ignore the vast majority of sounds we hear each day. Our neuronal networks are marvelous devices. They filter out the signals we do not need to consciously hear. So, although all sounds cause changes in neuronal activity within our auditory pathways, many of these sounds get filtered out by our neuronal networks before they reach the top of our brains where we consciously hear them. This automatically happens because minor meaningless sounds do not call forth any emotional reaction that would activate our autonomic nervous systems.

## Habituation—the Goal of Tinnitus Therapy

While your brain will immediately enhance certain sounds, there are other sounds that your brain has become so used to (the fancy medical term is "habituated to") so that you are not even aware of them. For example, suppose you move to a house that is on a main highway. At first, you hear all the traffic noise. Soon you accept it as a part of your new life. It is a constant background noise to everything you hear. Because it is not meaningful sound, you begin to ignore it. After a few months you realize that it doesn't bother you anymore. In fact, it doesn't even seem to sound as loud as it used to. Since it is meaningless noise, you are becoming habituated to it. Normally, unless it is particularly quiet where you are, you often don't even hear this noise any more.

### Habituation Hard for Hard of Hearing People

Incidentally, for those of us who have severe or worse hearing losses, it is difficult for us to habituate to sounds. Because we hear so few sounds, most sounds loud enough for our ears to detect enter our consciousness as warning signals—so we cannot just ignore them like people with normal hearing can.

Are the traffic sounds any quieter now? No. The traffic is still there day and night. What has happened is that your neuronal networks have filtered out these sounds since they are essentially neutral and meaningless to you. Instead of enhancing them, your neuronal networks have reduced these sounds so you do not hear them as loudly as you used to, if you can hear them at all. Now, you have to consciously listen for the traffic noise before you can hear it because you are thoroughly habituated to such sounds. Remember, this only occurs when such sounds do not have negative emotions associated with them.

You can do the same thing with your tinnitus. Since your reaction to tinnitus is a learned response, just like any other learned response, you can unlearn it. You need to weaken the conditioned reflex connections between your auditory, limbic and autonomic nervous systems before you can habituate to your tinnitus. This happens in two stages.

First, you must habituate your **reactions** by detaching the perception of your tinnitus from the negative responses of your brain. You do this by clearly understanding that you do not need to fear or be annoyed by your tinnitus. You have successfully done this when your tinnitus becomes just another background sound like fridge or traffic noise. It no longer annoys you although it is just as loud as it was before.

Second, you must habituate your **perception** of tinnitus by blocking (filtering out) any tinnitus-related brain activity before it reaches your level of consciousness. When you do this, your tinnitus actually fades into the background and often you will not even hear it.

Habituation is just the process of adapting to a stimulus through repeated exposure. Thus, you can define tinnitus habituation as an adaptation process of your auditory system that not only reduces how loud you now perceive your tinnitus, but also reduces your previously-held strong reactions to your tinnitus.[38]

In order to habituate to your tinnitus you need to totally put tinnitus out of your mind, not dwell on it.

When you habituate to your tinnitus, both your perception of your tinnitus, and your reaction to your tinnitus, is greatly, if not fully, diminished.[39] You know you have habituated to your tinnitus when your brain reclassifies tinnitus as an unimportant sound that you can safely and consciously ignore.

Therefore, when you habituate to both your perception of, and your reaction to, your tinnitus, you are seldom aware of your tinnitus. Furthermore, you are not annoyed by your tinnitus, even when you do perceive it. As a result, tinnitus ceases to have any real impact on your life. Instead of suffering from tinnitus, you move into the category of those people who just experience it.[40] What blessed relief!

---

**Chapter 3 Endnotes**

1 Hogan, 1998. p. 70.
2 Forstag, 2014. p. 19.
3 Moller, 2011. pp. 223-228.
4 Hogan, 1998. p. 65.p
5 Moller, 2011. pp. 113-120.

6 Bartels, 2007. p. 21.
7 Moller, 2011. pp. 149-155.
8 Sweetow, 2015a. p. 34.
9 Researchers Map Tinnitus in Human Brain During Surgery, 2015. p. 38.
10 Bartels, 2007. p. 25.
11 HearingReview.Com. 2015. p. 36.
12 University of Leicester, 2012. pp 1-2.
13 Kaltenbach, 2011. pp. 37-39.
14 Kaltenbach, 2011. pp. 37-39.
15 Hogan, 1998. p. 53.
16 Bauman, 2010b. p. 1.
17 Bartels, 2007. p. 20.
18 Bartels, 2007. p. 21.
19 Bartels, 2007. p. 25.
20 Moller, 2011. pp. 103-112.
21 Leaver, 2011b. pp. 1-2.
22 Levine, 2000. p. 6.
23 Zagolski, 2014. p. 27.
24 Zagolski, 2014. p. 27.
25 Moller, 2011. pp. 95-98.
26 Leaver, 2011b. p. 2.
27 Leaver, 2011b. p. 2.
28 Leaver, 2011b. p. 2.
29 Tinnitus: Is This What Happens When the Brain's Gatekeeper Breaks Down? 2011. p. 1.
30 Leaver, 2011b. p. 2.
31 Bartels, 2007. pp. 28-29.
32 Hogan, 1998. p. 72.
33 Hogan, 1998. p. 73.
34 Hogan, 1998. p. 74.
35 Hogan, 1998. p. 74.
36 Hogan, 1998. p. 81.
37 Auditory Disorders, 1997. pp. 1-2.
38 Tunkel, 2014. p. S22.
39 Sweetow, 2015a. p. 34.
40 Jastreboff, 1997c. pp. 1-5.

# Part II

# What Causes Tinnitus?

## Chapter 4

# The Many Causes of Tinnitus

There are many different things that result in tinnitus. We often refer to "causes" of tinnitus (what doctors call the etiology of tinnitus), but in fact we don't really know the specific cause of the common neurophysiologic kind of tinnitus.

For example, we may say that exposing our ears to loud noise "caused" our tinnitus. The noise probably caused some cochlear damage, but the noise itself did not cause our tinnitus. Technically, instead of "causes", we should use terminology that implies indirect causality, such as precipitating factors, events associated with tinnitus onset, tinnitus precursor events or tinnitus triggering events.[1] I prefer to use the term "associated with tinnitus" or "resulting in tinnitus" when I write about things that "cause" tinnitus.

In the following chapters in this section, we will look at the various classes of things that are associated with tinnitus, beginning with the four most common things

### Causes of Tinnitus

Here are the causes (onset factors) reported for tinnitus from 1,035 people.[2]

| Traumatic onset factor | % |
|---|---|
| Long-duration noise | 20 |
| Head injury | 12 |
| Explosive noise | 10 |
| Neck injury/whiplash | 9 |
| Brief non-explosive noise | 6 |
| Miscellaneous illnesses | 6 |
| Head and neck injury | 5 |
| Drugs, medications | 5 |
| Ear infections | 5 |
| Other ear problems | 5 |
| Colds/sinus infections | 5 |
| Stress | 4 |
| Surgery | 3 |
| TMD syndrome | 2 |
| Barotrauma | 1 |
| Sudden hearing loss | 1 |
| Allergies/hay fever | 1 |

that trigger tinnitus: exposing our ears to loud noises, taking various drugs, untreated hearing loss (often associated with aging), and negative emotions.

After that, in turn, we will look at tinnitus associated with the body (mainly the head and neck) and body movements (somatosensory tinnitus), various medical conditions that "cause" tinnitus, tinnitus associated with inner ear conditions, tinnitus associated with middle ear conditions, and end with tinnitus associated with various foods and other substances.

---

**Chapter 4 Endnotes**

1 Henry, 2010a. p.6.
2 Tinnitus Archive, 2004. p. 2.

## Chapter 5

# Loud Noise

Loud noise is the most common trigger of **preventable** tinnitus. A study of 1,687 people with tinnitus revealed that noise exposure accounted for one out of every four (24%) cases of tinnitus.[1]

When you expose your ears to loud sounds, typically your ears ring for a while after. That is tinnitus. This indicates that you are beginning to damage your ears. For example, about 55% of the people in one study remembered hearing tinnitus lasting from a few minutes to several hours or even days after exposing their ears to loud sounds.[2] If you continue to work, play or live around loud sounds, you may end up with permanent (and often annoying) tinnitus. It may take days, months or years (such as working in a noisy factory) for this to happen. At other times it can be instantaneous.

Permanent tinnitus can result from a single, sudden exposure to high levels of noise. For example, one man explained how he had put on a pair of earphones to play a computer game. What he didn't realize was that the volume was turned all the way up. Without warning, there was a loud trumpet fanfare that blasted his ears. His result—instant, permanent tinnitus before he could rip the headphones off. It can happen just that fast.

His ears had been ringing for ten weeks when he contacted me for help. He now also suffers from hyperacusis from this episode. (As you may recall, hyperacusis is where you perceive all normal sounds as much too loud—often so loud that they hurt.) Incidentally, very often noise damage not only results in tinnitus, but also in hyperacusis **and** some degree of hearing loss.

Another prime cause of tinnitus is sudden exposure to dangerously high levels of noise like explosions, gunfire and mortar rounds that people in the military or police forces often experience.

(It is interesting to note that, "through extensive neural research on rats with tinnitus, researchers have determined that the neural mechanisms underlying blast-induced tinnitus are substantially different from those underlying the common kind of noise-induced tinnitus. This is an important finding, as it suggests these two different types of tinnitus will require different therapeutic treatments.")[3]

However, it is usually **continued exposure to loud noises** over the years in noisy factories, mills and work areas; the exceptionally loud music in clubs, pubs and discotheques; the thumping boom car amplifiers; and noisy recreational pursuits that ultimately results in permanent tinnitus.

That is why those of you who work in noisy occupations or who are exposed to excessively loud sounds like military personnel, police officers, firefighters, carpenters, farmers, musicians, pilots, and mill workers are most susceptible to tinnitus. So too are you if you engage in such noisy recreational pursuits as shooting, riding motorcycles and driving snowmobiles. If you regularly expose your ears to excessive noise from loud concerts, iPods, MP3 players and such like, you also will likely have to put up with tinnitus later. So will you if you use loud tools such as chain saws, skill saws, leaf blowers, noisy lawnmowers, etc. around your house and yard without wearing ear protection. Therefore, avoid loud noise or protect your ears from loud noise. In your later years you will be glad you did!

**An Ounce of Prevention...**

If you are at high risk of developing clinically-significant tinnitus, you would be wise to attend a short informational session about tinnitus and its connection with your emotions **before** you develop tinnitus. (To find such a session, search for a tinnitus clinic run by audiologists in your area.) Just doing this could significantly decrease your risk of developing bothersome tinnitus because you can "short-circuit" any negative emotions connected to your tinnitus before they cause trouble. If you do this, you will still hear any resulting tinnitus, but it should not be much of a problem for you.[4] In any case, if you expose your ears to loud sound, you should wear effective ear protection so tinnitus won't develop in the first place!

You may find that tinnitus occurs immediately after you have been exposed to a loud noise. Most often, you get mild, temporary tinnitus, but it may be permanent. The length of time your tinnitus lasts and its severity generally increases each time you expose your ears to loud noise. Finally, one day you may discover that your tinnitus is now permanent and distressing.

**Tinnitus from Ear Syringing**

An audiologist asked, "I am a newly-qualified audiologist and frequently see patients that suffer from tinnitus. A number of my patients report that their tinnitus started after their ears were syringed. Why?"

You may be surprised to learn that having your ears syringed to remove wax can actually cause tinnitus. The same is true if you shower and aim a high-pressure shower-head directly into your ear canals. Actually, anything that violently moves your eardrums, whether water pressure or air pressure (from a loud noise), can result in tinnitus.

What happens is that the sudden forceful "squirt" of the water hitting your eardrum moves your eardrum in a similar manner as if you had heard a sudden loud noise like a gunshot. That is why, for some people, syringing or showering is the root of their tinnitus.

Note: Suctioning wax out can be just as bad if your eardrum is suddenly "sucked out", again imitating the movement of a sudden loud sound. The trick is to remove wax from your ear canal without making your eardrum move much in either direction if you want to avoid tinnitus from this cause.

If you shower using a low-pressure (reduced-flow) shower head, then letting the water squirt into your ear canals probably won't hurt your ears or cause tinnitus. I have done this for a couple of decades now, and it has not affected my existing tinnitus. Thus, the trick in avoiding tinnitus is to use a **gentle** spray, **not** a high pressure jet of water, whether syringing or showering.

When you expose your ears to loud noises, or perhaps suffer a blow to your head, cochlear damage and tinnitus often occurs. For example, you can get tinnitus from a severe blow to the head such as the blow you get from the airbags in a motor vehicle collision—not to mention the loud explosive sound as the air bag suddenly inflates. And as strange as it seems, a number of people have gotten tinnitus as a result of their doctors syringing the wax out of their ears too forcefully (See text box above). [5]

You can even get tinnitus from the ultrasonic cleaners and scalers dental hygienists sometimes use. In fact, "numbers of people report tinnitus after having their teeth cleaned by these devices".[6]

The tinnitus sounds caused by noise damage are many and varied. They may sound like ringing bells, chirping cicadas, a high-pitched whine, or roaring, hissing or fluttering sounds.[7]

## How Loud Is Too Loud?

There are two aspects to this question—how loud the sound is, and how long this loud sound lasts. Here are two rules of thumb.

1. A sudden burst of loud sound at 120 dB or higher can instantaneously cause ear damage.

2. Sustained sounds in the 80 to 110 dB range can cause hearing loss over a number of weeks, months or years.

The Occupational Safety and Health Administration (OSHA) in the US, and the Department of Occupational Health and Safety in Canada both have the same workplace standards; namely, you can expose your ears to an average of 85 dB for 8 hours. Then for every 3 dB increase in sound level, the time is cut in half.

The National Institutes of Health Consensus Development Conference (1990) in the US explained: "Sound levels of less than 75 dB(A) are unlikely to cause permanent hearing loss, while sound levels at 85 dB(A), with exposures of 8 hours per day, will produce permanent hearing loss over a period of ten years or more".

However, the United States Environmental Protection Agency (EPA) is probably closer to the truth when it says that an average of 70 dB per day (24 hours) will prevent any measurable hearing loss over a lifetime".

Therefore, keep your sound exposure to an average of 70 dB or less if you want to preserve your hearing until you die. And if you preserve your hearing like this, it's almost certain you won't get tinnitus from noise exposure either.

---

**Chapter 5 Endnotes**

1 Discovering and Understanding Tinnitus, 1997. p. 2.
2 Levine, 2000. p. 6.
3 Luo, 2014. p. 28.
4 Moller, 2011. pp. 575-596.
5 Levine, 2000. p. 7.
6 Mayes, 2010. p. 177.
7 Currie, 2005.

## Chapter 6

# Hearing Loss

Very often tinnitus and hearing loss go together. About 70% of people with hearing loss have tinnitus. And looking at it the other way, approximately 90% of the people with tinnitus have some degree of hearing loss.[1] One study revealed that of people with profound hearing losses, about 80% hear tinnitus.[2] The surprising thing to my mind is that about 20% are tinnitus-free.

The American Tinnitus Association is even more specific and reports that up to 90% of all people with tinnitus have some level of **noise-induced** hearing loss.[3]

Some researchers go by the 80/80 rule. It states that 80% of all people with tinnitus have sensorineural hearing losses, and that 80% of all people with sensorineural hearing loss have tinnitus.[4]

No matter which figures you accept, it is obvious that very often tinnitus and hearing loss go together. Since tinnitus and hearing loss often go together, it should be no surprise that tinnitus often is associated with the high frequency hearing loss that comes from aging.

Note that hearing loss can, and often does, result in tinnitus. However, the reverse is not true. Tinnitus is **never** the **cause** of hearing loss.[5]

Many people now think that our brains try to make up for the lack of normal sounds by producing tinnitus to fill the void. Their reasoning is wrong, but the result is correct—tinnitus unfortunately does fill the void.

Current thinking is that the neurons at those frequencies you no longer hear (or don't hear well at all) now have little/nothing to do. Since neurons don't like to be idle, they look over their shoulders at their neighboring neurons and begin doing what their neighboring neurons are doing. When enough neurons start doing the same thing when there is no real sound input, you end up with tinnitus. This is why tinnitus often (but not always) is at a frequency near the frequency of your greatest hearing loss. This shows that our brains can adapt and change their responses over time due to neural plasticity as we saw in Chapter 3.

Hearing loss does not always result in tinnitus, but it often happens that way. It is thought that the auditory system in your brain responds to your hearing loss by turning up its internal volume. Thus, you now perceive your tinnitus as louder.[6]

However, it could be that your hearing loss unmasks the tinnitus that was already there, but you did not hear it before because of the other sounds your ears were hearing.[7] It could also be that when you become aware of your hearing loss, it draws your attention to what you are hearing, and now you notice your tinnitus for the first time.

Apart from obtaining hearing aids **before** you develop tinnitus from straining to hear, there is not much else that you can do to prevent tinnitus once you have a hearing loss. Therefore, if you want to avoid tinnitus in the first place, avoid hearing loss, and if you want to avoid hearing loss, protect your ears from loud sounds.

---

**Chapter 6 Endnotes**

1 Tinnitus and Hearing Loss, 2011. p. 1.
2 Levine, 2000. p. 6.
3 American Tinnitus Association, 2002. p. 2.
4 Beck, 2015. p. 2.
5 Craggs-Hinton, 2007. p. 3.
6 Sweetow, 2015a. p. 34.
7 Levine, 2000. p. 6.

Chapter 7

# Prescription Drugs, Chemicals and Heavy Metals

The second most common trigger of **preventable** tinnitus is taking certain prescription and non-prescription drugs. Are you taking any of the medications that are known to trigger tinnitus? The book *Ototoxic Drugs Exposed* (see text box) lists more than 595 prescription drugs, herbals and chemicals that can trigger tinnitus. The shocking truth is that there are more than 560 generic drugs that are associated with tinnitus[1] spread over more than 1,200 brand names. (See the Appendix for a listing of all these drugs.) Such drugs can trigger tinnitus in the first place, make your existing tinnitus louder or trigger a new tinnitus sound.[2]

**Drugs That Can Cause Tinnitus**

There are hundreds of prescription and over-the-counter drugs from Abatacept (*Orencia*) to Zuclopenthixol (*Clopixol*) that can cause or trigger tinnitus or make your existing tinnitus worse. (See the Appendix for a comprehensive list of such drugs.)

The definitive book on this subject, *Ototoxic Drugs Exposed—Prescription Drugs and Other Chemicals that Can (and Do) Damage Our Ears* describes the ear-damaging (ototoxic) side effects of numerous drugs, herbs and chemicals. It lists 560+ drugs and 29 chemicals and heavy metals that are known to trigger tinnitus. If you think your tinnitus, or other ear problems, might have been caused by drugs, you might want to get this book. (See the back of this book for information on obtaining a copy of this invaluable book, or go to http://hearinglosshelp.com/shop/category/books/ and scroll down to the book on ototoxic drugs.)

The technical name for drugs that have side effects that can damage your ears is ototoxic drugs.

Ototoxic drugs typically damage the sensitive hair cells and/or underlying support cells in your cochlea and/or in your vestibular (balance) system. This can result in a number of side effects including tinnitus, hyperacusis, hearing loss and balance problems.

Some drugs are actually toxic to the ear and result in ear damage. Other drugs produce tinnitus as a side effect, supposedly without damaging the inner ear.[3]

Tinnitus usually appears first as a continuous high-pitched sound. The reason for this is that ototoxic drugs generally damage the hair cells at the base of the cochlea first—which is where the high-frequency sounds are detected and passed on to the brain.

Often tinnitus precedes or accompanies hearing loss from ototoxic drugs. In fact, tinnitus is the **number one** indicator that you may be doing damage to your ears. It also may be the **only** warning you'll ever get. Pay attention to it![4] If your ears begin to ring after you begin taking any drug, you should immediately report this to your doctor. You and your doctor should then decide what to do—whether to reduce the dose, change the medication or stop taking that medication altogether.

Tinnitus arising from taking ototoxic drugs may or may not be permanent.[5] The good news is that tinnitus resulting from taking certain ototoxic drugs is often temporary and goes away soon after you stop taking the drug (for example, *Aspirin*). Tinnitus from taking **Ibuprofen** may be temporary or it may be permanent. However,

**Will I Get Tinnitus From Taking a Given Drug?**

A man asked, "If tinnitus is listed as a possible side effect for a given drug, does one necessarily get tinnitus from taking it? Can I perhaps take it and not make my tinnitus worse and yet solve my medical problem?"

The answer is a definite "no" to the first question and a probable "yes" to the second question. Depending on your makeup, you may take a drug that has tinnitus listed as a side effect and not get tinnitus. In fact, most people that take drugs do not get tinnitus from taking them. Unfortunately, some do. Depending on the drug, it may be a very small percentage of those taking the drug that get tinnitus from taking it, or a much higher percentage.

The trick is knowing **before** you take a given drug into which group you are going to fall—the small unfortunate tinnitus group, or the large non-tinnitus group. Since there is no way of knowing ahead of time, you need to know of this possibility before you begin taking a given drug so you can decide for yourself whether you want to take this risk or not—especially if you already have bad tinnitus, and you don't want to do anything to make it worse.

tinnitus resulting from taking other drugs may be severe and permanent. For example, if you are taking an Aminoglycoside antibiotic, you are one of the lucky ones if it stops within a couple of weeks after you finish the drug therapy. For many people, this kind of tinnitus never goes away.

One of the treacherous things about tinnitus is that, if it is not very loud to begin with, or if you are quite sick, you may not even be aware of this warning signal until it is too late.

Tinnitus may show up very quickly after you begin taking an ototoxic medication, or it may take several days for it to become apparent. Thus, you may get tinnitus from the very first pill you take, or you may take a given drug for five years before tinnitus shows up. For example, tinnitus from loop diuretics (Furosemide) may start just minutes after you begin receiving it as an I.V. In contrast, tinnitus may not show up until two or three days after taking an Aminoglycoside antibiotic. With the Benzodiazepine class of drugs, tinnitus may only show up after you stop taking the drug after you have been on it for some years without developing tinnitus.[6] There is tremendous variability when it comes to drugs and tinnitus.

One question a lot of people ask is, "If an ototoxic drug causes tinnitus—then why doesn't my tinnitus go away when I stop taking the ototoxic drug?"

With a number of drugs, your tinnitus will go away in a couple of days to a couple of weeks after you stop taking the drug. Such drugs do not cause permanent damage to your ears.

Here is one explanation for why this occurs. Let's say a drug you are taking constricts the arteries going to your inner ears. The result is that less blood and oxygen reach your inner ears leaving the cells there "sick" (to use a fancy medical term). The result is tinnitus. When you stop taking the drug, blood flow returns to normal, your ears recover and your tinnitus fades away.

In contrast, some other drugs cause permanent damage or death to certain inner ear cells. Thus the resulting tinnitus is also permanent.

Another explanation for why tinnitus is permanent in one person and not in another has to do with how you deal with your tinnitus. Remember, tinnitus has both a physical and an emotional component. The above two scenarios only looked at tinnitus as a physical condition. Now let's see how the emotional component can affect the permanence of tinnitus. This can happen since your brain is "plastic" and can grow new connections between its various parts as situations change. If you take a certain drug and for whatever reason, whether physical or emotional, your brain develops new pathways for your tinnitus, then stopping taking that drug doesn't automatically destroy those connections, thus the tinnitus remains. (We discussed neural plasticity in Chapter 3.)

Think of a cloudburst that floods the land and carves out a new permanent channel for a river where none existed before. Stopping the rain doesn't change the new channel back to the old riverbed again. The river now flows permanently in a new direction.

This is similar to what can happen with your tinnitus when your emotions become involved. Stopping taking the drug doesn't affect these new connections. In order to get rid of your tinnitus in this case, you have to train your brain to quit using the new channels it has carved out and revert back to the old non-tinnitus channels. The good news is that you can modify these new connections as you'll see in Section III.

Tinnitus resulting from taking ototoxic drugs is generally high-pitched, continuous and occurs in both ears. However, certain ototoxic drugs produce distinctive tinnitus sounds. For example, tinnitus caused by Salicylates such as Acetylsalicylic acid (*Aspirin*) is generally a high-pitched or hissing sound and may sound like a continuous musical note.[7]

*Aspirin* can trigger tinnitus or make your existing tinnitus worse. Taking 6 to 8 adult *Aspirin* a day can cause ringing in your ears and temporary hearing loss.[8] As a general rule, the greater the blood serum levels of Acetylsalicylic acid (*Aspirin*), the worse the resulting tinnitus and/or hearing loss. Usually, but not always, the hearing loss and accompanying tinnitus are completely reversible within 24 to 72 hours after you stop taking this drug, but in rare cases, permanent hearing loss can occur.[9]

Although the rule of thumb is that you have to take 6 or more **adult** *Aspirin* a day to get tinnitus, some people are much more sensitive to *Aspirin* than that. For example, one lady with mild to moderate tinnitus noticed that her tinnitus had quickly increased until it was unbearable. Thinking about what had recently changed in her life, she realized that the only difference was that she had begun taking one **baby** *Aspirin* daily for heart disease prevention.

With her doctor's permission she stopped taking the *Aspirin* for one week and then began taking it again. She did this several times. Each time she stopped taking the *Aspirin*, her tinnitus loudness decreased, so she ultimately stopped taking the *Aspirin* in order to keep her tinnitus under control. Just one **baby** *Aspirin* a day had caused her unbearable tinnitus.[10] (For more on salicylate sensitivity, see the section "Salicylates in Foods" in Chapter 13.)

Tinnitus from taking Erythromycin can produce a "blowing," sound while loop diuretics (such as Furosemide) may produce a middle-frequency sound.[11]

Tinnitus from taking Quinine and related drugs generally sound similar to the tinnitus sounds resulting from taking *Aspirin*. Quinine (and its derivatives, including tonic water because of the Quinine in it) can produce temporary or permanent sensorineural hearing loss with tinnitus as the major symptom. In fact, some Quinine derivatives cause significant and long-lasting tinnitus. As a result, you should not take Quinine if you already have tinnitus.[12, 13]

The truth is, tinnitus is often caused or triggered by a wide variety of medicinal and prescription drugs such as anti-anxiety and anti-depression drugs, antibiotics, anti-malarial medications, blood-pressure controlling medicines, toxins ingested into the body, and heavy metal poisoning. In fact, heavy metal poisoning (mercury) from fillings in your teeth can cause tinnitus. This generally occurs when your dentist replaces your old fillings.[14]

---

**Chapter 7 Endnotes**

1 Bauman, 2010a. p. 46.
2 Compendium of Pharmaceuticals and Specialties, 2000. pp. 1589, 1669.
3 American Tinnitus Association, 2002. p. 2.
4 Bauman, 2010a. p. 46.
5 Haybach, 1998. p. 3.
6 Bauman, 2010a. p. 47.
7 Bauman, 2010a. p. 47.
8 Stanten, 1996. p. 16.
9 Disorders of the Inner Ear, 2000. p. 10.
10 Mayes, 2010. p. 107.
11 Haybach, 1999. pp. 33-34.
12 Disorders of the Inner Ear, 2000. p. 10.
13 Hain, 2001. p. 5.
14 Currie, 2005.

Chapter 8

# Negative Emotions

Many people don't realize the tremendous role that negative emotions such as **stress**, **anxiety** (including fear) and **depression** have on their tinnitus. Not only do these negative emotions predispose people to tinnitus in the first place, they also are significant in determining who will **suffer** from tinnitus and who will just **experience** it.

Severe tinnitus is associated with depression, anxiety, sleep disturbances, and other disabling symptoms that significantly impact a person's quality of life.[1] Thus, a relatively high proportion of people concerned about their tinnitus suffer from depression and/or anxiety. Furthermore, people who report sleep problems also tend to have the most severe tinnitus.[2]

Various psychological problems seem to predispose people to tinnitus, and thus may trigger tinnitus or make existing tinnitus worse. Factors such as stress, panic disorder, anxiety, depression, and emotional challenges seem to determine who will experience suffering from their tinnitus and who will not. This is because the emotional part of our brains (limbic system) largely controls how we experience our tinnitus, whether we suffer from it and how we gain relief from it.[3]

If you suffer from tinnitus, basically what happens is that your negative emotions become paired with the sound of your tinnitus. Your brain detects the tinnitus sound and then interprets it as either dangerous or threatening to the quality of your life.[4] If this happens you suffer from your tinnitus. If not, then you just "have" tinnitus, but it does not bother you much at all. This is why about two-thirds of all people with tinnitus do not suffer from it.[5]

Neural plasticity also explains why medical procedures on any part of your body (when there has been excessive pain and associated anxiety, fear or anger) can trigger tinnitus.[6]

Another key finding is that people who have experienced stress, panic disorder, anxiety, depression and/or emotional problems **before** the onset of their tinnitus will find it much more difficult to reduce their tinnitus than people who were happy before their tinnitus began. Therefore, caring for your emotional health **before** you ever experience tinnitus is just as important as working to reduce your tinnitus once you have it. Furthermore, if you now have tinnitus and any of the above emotional problems, it is important to treat these conditions as part of your tinnitus reduction program.[7]

According to Kevin Hogan, Ph.D., there are several personality traits that are found in a significantly greater percentage of tinnitus sufferers than in the general population. One, they have above average IQs, but are below average in their emotional coping skills. Two, they are introspective—thus when tinnitus intrudes, they notice it right away and because they ruminate on it, their tinnitus really begins to bother them. Three, they tend to be perfectionists, yet having, but not being able to control, their tinnitus shows that they are not perfect. Four, they generally are more sensitive about personal matters. Thus they tend to feel like a victim, tend to feel persecuted or picked on and have tendencies to hostile responses.

These personality traits not only can lead to severe tinnitus, but once the tinnitus has started, can act as causal factors in creating the feedback loops that keep tinnitus going and going and going.[8]

## Anxiety

People with tinnitus often suffer from anxiety. Being anxious can cause tinnitus by itself. Here's why. When you are riddled with anxiety or feel threatened in some way, you put your body into "fight or flight" mode. When this happens, your senses are heightened—including your hearing. This means that you actually hear better than you could a moment before when you were not in the "fight or flight" mode.

This instinct is definitely useful for survival, but not for reducing your tinnitus. In fact, it is exactly the opposite of what you need. Since you are now worried about your tinnitus, your emotional system kicks in and you perceive your tinnitus as even louder and more intrusive than you did before, or maybe you begin to hear tinnitus for the first time. This makes you even more anxious, and you feel threatened by your tinnitus.

Closely related to anxiety is panic disorder. According to one study, 56% of the people suffering from **panic attacks** also suffer from tinnitus.[9]

Unfortunately, if you tend to be high strung and anxious, you will also have a much more difficult time bringing your tinnitus under control than it if you are calm and laid-back.

Thus, if you are anxious all the time, the solution is also obvious. Learn to control your anxiety. You need to find a good counselor who can help you uncover the reasons for your anxiety so you can learn how to calm yourself down. Not only will this help your health in general, it will also help you to bring your tinnitus under your control.

## Stress

Note this well. Uncontrolled stress and tension often make your tinnitus worse. Hundreds of studies cite excessive **stress** as related to tinnitus annoyance and suffering. Excessive stress is highly correlated with tinnitus onset. In fact, "tinnitus is very often a manifestation of stress". As Barbara Jenkins reports, "The two things that exacerbate tinnitus more than anything else are stress and fatigue. Do all that you can to treat your body well so that your ears can heal as much as possible."[10]

The truth is, stress may be **the** most overlooked cause of tinnitus. More accurately, perhaps we should view stress as not the **cause** of tinnitus, but as a **prime aggravator** of tinnitus.[11] This is because stress helps create the right psychological environment for the onset of tinnitus.[12] "The thing which seems to separate the tinnitus patient from the non-patient is their level of stress." There is no doubt about it, stress and anxiety can make your tinnitus worse. Furthermore, tinnitus can make your stress and anxiety worse.[13] Thus, learning how to deal with the stress in your life can eliminate, or greatly reduce, tinnitus from this cause.

The hypothalamus (part of your limbic system) and related structures in your brain all play a part in causing tinnitus. This is because the hypothalamus, and related structures, are responsible for producing essential chemicals you need in order to function normally. Furthermore, shock, grief, and continuing stress severely affect your hypothalamus. When this happens, it does not produce these essential chemicals in normal quantities. The result is often severe tinnitus.

Tinnitus from stress may often be ringing, whistling or whizzing noises or may sound like rushing water.[14]

Note: People consistently describe how their tinnitus bothers them more when they are under stress. This may be due to an increase in tinnitus loudness, or because people focus more on their tinnitus when they are stressed. However, for some people, it could also be that stress acts through muscle tension (somatic modulation) to increase tinnitus loudness, since contractions of various muscles in the head and neck, such as clenching the teeth, furrowing the brow, or grimacing often accompany stress.[15] (For more on this see Chapter 9.)

## Depression

Psychiatric conditions are common in people with bothersome tinnitus. For example, researchers report that 48% to 60% of tinnitus sufferers are depressed.[16]

People who are unable to properly cope with the stress in their lives often sink into depression. In fact, depression is a common emotional effect of tinnitus for those who cope poorly with tinnitus. Thus they suffer from it. Interestingly enough, people not suffering from depression develop tinnitus less often.

Furthermore, studies reveal that depression **precedes** a significantly large number of tinnitus cases. Did you get that? If you are depressed, you are more likely to get tinnitus than the average person who is not depressed. Therefore, for a large number of people suffering from tinnitus, many were predisposed to tinnitus by **depression**, and before that, from severe **stress**.[17] Thus no matter how you slice it, tinnitus and depression seem to go together. Sometimes tinnitus causes depression and sometimes depression leads to tinnitus. Sometimes the one feeds on the other and thus creates a vicious cycle of increasing depression and increasing tinnitus.

It seems that depression in people with bothersome tinnitus is more than twice that of the national average (35% vs. 15%).[18] In a couple of other studies, around 60% of the people with tinnitus also suffered from depression vs. only 7% to 21% of the control groups.[19] This reveals that tinnitus is 300% to 800% more common in people that are depressed than in the general population.

In still another study, current depression was reported in 48% of tinnitus sufferers vs. 7% of the control group.[20] This again reveals that depression is much more common in people with tinnitus than in people without tinnitus. As you can see, tinnitus and depression often go together. Thus, effective tinnitus treatment needs to address **both** the tinnitus **and** the depression.

The good news is that once you escape from your depression, your tinnitus will generally become less perceptible.[21] That is why treating depression often reduces both the tinnitus volume and the distress you feel related to your tinnitus.[22]

Incidentally, tinnitus often troubles people between the ages of 50 and 65. Here's why. By this time, their bodies are aging and likely their hearing is also going. At this age, they are often anxious about the future, and this anxiety can lead to depression. In their depression, they focus unduly on their tinnitus.[23]

Therefore, if you are depressed, you would be wise to get your depression under control. As you do this, you will tend to find your tinnitus becoming less intrusive and more and more fading into the background.

---

**Chapter 8 Endnotes**

1 Lockwood, 2001a. p. 2.
2 Henry, 2010b. p. 24.
3 Hogan, 1998. p. 63.
4 Hogan, 1998. pp. 68-69.
5 Hogan, 1998. p. 79.
6 Moller, 2011. pp. 343-361.
7 Hogan, 1998. p. 60.
8 Hogan, 1998. pp. 108-110.
9 Hogan, 1998. p. 106.
10 Jenkins, 2014. p. 29.
11 Craggs-Hinton, 2007. p. 30.
12 Hogan, 1998. p. 97.
13 Beck, 2015. p. 3.
14 Currie, 2005.
15 Levine, 2000. p. 9.
16 Tunkel, 2014. p. S5.
17 Hogan, 1998. p. 64.
18 Leaver, 2011a. p. 33.
19 Hogan, 1998. p. 105.
20 Hogan, 1998. p. 105.
21 Hogan, 1998. p. 62.
22 Hogan, 1998. p. 102.
23 Hazell, p. 41.

Chapter 9

# Body (Somatosensory) Conditions

## Somatic Modulation of Tinnitus

Strange as it may seem, researchers have known for a long time that some people can control changes to their tinnitus by doing things such as moving their eyes, moving their jaws, turning their heads or applying pressure to parts of their bodies. Even bending over, which increases your blood pressure, can increase your tinnitus.[1] For example, Penny relates, "My tinnitus gets louder and the tone gets lower when I bend over or do anything that increases the flow of blood to my head".

Some people have the ability to control the loudness of their tinnitus just by clenching their jaws.[2] Anita explains, "My tinnitus also varies when I move my jaw muscles, like when eating. Opening and closing my mouth can make the pitch of my tinnitus vary. Even something like a yawn can set it off."

How and why this happens used to be a mystery. For many years, doctors thought tinnitus arose almost exclusively out of abnormal neuronal activity within the auditory pathways. However, they now know that tinnitus-related neural activity is much more complex and multimodal than they previously thought.

There are a number of triggers that can cause somatosensory tinnitus. Researchers have discovered that some people can cause tinnitus or change their tinnitus by the signals from various body sensors and motor nerves.

For example, if you had somatosensory tinnitus you might immediately change the loudness and pitch of your tinnitus—though only temporarily—by forcefully contracting the muscles of your head, neck, arms or legs; by eye movements—both horizontally and vertically; by pressing on certain trigger points on your face; by touching the skin on your hands/fingertips and certain places on your face; by moving your fingers or head and neck; or by pressing on your temporomandibular joints or the muscles that move your jaw from side to side.[3] One man explained, "I feel and hear a rumbling kind of tinnitus if I yawn or press the left side of my head/neck/face near the left ear."

If you can modulate (change) your tinnitus through body motion and/or body position, you are experiencing somatosensory (body) modulation of your tinnitus.

Somatosensory is just a fancy medical term that comes from the Greek word "soma"—body, and the Latin word "sensus"—to feel. Stedman's Medical dictionary defines somatosensory as a "sensation relating to the body's superficial and deep parts as contrasted to specialized senses such as sight". Thus, somatosensory tinnitus can be a side effect of activating touch and movement sensors in your body.

Somatosensory tinnitus is a good example of how the central nervous system (brain) integrates signals it receives from the auditory system as well as from non-auditory systems. This shows that there are connections between auditory neurons and somatosensory neurons. The result is that an auditory symptom like tinnitus may be changed when these somatosensory neurons are activated. Now you can see why your tinnitus can change when your brain receives various non-auditory signals.[4]

Somatosensory modulation of tinnitus includes changes in tinnitus loudness, changes in tinnitus pitch and changes in which ear you hear your tinnitus.[5] By far the most common are changes in volume—either louder or softer—with louder being much more common than softer.[6]

Incidentally, head and neck contractions change tinnitus more effectively than arm or leg movements. Whenever arm or leg maneuvers modulate or elicit tinnitus, head and neck maneuvers also do the same, but the reverse is not necessarily true. In fact, twice as many people can modify or elicit tinnitus with head and neck contractions as can people by doing arm or leg contractions.[7] The anatomic hierarchy follows this order—head, arm, leg.[8]

Although it is not commonly talked about, somatosensory tinnitus is actually fairly common. You may be surprised to know that about 70% of the people with tinnitus have some "trick" they've learned that changes the loudness of their tinnitus.[9]

In one study, 23% were aware that if they did certain things they could change their tinnitus. However, during the course of this same study, 68% ultimately found they had this capability although they had not previously known they could do it.[10]

In the above study, 41% found that they could increase their tinnitus by certain head and neck movements, while 17% found these same movements decreased their tinnitus temporarily. Also, 33% found they could increase their tinnitus by certain arm and leg movements, while 4% found these same movements decreased their tinnitus.[11]

Another study revealed that about one-third of the people in the study could influence their tinnitus with jaw movements or by putting pressure on their temporomandibular joints.

For example, one man reported, "I can reduce or increase my steady-state tinnitus by pressing quite hard on various parts of my jaw. Pressing the jaw into the joint tends to decrease the tinnitus, pushing my chin to one side tends to increase it. The effect is quite dramatic."

In one tinnitus clinic, about 20% of their patients could somatically modulate their tinnitus by head and neck movements or muscle contractions such as clenching their teeth together.[12] Of all the different maneuvers, clenching the teeth most commonly affected the pitch of a person's tinnitus.[13]

Somatosensory tinnitus seems to originate almost exclusively from the upper cervical (neck) and head regions. If your tinnitus is caused by myofascial trigger points (see the following section), you should be able to feel pain or knots in one or more of the affected muscles.

Here are the top 7 tinnitus-troublemaker muscles.

Jaw muscles that can contribute to tinnitus include:

1. **Masseter**: the muscles under your cheeks that you use for chewing.

2. **Temporalis**: the flat muscles between and above your eyes and ears.

3. **Pterygoid** (both medial and lateral): muscles behind your masseter muscles.

Neck muscles that can contribute to tinnitus include:

4. **Levator scapula**: muscles that connect the top of each shoulder blade to the top 4 vertebrae in your neck.

5. **Splenius capitus**: Two broad, strap-like muscles located in the back of your neck. They connect the base of your skull (behind your ears) to the vertebrae in your neck and upper thorax.

6. **Upper trapezius**: Muscles, one on each side, that connect the base of your skull and cervical vertebrae to the back of your collar bones.

7. **Sternocleidomastoid** (STIR-noe-KLY-doe-MASS-toid) (SCM): The two big muscles on each side of your neck. You can easily see them as they stick out when you turn your head sideways. Your SCM muscles go from your breastbone or sternum (sterno) to your collarbone or clavicle (cleido) to the bone behind your ears (mastoid).[14] If either SCM muscle gets out of balance, it can cause somatosensory tinnitus. [15]

If you have somatosensory tinnitus, you'll notice three things.

1. Your tinnitus is closely associated with factors relating to your head or upper neck. Not surprisingly, the most common site for somatosensory tinnitus is the area around your ears and particularly the area just below your ears where your SCM muscle joins the mastoid bone.

2. You most likely hear your somatosensory tinnitus on the same side as the somatic injury (pain, muscle tension).

3. Somatosensory tinnitus is normally (but not always) a high-pitched, constant ringing sound.[16]

Here's another interesting point. There are at least three factors that can cause your tinnitus to change in volume. They are:

- Psychosocial stress,
- High-intensity sound exposure,
- Head and neck somatosensory factors.

Thus, if your tinnitus is intermittent or has wide fluctuations in loudness or other qualities, and you have not exposed your ears to loud sounds, nor are under undue stress, then your tinnitus changes are likely from somatosensory modulation.[17]

For example, if your tinnitus is louder when you wake up, you may be grinding your teeth (bruxism) while you sleep. This somatosensory action could cause your tinnitus to be louder. On the other hand, if your tinnitus vanishes by the time you wake up, and then returns as the day progresses, a different somatosensory action may be taking place. In this case, it may be that muscle contractions required to hold your head upright are making your tinnitus louder, or you may be clenching your teeth under the stress of the day's activities. If you find that your tinnitus is louder after awakening from a nap in a chair, you may have stretched certain neck muscles as your head fell forward, backward or sideways while you were dozing—thus your louder tinnitus.[18]

Some studies have shown that electrically stimulating the skin in certain places of the body can modulate tinnitus. For example, researchers can cause somatosensory tinnitus by electrically stimulating the median nerve in your arm.[19] This indicates that what doctors call the "non-classical auditory pathways" are involved in such forms of tinnitus.[20] In fact, it seems that the non-classical auditory pathways figure prominently in various forms of somatosensory tinnitus.

So what exactly are the non-classical auditory pathways? The auditory nervous system consists of two parallel pathways. The first is called the classical pathway and the second goes by the name of non-classical pathway (otherwise called the extra-lemniscal pathway). These two pathways process information differently and go to different parts of the brain.[21]

The classical pathway is strictly for auditory information. It is narrowly tuned to sound frequencies. It processes auditory information as this information moves from the cochlea to the primary auditory areas in the brain.

In contrast, the non-classical pathway is more broadly tuned, is more diffusely organized and is more plastic as compared to the classical pathway. The non-classical pathway receives its information not

### Touch-Sensitive Nerves in Your Head and Neck May Cause Tinnitus

New research reveals that for some people with hearing loss, the tinnitus associated with hearing loss stems from over-active sensory nerves in the face and neck.[22] After hearing loss occurs, for some reason, touch-sensing nerves in the face and neck step up their activity in the brain. The result is that some neurons in the cochlear nucleus become hyperactive. This increased activity has been linked to tinnitus.

For these people, treatment for their tinnitus may be as simple as acupuncture targeted at the nerves in the head and neck. Acupuncture seems to be mostly effective in acute and recent tinnitus as well as in somatic tinnitus.[23] "There are many anecdotal reports of improvements in tinnitus as a result of acupuncture. Acupuncture can certainly reduce the stress and anxiety linked to tinnitus."[24]

These findings may also reveal why many people with temporomandibular joint dysfunction (TMD) also suffer from tinnitus.

only from the ears, but also from other sensory organs of the somatosensory system such as the tactile (sense of touch/feel) system and the visual system.[25]

The association between the auditory and the non-classical (somatosensory) pathways occurs due to connections in the dorsal cochlear nucleus of the brain. There multitasking neurons receive signals from both the auditory and the somatosensory pathways.

Because there can be this association between the auditory pathways and the non-auditory pathways, when abnormal interactions occur between the various systems connected to these pathways, the result can be somatic tinnitus.[26] Note that the shorter the interval between the stimulus of one pathway relative to the other, the greater the interaction between them.[27]

This explains the connection between various forms of "weird" tinnitus that affect the other senses such as somatosensory tinnitus and gaze-evoked tinnitus. This also explains why grinding your teeth can cause or modulate your tinnitus. It also explains how involving another sense can change your existing tinnitus.

## Myofascial Tinnitus

When you first see the term "myofascial", if you read it too fast you might think it refers to the muscles of the face. If you think this, you'd be wrong. (That would be the word "myofacial" without the "s"—if there was such a word.)

You don't want to mix up the words "facial" and "fascial". They are two entirely different words. The word "myo" (MYE-oh) does indeed refer to "muscle" (from the Greek mys—muscle), but the word "fascial" (FASH-ee-al) is not the same as the word "facial" (FAY-shul) referring to the face.

The fascia is a sheet of fibrous tissue under the skin. It is also a sheet of fibrous tissue that encloses muscles or groups of muscles and separates their several layers or groups. Thus, "myofascial" specifically refers to the fascia surrounding and separating muscle tissue.

Myofascial tissue occurs throughout the body—anywhere there are muscles, including muscles on the face (facial muscles). In fact, myofascial tinnitus actually arises from problems in the myofascial tissue in the facial (face) and cervical (neck) muscles, so it is easy to be confused if you don't watch for the presence or absence of the letter "s" in these words.

Now that we are clear on this, let's look at myofascial tinnitus and what causes it. In some cases, tinnitus is caused by myofascial dysfunction (MFD) of the muscles of the head and neck.

With appropriate treatment such as trigger point deactivation, specific exercises, and treatment of the underlying causes of the muscle dysfunction, professionals can reduce or even completely eliminate tinnitus from this cause.[28]

Myofascial dysfunction is characterized by:

- Tight bands of contracted muscle fibers,
- Myofascial trigger point nodules or "knots" (TPs) which are exquisitely-tender, discrete nodules within tense muscle bands,
- Muscle shortening and muscle stiffening with attendant limitation of range of motion,
- Motor abnormalities,
- Disturbed motor function,
- Sensory abnormalities,[29] such as local and referred pain.[30]

Note: Referred pain is where the trigger points are in one place and the associated pain is in another place.

Recent studies have shown a strong relationship between tinnitus and trigger points. For example, a person with tinnitus is nearly five times more likely than a person without tinnitus to have trigger points which often change the intensity or type of tinnitus heard when touched. As you would expect, muscles located near the head are the most likely to produce such changes in tinnitus.[31]

There is also a close association between tinnitus and pain. For example, people with tinnitus are almost three times more likely to experience pain. Furthermore, improvement in their tinnitus is directly related to similar improvements in their degree of pain. A similar direct relationship is found in people who grind their teeth (bruxism). Thus, people with pain in their face and mouth are more likely to have tinnitus.[32]

Myofascial dysfunction develops as a result of muscle abuse such as overuse (e.g. sitting for many hours with poor posture, and other poor work ergonomics); misuse (e.g. not chewing normally due to a dental problem); underuse; and trauma (e.g. whiplash). In addition, chronic tightening of the upper shoulder muscles from mental stress also plays a role.[33]

Trigger points in the masseter (the muscles under your cheeks that you use for chewing) and sternocleidomastoid (the two big muscles on each side of your neck) muscles can cause tinnitus of myofascial origin. Note: You can cause trigger points in your masseter muscles by clenching or grinding your teeth.[34]

Chronic poor posture with your shoulders rounded and your head forward promotes upper trapezius and sternocleidomastoid trigger points. You have two triangular-shaped trapezius muscles—one on each side of your upper back. These muscles cover your shoulder blades and extend from your neck to your mid-back.

Furthermore, head, neck, and upper shoulder muscular imbalances, and cervical spine mobility impairment may also promote trigger points in these muscles.[35]

Although pain is the best known symptom of myofascial dysfunction, it is also responsible for a wide variety of symptoms, especially in the head and neck. These symptoms often masquerade as disorders of the ear, nose, and throat. Tinnitus is one of these disorders. Tinnitus of myofascial origin may occur in one ear or in both ears.

There is no way to predict who might benefit from MFD treatment. For example, the tinnitus in people with severe hearing loss may completely go away with MFD treatment, while people suffering from tinnitus who have normal hearing may have no improvement with MFD treatment, and vice versa.

However, it seems that myofascial dysfunction treatment will more likely help you if:

1. You have only had your tinnitus for a short time (e.g. under two years vs. 10 - 20 years).

2. Your tinnitus accompanies other myofascial symptoms in your head and neck.

3. You tinnitus volume fluctuates in time with other myofascial symptoms in your head and neck.

4. Your tinnitus is more pronounced on the same side as your more prominent accompanying myofascial symptoms.[36]

The only certain way to determine if myofascial dysfunction treatment will help your tinnitus is to try it.

## Diagnosing Somatosensory Tinnitus

Unfortunately, somatosensory tinnitus is grossly under-diagnosed. Maybe this is because you can have both neurophysiologic and somatosensory tinnitus at the same time, or only have one or the other kind of tinnitus, and few health care professionals distinguish between these two kinds of tinnitus so just diagnose it as "tinnitus".

Thus, although few realize it, somatosensory tinnitus is actually very common. As many as 65 – 80% of people with tinnitus have somatosensory tinnitus to some degree or other. Therefore, notice whether you have temporary changes in your tinnitus when you move your jaw, open your mouth, clench your teeth, turn your head, or press on your temples, mandible, cheek, mastoid or neck with your fingertips.[37]

Somatosensory tinnitus is frequently caused by musculoskeletal disorders, of which myofascial pain syndrome is one of the most common. This syndrome is characterized by regional pain and myofascial trigger points.[38]

You can suspect that you have somatosensory tinnitus if at least one of the following things happened before your tinnitus began (or got worse). The more of the following symptoms you exhibit, the more likely you have somatosensory tinnitus.

1. You had head or neck trauma.
2. You notice your tinnitus is associated with clenching your teeth, moving your jaw or cervical spine.
3. You have recurrent pain in your head, neck or shoulders.
4. You have pain in your head, neck or shoulders that occurred at the same time as your tinnitus became noticeable, or both the pain and your tinnitus increased at the same time.
5. Your tinnitus increases when you exhibit poor posture, or when you are resting, walking, working or sleeping.
6. You intensely grind your teeth (bruxism) at times during the day or night.[39]

When taking your medical history, your healthcare professional should investigate whether you have any pain in your head, face, cervical spine and/ or in your shoulder girdle regions. In addition, he should assess your posture, the presence of any myofascial trigger points, and how your tinnitus changes with body movements or touch.[40] Typically, somatosensory tinnitus changes in loudness, pitch or localization whenever you move or touch your head or neck.

Furthermore, your healthcare professional should ask you whether your tinnitus started before, after, or simultaneously with any head or neck pain. This helps determine whether a muscle disorder is causing your tinnitus.

For example, your tinnitus may have started after a head or neck trauma, a dental procedure, cervical manipulation, or periods of intense bruxism (teeth grinding). You may also have noticed that your tinnitus changes during or after using your computer (poor posture), after using a different pillow, or those times when you feel more intense pain.[41]

When trying to determine whether you have somatosensory tinnitus or neurophysiologic tinnitus (the common kind of tinnitus caused by noise damage for example), the most important thing to notice is whether the origin of your tinnitus appears to be related to head and neck problems, rather than to ear problems.

Another indicator that you may have somatosensory tinnitus is if your audiogram shows normal hearing in both ears, or the same degree of hearing loss in both ears **and** your tinnitus is in only one ear, or your tinnitus is different in each ear.[42] This also applies if you have a normal audiogram but have both tinnitus and pain in your head or neck.[43]

## Temporomandibular Dysfunction (TMD)

Tinnitus from temporomandibular dysfunction is typically a type of somatosensory tinnitus.

You have two temporomandibular joints (TMJ), one on each side of your face in front of each ear. Your temporomandibular joint is the place where the temporal bone (**temporo**) of your skull and your lower jaw or mandible (**mandibular**) join—and that's how it got its fancy name.

Your TMJs move every time you chew, talk, swallow, smile or kiss. The TMJ is actually a sliding joint. This sliding action allows the pressure on this joint to be distributed throughout the joint and not just focused in one small area.

You also have a disc between these two bones, just like the ones between the vertebrae in your back. The two bones of the TMJ are held together by a series of ligaments—any of which can be damaged, just like in any other joint. A damaged TMJ ligament usually results in a dislocation of the disc, your lower jaw, or both.

Furthermore, the bones of the TMJ are connected by two main muscles. If your TMJ is not working correctly, either, or both, of these muscles may become painful and produce pain in the TMJ itself, or at the very least, abnormal movement of the lower jaw.

When one or both TMJ's are damaged in any way, the muscles in your head and neck automatically tense up, causing not only pain, but various clicking and crackling objective tinnitus noises,[44] and may also somatically modulate your existing tinnitus at the same time.

This happens to Penny. She relates, "When my tinnitus is bad it certainly changes with the movements of my jaw. When I'm doing my jaw exercises for my TMJ and I open my mouth wide, my tinnitus gets louder and the tone gets lower."

Some researchers emphasize the joint's role in TMJ-induced tinnitus and refer to it as TMJ syndrome. Others stress facial muscle tension as the key to the syndrome and describe it as myofascial pain-dysfunction syndrome. A recent report associated tinnitus with muscle dysfunction and not joint dysfunction.[45] This makes good sense. When the muscles are under tension, they distort the TMJ and one of the results is tinnitus—both the objective TMJ kind of tinnitus, and the subjective somatically-modulated kind of tinnitus we just discussed in the previous section.

Temporomandibular Dysfunction (TMD) can affect your ears and produce symptoms such as tinnitus (ringing in the ears), hearing loss that comes and goes, pressure or a blocked sensation in the ears, pain in the ears and dizziness.[46]

Along with the above ear problems, if you have TMD you may also experience headaches; pain in the face, eye or neck; blurred vision that comes and goes; frequent sore throats; difficulty swallowing; burning tongue; and tingling or numb sensations in the arms and hands.

Studies have shown a higher incidence of tinnitus in people with normal hearing who have TMD problems than in the control populations.[47] In fact, close to half of the people who have TMD have tinnitus as one of their symptoms.[48]

One test you can do is to clench your teeth. If it makes your tinnitus louder or changes its pitch (by somatically modulating your tinnitus), then there is almost certainly a relationship between your tinnitus, your TMJ and the muscles in your head and neck to some degree.[49]

One very common cause of TMD problems is stress.[50] Reducing stress allows the muscles to relax and thus reduces tinnitus from TMD. Cathy has an interesting warning system in place for when she is stressed. She explains, "When I clench my jaw, I get a squealing kind of tinnitus. In a way it's very handy because in the past I have broken some of my teeth from clenching too hard. Now I have a warning bell!"

## Gaze-Evoked Tinnitus (GET)

One of the more interesting kinds of somatosensory tinnitus is called gaze-evoked tinnitus (GET). Gaze-evoked tinnitus is a condition in which people can change the loudness and pitch of their tinnitus by looking to the far right or left of center,[51] and to a lesser extent, by looking up or down.[52]

Anita explains, "When I move my eyes side to side or up and down the pitch of my tinnitus goes up and my tinnitus gets louder. Then it returns to its usual loud, high-pitched steady sound." Anita's symptoms came after an operation to cut the auditory and balance nerves on one side of her head to stop her extremely bad vertigo and unbearably loud reverberations of all sounds.

Anita's experience is not all that uncommon. Doctors used to think that gaze-evoked tinnitus was rare, but now they are realizing it is much more common than they previously thought.[53] They now know that gaze-evoked tinnitus may develop after surgical removal of tumors of the auditory nerve, typically acoustic neuroma tumors.[54] Severing the auditory nerve can initiate various forms of cross-modal plasticity—where changes in the brain affect two or more senses—in this case resulting in gaze-evoked tinnitus.[55]

Interestingly enough, a lot of people with gaze-evoked tinnitus have a group of three symptoms, including gaze-evoked tinnitus, nystagmus (eyes jerking sideways) and facial nerve dysfunction.[56] These all can be side effects of acoustic neuroma surgery.

As was Anita's experience, people with gaze-evoked tinnitus find that the volume and pitch of their tinnitus is lowest when they look straight ahead and increases the more they look sideways.[57] Up and down gaze (down more than up) produces less consistent changes. Some people hear their basic tinnitus while their eyes are looking straight ahead. Others only hear tinnitus when they shift their gaze. One person noted, "Gaze-evoked tinnitus superimposes a different pitch of tinnitus on top of the background tinnitus I already have".[58] A number of people find that the loudness and pitch of their tinnitus remains constant during extreme lateral gaze (when their eyes are turned all the way to the left or the right), while others report theirs is transient.[59]

People with gaze-evoked tinnitus typically find that their tinnitus remains constant as long as they maintain a fixed lateral gaze,[60] but whenever they move their eyes, their tinnitus changes. This constantly-changing tinnitus is very hard to live with. As one person explained, "I found that continuous, steady tinnitus was relatively easy to tune out, but when my tinnitus was constantly changing, I thought it would drive me mad"![61]

Researchers have recently identified connections between tinnitus and eye movements. One study suggested that tinnitus is a complex phenomenon involving more than one site in each person's brain.[62] In fact, just the act of looking sideways activated an extensive neural network in the brains of the people in this study. Not only that, but each person differed somewhat in the places in their brains that were associated with increases in tinnitus pitch and loudness.[63]

Gaze-evoked tinnitus seems to be related to both visual and auditory brain activity. These two different brain areas normally communicate with each other to figure out which perception should receive priority.[64] For example, in people with normally-functioning ears, looking sideways suppresses auditory brain activity. By suppressing hearing during lateral gaze, our brains are telling us to pay attention to what our eyes are seeing.

However, when researchers mapped the brains of people with gaze-evoked tinnitus, they discovered that this usual balance between the visual and auditory parts of the brain wasn't present.[65] They believe this may explain why gaze-evoked tinnitus becomes louder when people with GET look sideways.[66]

## Nodding-Chime Tinnitus

Another rather unusual kind of somatosensory tinnitus is "nodding-chime" tinnitus. With this kind of tinnitus, when you nod or shake your head you hear a sound like chimes ringing. It's almost as if you have a bell (chimes) suspended in your head and when you move your head, the bell rings.

Hearing chimes when you nod or shake your head is not particularly common to be sure, but it is not unknown either. For example, one lady noticed that every time she shook her head she heard the pure tone "F". Another lady reported, "When I nod my head for "yes", or shake it from side to side for "no", I hear chimes. Kind of like those chime toys that babies have."

Still another lady explained, "For the past few weeks I've been hearing a chiming sound in my left ear if I shake my head fairly quickly side to side (as if saying 'no')".

A man had a similar experience. He explained, "For me, the note is slightly different for 'yes' and 'no'—'yes' is higher-pitched. I think I've experienced this for many years, but only started to notice continuous tinnitus at the age of 50, about 8 years ago. In addition to the nodding/shaking chimes, I get similar chimes when I jog."

What causes these mystery chiming sounds. One woman explained, "I started hearing 'chimes' in my head when shaking or nodding about nine months ago. It sounds a bit like wind chimes. It began when I had a sinus infection, and I thought it would go away after treatment, but it is still with me. I don't hear any other sound in my ears—it's only there when I shake or nod my head."

Another woman did a bit of experimenting on herself. She reported:

> I just tested myself by nodding my head vigorously. I confirmed that indeed, the movement changed the volume of my tinnitus, especially on the head upward movement of a "yes" head nod, and a leftward head movement in a "no" nod. (The "yes" movement yielded more dramatic results.) I have unilateral sensorineural loss in my right ear, with tinnitus that is not bothersome—it's simply "there".
>
> However, when I wear my hearing aid, it plugs that ear with the ear mold, and this somehow calls attention to my tinnitus—when I walk, I get a modulation of the tinnitus that reflects the rhythm of my footsteps. That's annoying.
>
> This is akin to my ability to "ding" my head—if I plug my right ear, and flick my finger just so around my cheekbone, I can produce a "ding" sound in my head. (Fun, huh?)

Instead of beautiful chimes, some people report unpleasant sounds. For example, one lady explained, "My weird tinnitus occurs when I shake my head up and down or side to side. It doesn't sound like chimes to me, but sounds more like static or buzzing."

Another lady reported:

> In addition to ongoing mild tinnitus, I experience movement-induced tinnitus as well. Unfortunately, the sound is not a pleasant chime tone, but a very startling loud buzz—like a noisy fly or bee right inside my ear! The first time I heard it I was terrified that an insect had flown into my ear and would sting me or get stuck and have to be removed surgically. The sound (so far) only happens when I shake my head from side to side to signify "no".

---

**Chapter 9 Endnotes**

1 Functional Magnetic Resonance Imaging, 2000. p. 1.
2 UB study finds that "crossed wires" in brain pathways controlling vision and hearing play a role in tinnitus, 2002. p. 1.
3 Moller, 2011. pp. 363-368.
4 Sanchez, 2011. p. 1089.
5 Levine, 2004. p. 123.
6 Levine, 2003. p. 3.
7 Levine, 2003. p. 3.
8 Lockwood, 2001b. p. 478.
9 UB study finds that "crossed wires" in brain pathways controlling vision and hearing play a role in tinnitus, 2002. p. 1.
10 Levine, 1999. p. 3.
11 Levine, 1999. p. 4.
12 Levine, 2003. p. 1.
13 Levine, 1999. p. 4.
14 Levine, 2004. p. 123.
15 Hobbs, 2014. p. 1.
16 Levine, 2004. p. 116.
17 Levine, 2004. p. 108.
18 Levine, 2000. p. 10.
19 Moller, 2011. pp. 363-368.
20 Moller, 2011. pp. 727-731.
21 Moller, 2011. pp. 51-68.
22 Nerves in Head and Neck Linked to Tinnitus, 2008. p. 60.
23 Moller, 2011. pp. 733-747.
24 Craggs-Hinton, 2007. p. 99.
25 Bartels, 2007. pp. 21-22.
26 Sanchez, 2011. p. 1090.
27 Rocha, 2015. p. 2.
28 Teachey, 2012. p. 1.
29 Teachey, 2012. p. 2.
30 Rocha, 2015. p. 1.
31 Rocha, 2015. p. 2.
32 Rocha, 2015. p. 2.

33 Teachey, 2012. p. 2.
34 Teachey, 2012. p. 2.
35 Teachey, 2012. p. 2.
36 Teachey, 2012. p. 2.
37 Sanchez, 2011. p. 1090.
38 Sanchez, 2011. p. 1090.
39 Sanchez, 2011. p. 1090.
40 Rocha, 2015. p. 1.
41 Rocha, 2015. p. 2.
42 Sanchez, 2011. p. 1090.
43 Rocha, 2015. p. 3.
44 Currie, 2005.
45 Levine, 2004. p. 116.
46 Klemons, 2010. p. 1.
47 Levine, 2000. p. 9.
48 Klemons, 2010. p. 1.
49 Hogan, 1998. p. 90.
50 Hogan, 1998. p. 92.
51 Lockwood, 2001a. p. 1.
52 Lockwood, 2001b. p. 472.
53 Lockwood, 2001b. p. 478.
54 Lockwood, 2001a. p. 1.
55 Moller, 2011. pp. 317-325.
56 Lockwood, 2001b. p. 478.
57 Lockwood, 1999. p. 1.
58 All About Tinnitus, 2001. p. 1.
59 Lockwood, 2001b. p. 478.
60 Lockwood, 2001b. p. 475.
61 Tinnitus Resources, 2002. pp. 4-5.
62 Lockwood, 2001a. p. 1.
63 Lockwood, 1999. p. 1.
64 Source of 'Ringing of the Ears' Extends Beyond Hearing Systems, 2001. p. 1.
65 UB study finds that "crossed wires" in brain pathways controlling vision and hearing play a role in tinnitus, 2002. p. 2.
66 Lockwood, 2001a. p. 2.

Chapter 10

# Medical Conditions

Conditions elsewhere in your body, besides your ears, may also trigger tinnitus. For example, high blood pressure (hypertension) and cardiovascular disease,[1] arthritis, anemia, multiple sclerosis and thyroid problems have all triggered tinnitus in some people. The results of head or dental surgery can result in tinnitus. Some hormonal changes can also trigger tinnitus.[2] There is even a higher incidence of tinnitus in people that have chronic pain.[3] Following are some of the more common medical conditions that can result in tinnitus.

## Allergies & Sinus Conditions

Allergies can trigger tinnitus. Penny writes, "Allergies play a big part in the level of my tinnitus. I couldn't walk into a library without having my tinnitus go off the charts—all because of dust." She adds, "Many people have allergic reactions to things and don't even know it's allergy-related. They don't connect what they ate with the level of their tinnitus, or what they smelled, or what plants they're surrounded by, or if there's mold out in their yard. When I'm in the presence of perfume, for example, my tinnitus gets louder—but this is only when I'm in an allergic phase."

Allergies can clog up your sinuses and middle ears much the same as a cold does. Many people with clogged sinuses experience tinnitus. This kind of tinnitus is typically caused by a thickening of the mucous in the middle ear.

In case you didn't realize it, your middle ears have mucous membranes lining them. These mucous membranes produce mucous which cleanses your ears. This mucous then drains out of your middle ears via the Eustachian tubes that connect your middle ears to the back of your throat. However if this mucous becomes too think and viscous, it won't drain away properly.

Unfortunately, the antibiotics and antihistamines people take in an effort to control their sinus infections and allergy conditions often cause the mucous to become too thick and viscous to easily drain away.

This kind of tinnitus may include clicking, crackling, gurgling or whirring sounds. You can either aggravate or relieve these noises by swallowing or blowing your nose, since there is often a negative pressure in your ears from your Eustachian tubes being plugged up.[4]

## Diabetes

Many, perhaps most, Americans are insulin resistant. Insulin resistance leads to Type II diabetes and in many cases, to tinnitus. As Barry Keate reports,

> There is a direct link between insulin resistance, diabetes, and tinnitus. Studies have shown that most people with tinnitus have one of these conditions and treating them with diet and exercise can result in a significant reduction in tinnitus symptoms.[5]

You may notice that the onset of your tinnitus was connected with your diabetes or hyperinsulinism (too much insulin in your blood). In fact, one recent study indicated that 84% of all people with subjective tinnitus of unknown origin had hyperinsulinism.[6] Furthermore, a Brazilian study of 498 people found that diabetes mellitus and hypertension were strong, independent risk factors for tinnitus.[7] Therefore, if you want to help prevent tinnitus, keep both your blood sugar and your blood pressure under control.

For example, the participants in a Brazilian study of tinnitus and insulin resistance were instructed to begin a diet suitable for diabetics. They began a two-year diet designed to return their insulin to normal levels. Here are the results.

> Of the original 80 participants who joined the study, 59 adhered to the diet and 21 did not. The likelihood of having decreased tinnitus symptoms was **five times greater** in those who kept to the diet (76%) than those who did not (14%).
>
> Specifically, of those who followed the diet for at least two years, 24% had no improvement, 22% had some improvement, 39% had clinically significant improvement and 15% had complete resolution. In all, 74% had improvement and, of those, 54% had significant improvement or total resolution of their tinnitus.[8]

If you already have tinnitus, and have not been able to find the cause, it may very well be that your tinnitus is the result of insulin resistance and/or diabetes Type II. Have your doctor check you out for these conditions, and if your blood sugars are off, take corrective action by changing your diet (eliminate processed foods and grains and add unprocessed, raw nuts and vegetables to your diet). Also, get more exercise, or maybe you need to start exercising in the first place. You have even odds (a 50% chance) of having significant improvement in your tinnitus when you do this.

## Head Trauma (Blow to the Head or Whiplash)

A blow (trauma) to the head can cause instant tinnitus, especially a blow that hits your outer ear. Sometimes this can result in a perilymphatic fistula—a tear in the round or oval window that separates your middle and inner ears. This allows perilymph to leak from your inner ear into your middle ear. The resulting hearing loss tends to be in the high-frequencies. As a result, the tinnitus is often a high-pitched hissing or cricket-chirping sound. Unfortunately, patching this "hole" by surgery typically does not cause the tinnitus to go away.[9]

Other causes of post-traumatic tinnitus include temporal bone fractures (a type of skull fracture), labyrinthine concussion (causing damage to your inner ear), ossicular chain disruption (affecting the tiny bones in your middle ears), barotrauma (sudden changes in pressure) or noise trauma.[10]

Note that a blow to the head from any cause can knock your upper neck vertebrae "out" and also cause somatosensory tinnitus which we discussed in Chapter 9.

## Barotrauma

Barotrauma is damage to your ears caused by sudden changes in air pressure. Barotrauma can occur from water sports such as diving from a diving board and scuba diving. It can also occur with rapid changes in altitude such as when flying, especially in non-pressurized planes.

If you have large vestibular aqueduct syndrome (LVAS), you may be very susceptible to barotrauma and the resulting hearing loss and subjective tinnitus.[11]

If your tinnitus comes on right after any rapid changes in air pressure, you should suspect barotrauma as the trigger.

## Fatigue

When you are tired often your tinnitus will get worse. However if you become severely overtired, your tinnitus may suddenly become a loud roar and scare you silly! This happened to Lenora. She explained:

> Since being overly fatigued due to taking an overnight job in addition to a 9 A.M. to 5 P.M. job, my tinnitus has gone from a very mild ringing noise to a severe engine motor noise. This had never happened to me before until I took this overnight job. It only occurs when I am severely, and I mean severely, overtired.
>
> It is a very loud motor engine type noise—a loud rumbling noise—something like a washing machine in my head. I take my hearing aid off, and it's there so I know I am not hearing an airplane or something. It was so loud it scared me half to death!

I explained to Lenora that she needed more sleep and these scary sounds would go away. Six days later, she told me:

> After getting much, much, much needed rest, yes indeed, I am doing ever so much better. Oh my goodness, what a relief! I will make sure I get my rest from now on![13]

**"Charlie"**

Although it may seem unlikely, you can actually make friends with your tinnitus—at least some of the time. For example, Melanie, Rosemary and I have a tinnitus-friend we call "Charlie". He comes to remind us we are tired and it's time for us to hit the sack.

Here is how Rosemary describes her "Charlie". "As I am writing these words, I have a persistent low-pitched hum in my left ear. It comes in the evening after a busy day and tells me that it is past my bedtime. 'Ah!' I say to myself, 'There's Charlie again. I suppose I should knock it off.' 'Charlie' acts like a welcome built-in warning system—an alarm clock in reverse."[12]

Melanie and I each have a "Charlie" too. To us he is a low-pitched rumbling sound. We typically only hear him when we are tired and know we should go to bed.

I've had similar experiences when I am grossly overtired. All of a sudden I hear a roaring sound like a freight train bearing down on me. It sounds like the train will come crashing though the wall it is so loud. It's scary. The solution is simple. Just go to bed—now!

That's how easy it is to get rid of this particular kind of loud, roaring tinnitus. Just hit the sack and get a good night's sleep!

# Pulsatile Tinnitus

Pulsatile tinnitus, as its name implies, is a type of tinnitus that typically, but not always, pulsates in time to your heart beat. In a few cases, pulsatile tinnitus is a phantom sound that can only be heard by you (subjective tinnitus). However, normally a doctor can hear your pulsatile tinnitus though his stethoscope (objective tinnitus).[14]

No matter what causes it, pulsatile tinnitus can create the same kinds of negative reactions as other forms of tinnitus, including frustration, anxiety, annoyance, depression and insomnia.[15]

Pulsatile tinnitus is not all that common. Only about 3% to 10% of the people reporting tinnitus experience pulsatile tinnitus.[16] Interestingly enough, you usually only hear your pulsatile tinnitus in one ear.[17]

## Sounds of Pulsatile Tinnitus

Pulsatile tinnitus sounds are rhythmic pulsing sounds. They may be drumming, beating, pounding, throbbing, pulsating or fluttering sounds that are synchronous with your heart beat.[18] In addition, pulsatile tinnitus may produce a lower-pitched thumping or booming sound, a rougher blowing sound that is coincidental with respiration, or a clicking, higher-pitched rhythmic sensation. Pulsatile tinnitus may have single beats, or biphasic beats (like the clip-clop of a horse), or it may even make a swishing or swooshing sound.[19]

Harry hears a whooshing sound in his ears each time his heart beats. He can stop it by pressing on the artery on the left side of his head. What had happened in Harry's case was that a vein and an artery had grown "feelers" and had merged, and Harry was hearing the increased blood flow though these new blood vessels.

Incidentally, blood flowing through arteries and veins each have their own characteristic sounds. Arterial "bruits" are beating sounds of blood rushing though arteries. Venous "hums" are the sounds of slower blood flow in veins.

Tanya's pulsatile tinnitus is a very high-pitched and loud ringing sound that beats in time with her heartbeat.

Ron hears a zing, zing, zing at the same speed as his heartbeat. He explains, "It just came on when I was shaving one morning. When it's good, I can only hear it when I put my head back. When it's bad, I get other tinnitus sounds with which the zinging seems to compete."

Some people even hear their pulsatile tinnitus as a squeaking sound. One lady reported, "I hear my pulse as a 'squeak' frequently. It is only on my left side, but it is very annoying." Karen explained, "I have recently begun hearing a squeaking in my right ear that is in time to my pulse". Jeffrey related, "In the past couple of months I've been hearing a 'squeaking pulse' sound in both ears at night, generally when lying in bed and predominately on the side where my head touches the pillow"; while Terry declared, "I have squeaking in my right ear. It's very irritating. It has been doing that for more than a year now."

## What Causes Pulsatile Tinnitus?

There are at least 25 different known causes of pulsatile tinnitus. However, most cases of pulsatile tinnitus that are strongly associated with the timing of the heart beat are most likely related to blood flow, or a malformation of the arteries and/or veins located in or near your ears, either on the surface of your head or just inside your head.[20]

For example, there is a rich blood supply in the lining of your middle ears. Your inner ears also have their own blood supply. The large carotid artery passes close to the cochlea and the jugular vein runs very close to your ears. Any of these can become noisy for a variety of reasons and create a pulsating kind of tinnitus.[21]

The three most common causes of pulsatile tinnitus,[22] which account for about two-thirds of all cases diagnosed, are:

**Benign Intracranial Hypertension** syndrome (BIH): BIH accounts for 39% of all diagnosed cases of pulsatile tinnitus. Benign intracranial hypertension is increased pressure of the fluid that bathes your brain. In addition to tinnitus, the syndrome includes headaches, blurred vision and menstrual irregularities in obese women.[23] It is more common in young, overweight women.

**Carotid Artery Disease** (CAD): CAD accounts for 17% of all diagnosed cases of pulsatile tinnitus. Carotid artery disease is the atherosclerotic build up of cholesterol on the walls of the large carotid arteries in your neck. This reduces the space inside the arteries, thus leading to turbulent blood flow that can be heard as pulsatile tinnitus. Sometimes this is called "carotid stenosis."

**Glomus Tumors**: Glomus tumors account for 12% of all diagnosed cases of pulsatile tinnitus. Glomus tumors are non-cancerous (benign) growths (abnormal masses of blood vessels) in or near the ear.[24]

In addition to the above three major causes of pulsatile, there are at least 22 other causes that together account for 23% of the diagnosed cases of pulsatile tinnitus. Here are a number of them.

**Turbulent blood flow**: This is similar to Carotid Artery Disease, but occurs in arteries other than your carotid arteries. This can happen when your arteries harden (atherosclerosis). With atherosclerosis, a build-up of cholesterol on the inner lining of the arteries partially blocks your arteries. This prevents blood from flowing smoothly. This flow then becomes noisy in the same way that a smoothly-running river becomes noisier at a set of rapids. You hear this extra noise as pulsatile tinnitus. Pulsatile tinnitus in older people is often due to this cause.

**Increased blood flow in different blood vessels**: This often happens when a certain blood vessel narrows. To compensate, neighboring blood vessels have to carry extra blood and this extra flow generates more noise, especially if they are nearer to your ears than the partially-blocked blood vessel. Incidentally, if you can change the intensity of your tinnitus when you turn your head, your pulsatile tinnitus is likely caused in a vein rather than an artery.[25]

**Emissary vein**: If you can stop your pulsatile tinnitus by pressing around your ear somewhere, then an emissary vein is likely causing your tinnitus.[26] (Emissary veins connect the dura mater surrounding your brain to your scalp).

**High blood pressure**: High blood pressure makes the blood flow faster and thus produces more noise.

**Twisted arteries**: Can cause turbulent (noisy) blood flow.

**Aneurysm in an artery**: If the pulsatile tinnitus starts suddenly and you have pain on one side of your head or neck, you may have a carotid aneurysm (a ballooning or swelling of a place in an artery).[27]

**Arteriovenous fistulae**: These are abnormal connections between an artery and a vein. Normally arteries carry blood from your heart to your body, and veins carry blood from your body back to your heart and lungs to get re-oxygenated. Sometimes "feelers" grow out from the capillaries and join to veins. This diverts blood from the arteries to the veins and results in increased blood flow with the resultant increase in noise.

**"High-riding" carotid artery**: This is a carotid artery that is closer to your ears than normal.[28]

**General increase in blood flow**: If you exercise strenuously, you may have increased blood flow throughout your body including around your ears.

**Perforated ear drum or middle ear infections**: With either of these conditions, you may become more aware of sounds inside your body as they are no longer masked by external sounds.

**Sensitive hearing (hyperacusis)**: Your brain may become more aware of normal noises in your blood vessels.[29]

**Patulous (Open) Eustachian tubes**: One of your Eustachian tubes (connecting your throat to your middle ears) may be "stuck" open so you hear breath sounds.

**Palatal muscle spasms**: Small spasms in the muscles of the soft palate. For example, a rapid clicking sensation with pulsatile tinnitus may be due to the contractions of the middle ear and muscles of the soft palate.[30]

**Stapedial muscle spasms**: The stapedius is the tiny muscle attached to the stapes [stirrup] bone in your middle ear.[31]

These latter three conditions (patulous Eustachian tubes, palatal myoclonus [myoclonus is just a brief, involuntary twitching or spasm of a muscle or a group of muscles] and stapedial muscle spasms [middle ear myoclonus]) are sometimes called pseudo-pulsatile tinnitus since this twitching may seem like it is pulsing in unison to the heartbeat and thus may mimic pulsatile tinnitus.

Sometimes several factors may combine to cause your pulsatile tinnitus. For example, you may have high blood pressure coupled with atherosclerosis causing turbulent blood flow with the resultant increase in noise.[32]

In addition to the above, there are many cases of pulsatile tinnitus that defy diagnosis and identification of the causative agent.[33] These account for between 9% and 30% of the cases doctors encounter.[34]

## Treating Pulsatile Tinnitus

If you have pulsatile tinnitus (or pseudo-pulsatile tinnitus), you should have a thorough medical evaluation to locate the cause, if possible.

The cure rate for pulsatile tinnitus is quite high once your doctor locates and identifies the exact problem.[35] For example, surgery on glomus tumors is generally successful with only a 5% recurrence rate.[36]

If your tinnitus is from turbulent blood flow, your doctor may correct it using angioplasty (a tiny balloon to press open a partially blocked blood vessel) or stenting (inserting a new artificial blood vessel wall).[37]

Some causes, such as high blood pressure may be fairly easy to treat. Other conditions may be successfully treated with drugs or surgery, leading to a reduction in pulsatile tinnitus.[38]

---

**Chapter 10 Endnotes**

1 Tinnitus Association of Calgary.
2 Info-Tinnitus, Causes and Factors in the Hearing System, 1990.
3 Mayes, 2010. p. 173.
4 Currie, 2005.
5 Keate, 2016. p. 1.
6 Hogan, 1998. p. 83.
7 Gibrin, 2013. p. 19.
8 Keate, 2016. p. 1.
9 Levine, 2000. pp. 7-8.
10 Moller, 2011. p. 511.
11 Bauman, 2002a. p. 5.
12 McCall, 1991. p. 166.
13 Bauman, 2011b. p. 83.
14 Johnson, 1999. p. 1.
15 Pulsatile Tinnitus, 2001. p. 2.
16 American Tinnitus Association, 2002. p. 2.
17 Pulsatile Tinnitus, 2001. p. 1.
18 Currie, 2005.
19 Johnson, 1999. p. 2.
20 Johnson, 1999. p. 2.
21 Pulsatile Tinnitus, 2001. p. 1.
22 Johnson, 1999. p. 5.
23 Levine, 2000. p. 3.
24 Pulsatile Tinnitus, 2001. p. 1.
25 Levine, 2000. p. 3.
26 Levine, 2000. p. 3.
27 Levine, 2000. p. 3.
28 Johnson, 1999. p. 1.
29 Pulsatile Tinnitus, 2003. p. 2.
30 Schleuning, ~2003. p. 1.
31 Johnson, 1999. p. 2.
32 Pulsatile Tinnitus, 2001. p. 1.
33 Johnson, 1999. p. 1.
34 Moller, 2011. pp. 467-475.
35 Johnson, 1999. p. 2.
36 Johnson, 1999. p. 6.
37 Johnson, 1999. p. 3.
38 Pulsatile Tinnitus, 2001. p. 2.

Chapter 11

# Inner Ear Conditions

Certain inner ear conditions may also trigger tinnitus. For example, Anita has weird tinnitus, caused by surgery to cut her auditory and balance nerves on one side to stop her extremely bad vertigo and unbearably loud reverberations of all sounds. She explains, "The pitch of my tinnitus gets louder with every sound I hear. Every word or sound I hear makes a short staccato sound of the high pitched tinnitus sound as it reverberates in my head like the sound of an old fashioned typewriter key clacking on the paper."

Another person wrote, "After my surgery, the tinnitus in the deaf ear got worse. Apparently it is not unusual for someone who suddenly loses their hearing in one ear to have their tinnitus dramatically increase."[1]

There are a number of inner ear conditions that can cause tinnitus. Some are relatively common. Others are much less common such as superior canal dehiscence. Superior canal dehiscence is typically a hole in the bone in the upper semi-circular canal in your vestibular (balance) system that can result in tinnitus as well as balance problems.[2]

The truth is, almost anything that can go wrong with your ears or in your auditory system can trigger tinnitus. Following are some of the more common inner-ear conditions that can result in tinnitus.

## Auditory Nerve Damage/Acoustic Neuromas

Tinnitus may be the result of any kind of damage to the auditory nerve. For example, it could be the result of poor nerve function due to pressure on it from surrounding tissues. Furthermore, blood vessels pulsing against the auditory nerve (microvascular compressions) can also result in tinnitus.[3]

A more common scenario resulting in tinnitus is an acoustic neuroma (sometimes called a vestibular schwannoma).[4] Acoustic neuromas are benign (non-cancerous) tumors that grow on your auditory nerves—usually only affecting one ear at a time (unless you have a condition called neurofibromatosis, Type II). Although they are non-cancerous (and are often slow growing), you need to seek medical attention as they can continue to grow and eventually "squish" your brain, and in extreme cases, result in death.

If acoustic neuromas are caught soon enough and removed while they are small, you may be left with some hearing loss and tinnitus from the damaged auditory nerve. However, if they are too big, the only solution is to cut them out, and in the process sever the auditory nerve. You are then left totally deaf on that side, and may also be left with a severe case of tinnitus as well. The tinnitus sounds caused by auditory nerve damage may include high-pitched ringing bell sounds, or whistling, roaring or buzzing sounds.[5]

Tinnitus is a common symptom in people with acoustic neuromas. In 70 - 80% of the people with acoustic neuromas, their tinnitus is on the same side as the tumor. In 10% of people with acoustic neuromas, it is the principal symptom indicating the presence of the tumor. Around 14% of the people with acoustic neuromas have moderate to severe tinnitus. By the time an acoustic neuroma causes hearing loss, about 95% have already experienced tinnitus. About 50% of the people with balance symptoms from acoustic neuromas also experience tinnitus.[6]

## Meniere's Disease

Meniere's disease is an inner ear disorder that causes a person to experience episodes of vertigo, dizziness, nausea, ear pressure, fluctuating hearing loss and tinnitus.[7] Hearing loss associated with Meniere's disease, at least initially, is a low-frequency loss and thus the tinnitus associated with Meniere's disease is often a lower-pitched

**The Agony of Meniere's Disease**

If you have Meniere's disease or suspect you might have it, you will find a lot of good information in the book *The Agony of Meniere's Disease—Please Make My World Stop Spinning*. (See the back of this book for information on obtaining your copy of this helpful book or go to http://hearinglosshelp.com/shop/category/books/ and scroll down to the book on Meniere's disease.)[8]

roaring sound.[9] As the disease progresses and hearing loss increases, tinnitus tends to become louder[10] and more variable in its description.[11]

A typical attack of Meniere's disease may be preceded by ear pressure (a feeling of fullness in the ears) or aching in one or both ears, fluctuating hearing and loud tinnitus noises.

Most Meniere's disease sufferers are generally symptom-free between acute attacks, except for the tinnitus, which is always there.

## Viral Ear Infections

Viral ear infections can cause tinnitus. Herpes zoster oticus is one such virus, so is Varicella, the chickenpox virus. You may have severe ear pain in addition to tinnitus and often hearing loss and balance problems too.[12]

## Natural Auditory Feedback

If all the above sources of tinnitus aren't enough, recent studies have shown that our ears also have a natural auditory feedback system. Even in the absence of sound, there is continuous background auditory system activity. This means that our auditory systems continually send sounds to our brains. If it is quiet enough, we may hear this perfectly-natural background activity as tinnitus.

---

**Chapter 11 Endnotes**

1 All About Tinnitus, 2001. p. 2.
2 Tunkel, 2014. p. S11.
3 Moller, 2011. p. 327.
4 Tunkel, 2014. p. S11.
5 Currie, 2005.
6 Moller, 2011. pp. 681-686.
7 Bauman, 2011a. p. 11.
8 Bauman,, 2011a.
9 Levine, 2000. p. 6.
10 Moller, 2011. pp 311-316.
11 Levine, 2000. p. 7.
12 Levine, 2000. p. 8.

Chapter 12

# Middle Ear Conditions

There are a number of middle-ear conditions that can result in tinnitus. For example, many people, including children, experience tinnitus along with a middle ear infection (otitis media) or a sinus infection. Generally, the tinnitus will lessen and gradually fade away once the infection clears up.

Often middle-ear surgery to restore hearing can cause tinnitus to improve. However, tinnitus can also be an unwanted side effect of middle-ear surgery.[1]

Here are some causes of tinnitus originating in the middle ear.

## Otosclerosis and Middle Ear Calcification

Otosclerosis (OH-toe-sklair-ROW-sis) is an inherited condition that causes abnormal, spongy bone growth on one or more of the tiny bones in your middle ear that usually fixes the stirrup (stapes), the third bone in your middle ears, to the oval window of your cochlea. Because the stapes then no longer vibrates freely, you end up with a hearing loss. About 75% of the people with otosclerosis also have tinnitus to some degree. In fact, the first symptom of otosclerosis is often tinnitus.[2]

If your body chemistry is off, high acid levels can also cause a somewhat similar calcification of the bones in your middle ears. This calcification often occurs in older people and results in tinnitus. The tinnitus most commonly associated with high acid levels includes buzzing, hissing and humming sounds.[3]

# Muscle Contractions in the Middle Ear

## Ear Drum (Tympani) Conditions

If your ear drum has suffered physical damage or perforation, you may experience a humming or a buzzing kind of tinnitus as it vibrates. You can even get tinnitus as a result from swelling in your ear canals.

You can also have a fluttering/buzzing kind of tinnitus if anything in your ear canal touches your eardrum. For example, if ear wax touches your eardrum sometimes it can make an unusual kind of tinnitus as your eardrum rapidly and rhythmically vibrates from the wax touching it.

This happened to me only once that I can remember. I had put my hearing aids on and immediately heard a strange loud buzzing and fluttering sensation in one ear. I thought one of my new hearing aids was acting up so I took it off again. The buzzing continued. I knew right away what the problem was. As I was putting on that hearing aid, the ear mold had pushed a chunk of wax against my eardrum, thus causing the unusual but instant tinnitus. I cleaned out my ear and that buzzing/fluttering tinnitus stopped immediately.

You may also hear coarse intermittent sounds in one ear, coincident with jaw or head movements, if you have a foreign body such as cerumen (wax), water (or other liquids) or a hair resting against your eardrum.[4] With this kind of tinnitus, simply remove the offending wax and/or foreign matter and the tinnitus should stop.

## Stapedial Muscle Contractions

A fluttering kind of tinnitus is often the result of abnormal stapedius muscle contractions. (Normally the stapedius muscle automatically pulls your stapes [stirrup] backwards [away from your oval window] in response to sudden loud sounds to help protect your ears.) This fluttering kind of tinnitus only happens in one ear at a time.

If the fluttering is associated with facial movements, then stapedial contractions are highly likely to be causing the fluttering sound. This is most commonly seen after recovery from Bell's palsy, or facial paralysis on one side. When the affected side of the face contracts, the stapedius muscle on that side also contracts due to aberrant facial nerve regeneration.[5]

## Tensor Tympani Muscle Contractions

The tensor tympani muscle is one of the two tiny muscles in your middle ears. (The other is the stapedius muscle mentioned above.)

The tensor tympani muscle reacts to sudden loud sounds. Its job is to pull the tiny malleus (hammer) bone away from your eardrum (tympani), thus tensing your eardrum (hence its name tensor tympani). This reduces the volume of sounds that are transmitted to your inner ears, which helps protect your delicate inner ear structures from noise damage.

When everything is working properly, you aren't even aware you have two tensor tympani muscles working for you. Their actions are totally automatic.

However, if you have hyperacusis (where normal sounds are now abnormally loud), and also have misophonia (where you have negative emotional reactions to certain specific sounds), increased (abnormal) activity develops in the tensor tympani muscle, which you experience as a type of tinnitus.

Your tensor tympani muscle may cause two kinds of tinnitus. You may experience a series of clicks as your tensor tympani muscle rapidly contracts and relaxes. You may also experience rhythmic sensations such as your eardrum fluttering. This occurs when the tensor tympani muscle continually and rhythmically contracts and relaxes.[6]

The good news is that if you get your hyperacusis and misophonia under control, often this kind of tinnitus also goes away.

## Patulous Eustachian Tubes

If your Eustachian tubes do not work properly you may experience some strange tinnitus sounds. Here's why.

Your Eustachian tubes have four functions.

1. They equalize the air pressure in your middle ears to the outside air pressure. Your Eustachian tubes are normally closed, but they open momentarily when you swallow, yawn or sneeze and allow the air pressure to equalize.

2. They allow unwanted fluids (mucous, etc.) to drain out of your middle ears and into your throat.

3. They normally prevent unwanted stuff from your mouth (food, mucous, etc.) from getting into your middle ears.

4. They, and this is where the tinnitus sounds come in, prevent both the sounds of your breathing and your voice from taking a short-cut and going directly to your ears from your throat.

If your Eustachian tube(s) stays open, (this is called patulous [PAT-you-lus] Eustachian tube), you may hear your breath sounds as a blowing, roaring or whooshing tinnitus, synchronous with your breathing. Your voice will also sound loud, distorted and have an annoying reverberating echo. This is called autophony.

Among the things that can cause patulous Eustachian tube are pregnancy, taking nasal decongestants, fatigue, stress, weight loss[7] and having the top two vertebrae in your neck (C1 & C2) out of proper alignment.

If your C1 and C2 vertebrae are out of alignment, the health care professional to see is a special kind of chiropractor called an upper cervical chiropractor (http://www.upcspine.com/prac1.asp).

If your patulous Eustachian tubes result from other causes, then you probably should see an ear specialist (ENT doctor).

---

**Chapter 12 Endnotes**

1 Moller, 2011. pp 663-668.
2 Moller, 2011. pp 285-291.
3 Currie, 2005.
4 Levine, 2000. p. 3.
5 Levine, 2000. p. 3.
6 Bauman, 2013, p. 2.
7 Currie, 2005.

Chapter 13

# Certain Foods (and Other Substances)

Specific foods such as red wine, grain-based spirits, cheese and chocolate can trigger or increase tinnitus in some people.[1] Penny finds that wine, vinegar and certain spices affect the loudness of her tinnitus. She also finds that any foods containing mold will make her tinnitus louder. Obviously, this includes many cheeses. Surprisingly it also includes canned juices because manufacturers are allowed to include a certain amount of moldy fruit in their canned products.

Drinking alcohol may exacerbate your tinnitus. In fact, in one study, 38% of current tinnitus sufferers were found to have had a past dependence on alcohol—about three times as high as in the control group.[2]

Interestingly enough, although alcohol may increase the tinnitus levels in some people, especially those who find that alcohol stimulates them, it can also reduce the tinnitus volume in those people who find that drinking alcohol has a calming effect.[3]

Nicotine affects your vascular system by narrowing your blood vessels. Thus, less blood (and oxygen) gets to your ears. This can trigger tinnitus or make your existing tinnitus worse.[4] Some people have reported that once they stopped smoking, their tinnitus improved or even disappeared.[5]

Other things of which to beware include monosodium glutamate (MSG),[6] marijuana and some spices.[7] For example, Sue finds that eating hot spices such as chili peppers, hot salsa and hot paprika make her tinnitus louder.

Is your tinnitus sensitive to caffeine, a high "junk food" diet (which can increase your blood pressure and thus your tinnitus) or excess sodium intake?

Cutting out these may also eliminate or reduce the severity of your tinnitus, not to mention improve your overall health. (Remember caffeine is not only found in coffee, but also in tea, many of the most popular soft drinks, chocolate and in some prescription and non-prescription drugs.)[8]

For some people eating citrus fruits such as oranges and grapefruit seems to increase their tinnitus. After eliminating citrus from their diets, these people report a decrease in their tinnitus.[9]

For good health you should consider reducing your sodium (salt) intake, eliminating refined sugars, including high-fructose corn syrup, and increasing your consumption of whole, raw foods such as vegetables, nuts and seeds. These steps not only help improve your overall health, but also can also help reduce your tinnitus and related stress.[10]

**Caffeine Linked with Lower Levels of Tinnitus**

Although caffeine is associated with increased tinnitus in some people, it may also help reduce the incidence of tinnitus in other people. For example, in one study, researchers found lower rates of tinnitus in younger and middle-aged women who had higher caffeine intake. "Specifically, researchers reported that, when compared with women with caffeine intake of less than 150 mg/day (about 1½ 8-ounce cups of coffee), the incidence of reported tinnitus was 15% lower among those women who consumed 450 to 600 mg/day of caffeine (4½ to 6 8–ounce cups of coffee). The majority of caffeine consumed among the women was from coffee and the results did not vary by age."[11]

Note that the incidence of tinnitus is only 15% lower, but, if you want to try it out, drink more coffee and see if it reduces your incidence of tinnitus. If it doesn't and makes your tinnitus worse, then you know you need to cut out caffeine, not take it.

## Salt (Sodium)

Salt (basically the sodium component in salt) can have an immediate effect on your tinnitus and can make your existing tinnitus worse. Excess salt constricts blood vessels, which in turn, increases blood pressure and reduces blood flow to your ears. In some people, this increased blood pressure is directly linked to their increased tinnitus.

One man explained, "It seems like if I eat out and ingest larger amounts of sodium, my tinnitus goes off the rails." Another man explained, "I have learned that when I have a salty meal my tinnitus gets worse for several hours. The next day it will improve, providing I haven't taken more excess salt."

These people are sensitive to larger amounts of sodium in their diet. Restaurant food not only contains salt added by the cook, but often also contains "hidden" sodium such as monosodium glutamate (MSG), a flavor enhancer. The MSG added to food by the chef contains considerable sodium—represented by the "S" in the acronym MSG.

Furthermore, there are high levels of salt in most processed and pre-packaged foods. For example, a can of soup typically contains more sodium than the recommended daily allowance for an adult person.

Thus you have to be aware of all the salt you ingest. Barry Keate, the CEO at Arches Natural Products, explains, "I speak with many people who are beset with serious tinnitus but don't make the connection between blood pressure and tinnitus loudness. Many of these people will chow down on chips and other salty snacks, at the same time bemoaning the ringing in their ears. When salt intake is reduced, many of these same people report a lessening of tinnitus sounds."[12]

## Sugar

Few people seem to realize that sugar and tinnitus can go hand in hand. The more sugar you have in your system, the louder your tinnitus may become. One person explained, "I've had tinnitus for about two years. It can be a real problem, especially when I don't watch the sugar intake in my diet. If my system is loaded with sugar, it leads to louder and more intense tinnitus."

In one of their Fact Sheets, the American Tinnitus Association reported, "Some people find that foods with high sugar content make their tinnitus louder.[13] Therefore, monitor how you respond, and find a healthy balance where you do not eliminate all the foods that you love, but also where you do not unnecessarily exacerbate your tinnitus."

Too much sugar is bad for your body as a whole (think diabetes), not just your ears, so you should watch your sugar intake anyway. In fact, "for many years scientists have spoken of a connection between tinnitus and sugar metabolism disorders such as diabetes. Indeed, studies have shown that a massive 84 - 92% of people with tinnitus have a sugar metabolism disorder called hyperinsulinemia, which means that there is too much insulin present in the blood relative to the level of glucose."[14] "Too much insulin in the blood is the first step on the slippery slope to type II diabetes."[15]

If your tinnitus is a result of "sugar problems", here's some good news for you. "When people with tinnitus follow a diet suitable for diabetics, their head noises can drastically reduce or even disappear."[16]

Even hunger can cause your tinnitus to increase. Penny explains, "When I'm hungry my tinnitus gets louder. My doctor says it's because my blood sugar level drops. About 40 minutes after I eat, my tinnitus gets softer again."

## Salicylates in Foods

Salicylate is the main component of a number of drugs, the most common being Aspirin (acetylsalicylic acid), a known ototoxic substance. Ingesting too much salicylate can result in tinnitus.

Near the beginning of this chapter, I mentioned a number of substances which are listed as causing tinnitus. However, striking by their absence are a number of common herbals that contain salicylates (sah-LISS-ih-lits), and thus you would think should be listed here, but are not.

A lady wondered about that too. She asked, "Do you know about the ototoxicity of various foods. I read that tea is high in salicylates, as are also a lot of fruits. Does this mean that drinking/eating these things can make my existing tinnitus worse?"

As attested by the lack of such foods in the above listings, the short answer is typically "no". It is true that salicylates occur naturally in a good number of foods such as fruits, vegetables, dried spices, tea and food flavorings in quite high concentrations, but reports of resulting tinnitus are almost non-existent.

With few exceptions, people that ingest foods containing salicylates never notice any change in their tinnitus, and thus these foods are not reported to cause tinnitus. Why?

Maybe we need to ask, "Can we ingest sufficient amounts of salicylates in our foods to cause the typical ototoxic side effects of tinnitus, reversible hearing loss, dizziness and vertigo?"

People on the average "Western diet" naturally ingest an estimated 10 to 200 mg. a day of salicylates. In comparison, the average dose of (adult) *Aspirin* contains a whopping 650 mg. of Salicylic acid per pill, while a baby *Aspirin* contains just 81 mg. of Salicylic acid.

Conventional wisdom says that a person has to take around 5 or 6 **adult** *Aspirin* tablets a day before they get tinnitus, or notice a change in their existing tinnitus. Although this is generally true, a few people actually get tinnitus from just taking a single baby *Aspirin* a day, so you need to learn exactly what the salicylate tolerance is for your own body.

Let's compare the salicylate content of a few foods that are high in salicylates to a person taking a single baby aspirin (81 mg.) a day. Here's how it stacks up.

Curry powder has the highest salicylate content of any food—218 mg. per 100 g.[17] To get 81 mg. of salicylate, you would have to ingest 1.31 oz. of Curry powder at a sitting (if you could stand it)! If you wanted to consume the equivalent amount of salicylates contained in 6 adult *Aspirin*, you'd have to choke down almost 4 **pounds** of pure curry powder. It's just not going to happen!

Raisins are high in salicylates (6.62 mg. per 100 g.). To even get just one baby's aspirin worth of Salicylic acid, you'd have to eat about three pounds of raisins. And to get the equivalent salicylates contained in 6 adult *Aspirin*, where tinnitus typically starts to be noticeable, you'd have to gorge yourself with 144 **pounds** of raisins—at one sitting mind you!

Almonds are also considered high in salicylates at 3 mg. per 100 g. To get one baby's aspirin worth of Salicylic acid, you'd have to chomp your way through 6 pounds of almonds at one sitting! I eat a handful of almonds almost every day—but one handful (less than 1 ounce) is a far cry from the 288 **pounds** of almonds I'd have to gobble to begin to have a change in my tinnitus from eating almonds.

Some people are worried about getting tinnitus from eating tomatoes. Tomatoes have 0.13 mg. of salicylates per 100 g. Therefore, to get even one baby's *Aspirin* worth of Salicylic acid, you'd have to stuff yourself with a whopping 134 pounds of tomatoes at one sitting! If you wanted to get the equivalent salicylate content contained in a single adult *Aspirin*, you'd have to devour more than half a ton of tomatoes—again, all at one sitting. In order for you to get tinnitus from the salicylate content in tomatoes (the equivalent of 6 adult *Aspirin*), you'd need to engorge yourself with 3 **tons** of fresh tomatoes at one sitting—and by then tinnitus would be the least of your worries!

Thus, even though you eat natural foods that are high in salicylates, you physically could not ingest enough salicylates from these natural foods each day to either cause tinnitus, or affect your existing tinnitus, unless you are super-sensitive to salicylates.

So feel free to eat your tomatoes, feast on broad beans, lace your food with curry powder and garlic, and drink your green tea—all in moderation of course—and you won't have to worry that these foods will cause your tinnitus to get worse.[18]

## Salicylate Intolerance (Salicylate Sensitivity)

After having told you to feel free to eat all the foods you want that contain salicylates because they should not cause tinnitus or affect your existing tinnitus, I need to add a word of caution. The foregoing only applies if you do not have a special sensitivity to salicylates—known as salicylate intolerance. If you do, then even the normal amount of salicylates contained in foods can be too much for your body to tolerate.

Therefore, the few people with salicylate intolerance need to avoid foods containing salicylates, or they stand a good chance of getting tinnitus or making their existing tinnitus worse—not to mention experiencing a number of other nasty side effects.

Lana has tinnitus. She also discovered that she has salicylate intolerance, which explains her fluctuating tinnitus when she eats certain foods. She writes, "I have learned to control my tinnitus by avoiding high-salicylate foods and steering clear of all teas, including herbal teas as they contain high levels of salicylates. I also avoid herbs and spices."

Sharon also has salicylate intolerance. She explained, "I, too, suffer from tinnitus. Until I was diagnosed with salicylate intolerance I was not able to control my tinnitus. Now, through avoiding salicylate-containing foods, my tinnitus is manageable. It is frustrating and time consuming needing to be aware of, and eat, a salicylate free diet."

Salicylate intolerance is not an allergic reaction—rather it is a pharmacological reaction to the chemical components in foods (much like experiencing the side effects of taking drugs). In contrast, an allergy is an immunological reaction to food proteins no matter how much or little you ingest.

Some people with salicylate intolerance are more sensitive than others to salicylates and will react to smaller doses, while others are less sensitive and will only react to larger doses of salicylate-containing foods.[19] Reactions to salicylate intolerance may be immediate or delayed for some hours.

Salicylates also have a cumulative effect in the body and build up over time. This means that a person with salicylate intolerance may be able to tolerate a small amount of salicylates, but will experience negative side effects after excessive exposure.[20]

This is sometimes called the "bucket theory". Imagine that there is a bucket in your body. If the bucket is nearly empty, you would have no symptoms. However, as you are exposed to more and more salicylates, the bucket begins to fill up, yet you still don't experience any reactions. All this changes when your bucket nearly fills up. At this point you will start to see reactions to the salicylates. If your bucket fills to overflowing, you will experience severe reactions. These reactions will become less over time as your bucket slowly empties as you avoid ingesting more salicylates.[21]

In addition to tinnitus, ototoxic reactions to salicylate intolerance may include dizziness, vertigo, balance problems and hyperacusis.[22]

If you have salicylate intolerance, you will have to watch your intake of almonds, apples, apricots, blackberries, blueberries, cherries, cucumbers (and pickles), currants, eggplant, gooseberries, grapes (raisins), nectarines, oranges, peaches, peppers, pineapple (fresh), plums/prunes, radishes, raspberries, strawberries, tomatoes and a bunch of other foods and spices.[23] In addition, salicylates can be found in many medications, perfumes and preservatives.

---

**Chapter 13 Endnotes**

1 Discovering and Understanding Tinnitus, 1997. p. 3.
2 Hogan, 1998. p. 107.
3 Coleman, 2009. pp. 164-165.
4 American Tinnitus Association, 2002. pp. 3-4.
5 Craggs-Hinton, 2007. p. 89.
6 Tinnitus Association of Calgary.
7 Info-Tinnitus, Causes and Factors in the Hearing System, 1990.
8 Information About Tinnitus, 1988.
9 Coleman, 2009. p. 166.
10 Craggs-Hinton, 2007. p. 80.
11 HearingReview.Com, 2014, p. 46.
12 Keate, 2010a. p. 2.
13 American Tinnitus Association, 2002. p. 4.
14 Craggs-Hinton, 2007. p. 84.
15 Craggs-Hinton, 2007. p. 84.
16 Craggs-Hinton, 2007. p. 85.
17 Swain, 1985. p. 954.
18 Bauman, 2010a. p. 662-663.
19 Salicylate Sensitivity—Info4, 2011. p. 1.
20 Salicylate Sensitivity—Info2, 2011. p. 1.
21 Atkinson, 2008. p. 4.
22 Salicylate Sensitivity—Info3, 2011. pp. 1-2.
23 Atkinson, 2008. p. 5.

# Part III

# Things You Can Do to Take Control of Your Tinnitus

## Chapter 14

# Steps to Treating Your Tinnitus

You have learned what tinnitus is and a good number of things that cause, trigger or are associated with tinnitus. Now, you are ready to learn how to take control of your tinnitus and habituate to it, and if possible, eliminate your tinnitus.

However, before we even get started, note that about 10% of people with the common neurophysiologic kind of tinnitus find that nothing seems to help them. Dr. Jastreboff, the father of Tinnitus Retraining Therapy (TRT), with rare insight, explains why.

He reports that 82% of patients experience clear improvement, with approximately 90% of patients reporting at least some improvement. "Regarding the remaining 10%," he explains, "I have learned to predict when TRT will or will not be successful." You will not successfully habituate to your tinnitus if:

1. You take large doses of benzodiazepine drugs such as Alprazolam (*Xanax*). (His definition of a "large dose" is 1.5 mg or more per day.) Benzodiazepines prevent neural plasticity and hence any habituation to tinnitus. (See the section on "Anti-Anxiety Drugs (Benzodiazepines)" in Chapter 26, "Medical Remedies", for more on this.)

2. You use your tinnitus and/or hyperacusis as a means of getting social attention. If you need to feel victimized, your tinnitus will never get better because you do not want to put an end to what makes you feel special.

3. You do not want to get better for financial reasons, so that you can continue to receive health care benefits for example. If you have a financial interest in your tinnitus, you will find it most difficult to

> habituate to your tinnitus. Thus, if you are a litigant involved in a car accident that caused or exacerbated your tinnitus, or are involved in a case where a medical or dental procedure caused or exacerbated your tinnitus, you will find it almost impossible to habituate to your tinnitus. This is because you are emotionally involved with your tinnitus and are thinking about your tinnitus all the time as a result of the ongoing litigation.[1,2]

If you fall into any of the above classes, you need to address those issues now—before you read further—if you ever want to gain control over your tinnitus.

For the rest of you, there is hope. You can start on the road to gaining control over your tinnitus, beginning now.

## Clinical Practice Guidelines

When you first notice your tinnitus, you should figure out what you need to do to effectively deal with your tinnitus. This is where triage comes in—prioritizing your tinnitus treatment needs and options. You can do this yourself with the help of this book, or you can go to a health care professional who hopefully will examine you, note your various symptoms, and then refer you to the appropriate health care professional(s) for treatment.

At least, this is what should happen when you go to a health care professional. However, in the past, too often this didn't happen.

What actually happened went more like this. You, like millions of people before you with tinnitus, asked yourself the age-long question, "Whatever can I do to get rid of this infernal racket in my head?" You considered this to be a medical problem, and thus, quite logically, you went to your doctor.

Your doctor examined you, and because he typically couldn't find a **medical** problem as the source of your tinnitus (unless you had something like pulsatile tinnitus), and because he didn't know much/anything about effective tinnitus treatments, he simply advised, "There is nothing that can be done. You will just have to learn to live with your tinnitus."

For tinnitus sufferers, this advice gave them absolutely no hope. It just sentenced them to constant, mind-rending, nerve-wracking tinnitus until the day they died. That's the bad news.

Now for the good news. If you are reading this, you are truly blessed. Why? Because today there is hope. There are now several tools in the fields of sound therapy, audiology, medicine and psychology to help you in your efforts to gain control over your tinnitus and to shift it from "bothersome" to "non-bothersome".

Depending on your particular kind of tinnitus, you can work alone, or work together with your health care professional, in order to bring your tinnitus under your control so it won't bother you anymore! Isn't that great news?

Furthermore, to ensure that your doctor doesn't give you the false "there's nothing that can be done" line, recently, ear specialists came up with a document called *Clinical Practice Guideline: Tinnitus.*[3] This document details what health care professionals should do when they encounter you—a sort of "best practices" guideline for tinnitus so you get effective help and are not just "brushed off".

This guideline represents the best judgment of a team of experienced researchers after looking at the scientific evidence available for treating tinnitus.[4] Having said that, this guideline is not intended to supersede a health care professional's judgment. Rather, health care professionals should view it as a good starting point if they don't have a proven better treatment for a specific person with tinnitus.[5]

Also note that the researchers put this guideline together specifically to treat only those people with persistent, bothersome tinnitus. They define "persistent" as bothersome tinnitus that has lasted for more than six months.

If you have had tinnitus for less than six months, or your tinnitus does not bother you all that much, you can still follow its principles. Use it for triage—where you look at all the factors that may be related to your tinnitus, prioritize them and seek treatment for them in order of their priority if you need help in dealing with your tinnitus.

When encountering a person with tinnitus, according to this guideline, whichever health care professional you see first should:

1. Perform a targeted history and physical examination in order to identify conditions that, if promptly identified and managed, may relieve your tinnitus.

2. Obtain a prompt, comprehensive audiologic examination if you have tinnitus that is unilateral, persistent (greater than six months), or associated with hearing difficulties.

3. Determine whether you have bothersome tinnitus of recent onset, or whether you have had tinnitus for more than six months, in order to prioritize what treatments you may need.

4. Teach you (if you have persistent, bothersome tinnitus) how to effectively deal with your tinnitus.

5. Recommend you have a hearing aid evaluation.

6. Recommend you have cognitive behavior therapy if you have persistent, bothersome tinnitus.[6]

## Quick Guide: Where Do I Go If I Have Tinnitus?

When you first realize you have tinnitus, you immediately worry about this strange new sound in your ears. You ask yourself, "What should I do now?" or more likely, "Which health care professional should I see?"

Below is a decision-making process to help you make the best decision you can based on what you know about the origin of your tinnitus; what you know about the kind of tinnitus you are experiencing; and what you know about any other physical or psychological conditions you are experiencing at this time.

A quick triage would be:

A. Go to emergency care, to your doctor, or to an otolaryngologist (commonly called an ears, nose and throat doctor [ENT]) **immediately** if you have any of the following:

- Injury to your body. (Tinnitus is often associated with injuries to your head and/or neck.)
- Weakness or paralysis of any muscles in your face. (You may have had a stroke that is also causing your tinnitus.)
- Sudden unexplained hearing loss in one or both the ears. (You may have a blood clot in your ears, a tumor, a virus, etc. that needs to be checked immediately by a doctor.)

B. Go to emergency care or to a mental health clinic **immediately** if you have either of the following:

- Extreme anxiety or depression.
- You are planning to commit suicide and have the means to do it.

C. Go to an ENT doctor or to a physician as soon as possible if you experience any of the following:

- Your tinnitus pulses in time with your heartbeat. (You have pulsatile tinnitus related to a vascular problem.)
- You have pain in your ear, your ear is draining or there is a foul odor coming from your ear. (You likely have an ear infection causing your tinnitus.)
- You have vertigo. That is, you feel you are moving or spinning or the room is moving or spinning when neither is happening. (You have a damaged vestibular [balance] system.)

D. If you have tinnitus and all of the following are true, then you probably don't need to go to a doctor at this point:

- Your tinnitus is a constant sound that does not pulse with your heartbeat.
- You do not have ear pain, drainage from your ear, or a foul odor coming from your ear.
- You do not have vertigo.
- You do not have weakness or paralysis of any muscles in your face.
- You do not have sudden unexplained hearing loss.[7]

If you fit "D" above, it is unlikely you have an emergency situation. You can take your time to figure out your next step.

## Treatment Options—Choosing the Right Treatment for Your Tinnitus

Since there are a number of kinds of tinnitus that are triggered by a wide variety of conditions, it should come as no surprise that there are also a number of different ways to treat your tinnitus.

For example, you should seek medical attention to rule out any number of diseases or conditions that could be causing your tinnitus such as anemia, diabetes, acoustic neuromas, superior canal dehiscence,[8] otosclerosis, high blood pressure, allergies, arthritis, multiple sclerosis or thyroid problems.

In a **few** cases, the cause may be as simple as wax touching your eardrum. Your family doctor can quickly remove this and put an end to this kind of tinnitus.

## Eliminate Tinnitus Triggers

Consider what triggers your tinnitus. Can you make some lifestyle changes to reduce your tinnitus? For example, are you wearing ear protectors when you are around loud noises? Loud sounds can aggravate your tinnitus and make it louder.

If you already have tinnitus, you should avoid loud sounds at all costs. This may eliminate your tinnitus, reduce its severity or at the very least, prevent it from getting worse.

Are you eating properly? Are you getting enough exercise? These things may have an effect on your tinnitus.[9] However, there is no solid scientific evidence that any special diet will help your tinnitus once you have it. Many people follow rigid diets that reduce their quality of life. In the past, dietary advice was often given because there simply wasn't anything else.[10]

Having said that, as we saw in Chapter 13, there are a number of specific foods and other substances that can trigger your tinnitus or make your tinnitus worse. Learn to avoid these things in the future.

After considering the possible causes that triggered your tinnitus, unless they can provide a path towards treatment, don't dwell on questions such as "Why me?" or "Why tinnitus?" Doing this just keeps your mind focused on your tinnitus. Instead, focus your attention on the loves of your life. Live a happy, productive life and let your tinnitus slowly fade into the background on its own.

## No One Tinnitus Treatment Works for Everyone

Note this well. There is **no** one universal treatment for tinnitus (and there **never** will be). No one treatment works for everyone, but the good news is that every treatment in this book works for someone.

Therefore, try various approaches. Don't just stick with one method. Those people that use multiple methods have better success than those who just try one "pet" method. Remember, there isn't just one way to reduce your tinnitus. In fact, there isn't even a single "best" way.[11]

The many complex factors inherent in tinnitus explain why certain tinnitus treatments work for some people but not for others. Each method has its uses for given people with specific kinds of tinnitus.

Not only are there a variety of totally-different tinnitus treatments, there are also a number of different health care professionals that treat each of these different kinds of tinnitus.

For example, the health care professional that treats pulsatile tinnitus (a medical doctor—likely a vascular surgeon) is different from the health care professional that treats somatosensory tinnitus (a physiotherapist, massage therapist or upper cervical spine chiropractor). The health care professional that typically treats middle ear tinnitus (an ENT specialist) is different from the health care professional that treats the common neurophysiologic kind of tinnitus (an audiologist and/or psychologist).

Even in these broad tinnitus groups, there are a number of different treatments based on the specific cause of your tinnitus. For example, if you have neurophysiologic tinnitus caused by taking ototoxic drugs, the treatment may be to stop taking the culprit drug and have your medical doctor switch you to a drug that doesn't cause tinnitus. However, if your neurophysiologic tinnitus is caused by noise exposure, you'd likely see an audiologist to learn how to take control of your tinnitus.

Furthermore, be aware that you may have more than one kind of tinnitus at the same time. Thus, you may need to see different health care professionals for different tinnitus treatments.

Oftentimes, when tinnitus appears, it does not stand alone. You may have one or more health conditions associated with it. Thus, it is important to seek treatment for the "whole you", not just your tinnitus. This is because if you treat the underlying causes of your other associated conditions, you may find your tinnitus goes away in the process.

For example, as you have already learned, tinnitus often accompanies hearing loss—whether you realize you have hearing loss or not. You may think that your tinnitus just suddenly appeared for no reason at all. But the truth may be that your tinnitus is accompanying a high-frequency hearing loss that you are not even aware you have. Treating the hearing loss (perhaps with hearing aids) can result in your tinnitus fading into the background. Thus treating the primary cause (hearing loss) allows the secondary condition (tinnitus) to "fix itself".

Another example. You get tinnitus as a result of head trauma—perhaps from being in a motor vehicle accident. The underlying cause could be that your C1 and C2 vertebrae (the top two vertebrae in your neck) were "knocked out" of proper alignment from whiplash. Rather than seeking someone to treat your resulting tinnitus, a better course of action would be to seek out an upper cervical spine chiropractor to realign your neck (explained in the section on "Chiropractic Treatments" in Chapter 20), and, in the process, quite likely your tinnitus will disappear on its own.

Yet another example. If you have diabetes, or pre-diabetes, you may develop tinnitus. Rather than specifically focusing on ways to treat your tinnitus, a better course of action in this case would be to treat your diabetes. Again, your tinnitus may go away on its own without any need for specific treatment.

Here are some questions to help you zero in on the likely cause of your tinnitus, and thus, give you clues as to which kinds of treatments probably will be the most successful. In turn, this will indicate which health care professional(s) you need to see.

1. Did you recently (in the last two weeks or more) begin taking any new drug or medication, or increase the dose on any existing medication? (If so, your tinnitus may be caused by that drug.)

2. Have you been under undue stress lately, or really anxious or depressed? (Any of these can cause tinnitus or make your existing tinnitus worse.)

3. Is your face or neck "tight" (you have pain or a stiff neck). (You may have somatosensory tinnitus.)

4. Do you have pain in the muscles of your face or neck? (Again, you may have somatosensory tinnitus.)

5. Do you have pain in your jaw or temporomandibular joint. (This too can result in a type of somatosensory tinnitus.)

6. Does your tinnitus change in volume or pitch when you press on the muscles of your face near your ear, or if you turn your head from side to side. (This is also related to somatosensory tinnitus.)

7. Did you experience any head trauma, blow to the head, or whiplash in the weeks or months before your tinnitus began? (Another cause of somatosensory tinnitus.)

8. Does your tinnitus get louder if you eat certain foods? (Your tinnitus may be sensitive to certain foods.)

9. Is your tinnitus related to your allergy flare-ups? (Get your allergies under control to control you tinnitus.)

10. Did your tinnitus begin after you exposed your ears to loud sounds (nightclubs, rock concert, explosion, gunshot, auto racing, noisy tools, etc.)? (You probably have noise-induced tinnitus.)

11. Have you noticed any change in your hearing? or more difficulty in hearing in noisy situations? (Your tinnitus may be a result of hearing loss.)

12. Does your tinnitus change in pitch or volume when you move your eyes right or left, or up or down? (You have gaze-evoked tinnitus.)

13. Does your tinnitus sound like wind-chimes when you nod or shake your head? (You have nodding-chime tinnitus.)

14. Do you have diabetes? (You may have diabetes-related tinnitus.)

15. Do you get a loud roaring tinnitus when you are very tired? (You need more sleep.)

16. Do your eardrums seem to flutter? Or do you hear a clicking or fluttering sound that seems to come from deep in your ears? (You may have tinnitus due to tensor tympani dysfunction.)

17. You don't have a clue where your tinnitus came from. It just "appeared" one day. (Try any of the general tinnitus treatments.)

## Put Yourself in the Driver's Seat

If you get tinnitus, you need to take control of your tinnitus yourself and work to habituate to your tinnitus. Treating tinnitus, for the most part, is not what a health care professional does **to** you, or even for you, but what you do **for** yourself to bring your tinnitus under your control.

If you just let health care professionals do things **to** you, you do not take control. Instead, you are passive and typically feel like a victim. And just as typically, you act like a victim. The result is that your tinnitus controls you. Therefore, do not become a victim of self-pity. You will just hurt yourself, your family and your friends, and you will lose your drive to overcome your tinnitus.

That is why you need to take active control of your tinnitus treatments. As tinnitus researcher Fatima Husain, Ph.D. explains, people "should—and very often do—control the management of their own tinnitus".[12]

She further explains, "I would suggest that patients adopt habits or activities that increase a sense of control and enhance their self-efficacy. Reaction to tinnitus is both physiological and psychological," so use every tool in your tinnitus toolbox. The specific things that help you may be unique to your tinnitus, so you need to think about what things might work for you.[13]

**The Hawthorne Effect**

Just taking action can sometimes help improve your tinnitus. This is known as the Hawthorne Effect. This effect occurs when people experience a sense of relief or improvement just because someone is (finally) doing something for them. For example, the hope offered by a kind professional who takes the time to explain your tinnitus might help you feel better about your tinnitus, regardless of any treatment undertaken.[14]

## Learn All You Can About Your Tinnitus

As you can appreciate, "A major step in gaining control and managing your tinnitus is access to good information about tinnitus"[15] like you will find in this book.

One of the first things you should do is to learn as much as you can about your tinnitus. Once you know at the conscious level that tinnitus is not a life-threatening problem, and therefore nothing to fear, it becomes something over which you can gain a great deal of control. This alone can reduce your stress level and thus your tinnitus.

Remember, if you are fearful of your tinnitus you cannot habituate to it. Understanding your tinnitus helps dispel this fear, and that is half the battle won right there. Reading this book is a great way to start. See "Sources of Help" for other good resources on tinnitus. You also might want to follow up on any footnote references that catch your eye. Then, too, there is a tremendous amount of information available on the Internet that can help you. Talk to fellow tinnitus sufferers, whether in person, in a tinnitus support group, or via the Internet. As a tinnitus sufferer, you are not alone. There are a lot of us who are hearing something similar to what you hear.

Once you have learned all you can about tinnitus, sit down and analyze how your tinnitus affects your behavior. Look at the things you do that make your tinnitus worse. Such things are negative behaviors. Cut them out. Now look at those things you can do that make it easier to cope with your tinnitus. These are positive behaviors. Do these things.[16]

The rest of this book details a number of things you can do to help yourself. Try a number of them at the same time, or choose one that tickles your fancy. The important thing is that you do something. This puts you in control. Now you are no longer a victim of your tinnitus.

Therefore, use those methods that either eliminate your tinnitus, make your tinnitus easier to tolerate, or stop it from negatively affecting your life. Come up with a personalized plan to manage your tinnitus. This way, instead of being obsessed with the idea of a miracle pill or cure, you will be actively involved in carrying out your own tinnitus reduction strategy. Even if you do not eliminate your tinnitus, your actions will make your tinnitus easier to live with.[17] Look at it this way. Accept your present tinnitus as your base line. If something you try decreases your tinnitus, that is a plus—a success. If it doesn't make any difference to your tinnitus, you are no worse off, so try something else.

As you read through the following ways of controlling your tinnitus, it might be helpful to note what has worked for people who have suffered from their tinnitus. In a survey of American Tinnitus Association members, a whopping 45% of people with tinnitus found their best coping strategy was to focus on things other than their tinnitus and thereby ignore their tinnitus (and thus habituated to their tinnitus). Another 24% masked it with background sounds (TV, radio, sound machines, etc.). In addition, 5% used relaxation techniques, 7% tried drugs, 8% used miscellaneous techniques, while 9% found that nothing had helped them so far.[18]

Notice that the things that worked the best were things where you have to take active control.

## Grieve for Your Tinnitus

One day a stranger called tinnitus suddenly invaded your life—unwanted and unbidden to be sure—and you are powerless to make him leave. You have lost—perhaps forever—the silence you once enjoyed. This knocks you out of the driver's seat. Thus you need to grieve so that you can ultimately gain control over your tinnitus.

When dealing with tinnitus, people often move though various stages of grieving. We can break this process down into three simple stages: disbelief, distress and caring.[19]

The disbelief stage often starts with the diagnosis of tinnitus that is not expected to go away. In this stage you think, "This can't be true" or "Why me?" This disbelief is a common reaction and may last one or two months.

However, your tinnitus persists. Now you enter the distress stage. In the distress stage you experience various negative emotions such as sadness, worry and anger. These emotions and feelings can be intense, prolonged and can seem overwhelming.

During this stage you become focused on your tinnitus. Your negative emotional reactions build up. This stage usually lasts about four months, but it can last much longer if you don't seek out, and receive, appropriate help and reassurance about your tinnitus.[20] The longer you stay in this stage, the stronger the negative bonds you build up. This just makes it that much harder to get your tinnitus under control when you finally reach the next stage.

In the third caring stage, you will still have disbelief and moments of pain, sadness, worry or anger, but now you will have more interest in what is going on around you. You will start planning ahead. This is the stage where you can actively start using coping strategies and treatments so that your tinnitus moves away from being the central focus of your life.[21] When you learn and use effective coping strategies, you will show significant improvement in your well-being.[22]

**Grieving for Your Hearing Loss (Tinnitus)**

If you need more information about the grieving process and how you can work through the various stages of grieving, you may find that reading the short, effective book *Grieving for Your Hearing Loss—The Rocky Road from Denial to Acceptance* will help you. Just substitute the word "tinnitus" for the words "hearing loss" as you read this little book. See inside the back cover for information on obtaining your copy of this most helpful book or go to http://hearinglosshelp.com/shop/category/books/ and scroll down to the book on grieving.

Successfully caring for your tinnitus doesn't mean fixing it or making your life perfect. Care means building coping strategies into your daily activities and routines.[23] First you must accept your tinnitus. Then you can learn how to successfully deal with it.

## Don't Go It Alone—Seek Emotional Support

If you have annoying tinnitus, you need emotional help and support. Each person reacts to tinnitus differently because of differences in personality, defense structures, social factors, severity of tinnitus and related hearing problems. Therefore, you may need individual counseling for anxiety, depression, withdrawal, anger, irritability, feelings of helplessness and problems with sleeping, since these emotional disturbances can significantly disrupt your everyday life. You may also benefit from counseling for relationship problems due to your preoccupation with your tinnitus, withdrawing from others and to a lesser extent suicidal thoughts.

Typically, by itself tinnitus does not lead to depression and suicide. Actually, it's more often the other way around. Tinnitus is often a symptom of long-standing severe depression, which can sometimes result in suicide. Certainly, tinnitus can make depression worse. From time to time, many depressed people feel suicidal because of various things (including tinnitus), but few of them actually carry it out.[24]

Some people are angry and feel guilty about their treatment (or lack of treatment) for their tinnitus. Fear, anger and guilt are powerful emotions that enhance conditioned reflexes. As a result, you focus your attention on your tinnitus. However, your tinnitus will likely improve if you overcome these feelings, and stop dwelling on thoughts of injustice.[25]

If you have tinnitus and are married or live with someone, often it is good to seek counsel as a couple. You need the support of family or close friends. Just as important, the other person needs to understand what is going on in your life. This mutual emotional support, help and comfort is very important to your emotional well-being. It reassures you that you are loved, cared for and valued in spite of your tinnitus.

If you have just realized you have tinnitus, it is normal to be concerned and anxious about it. Unfortunately, too often well-meaning people fuel your fears by inadvertently giving you poor advice. Such advice is really a form of "negative" counseling. It includes such things as telling you to have a doctor check you for a brain tumor. Or worse still, telling you it is basically a psychiatric condition (which you interpret as meaning, "I am a mental case").

Another form of negative counseling comes from many doctors who still advise, "There is nothing that can be done for your tinnitus. You will have it for the rest of your life, so you might as well learn to live with it."

This negative reinforcement of your tinnitus causes you more problems. For one thing, the resulting fears and anxieties activate your autonomic nervous system. Your brain now actually tunes your neuronal networks to better detect your tinnitus. As a result, you are more and more aware of it. This gives rise to more negative emotional responses. You become increasingly annoyed with your tinnitus. This is how false information and negative counseling actually can make your tinnitus worse. You need the truth about tinnitus for "the truth shall set you free".

When you realize the truth about tinnitus, you usually feel more in control, and feel less threatened by it. In reality, at this point you are well on your way to successfully dealing with your tinnitus whether you realize it or not.[26]

A great means of help and support is to join a tinnitus self-help group such as the American Tinnitus Association (ATA) or the Tinnitus Association of Canada. Some groups meet locally. If there is no local group in your area, you can join on-line tinnitus support groups. Often hearing loss groups double as tinnitus support groups since many people have both conditions at the same time. Two such nationwide groups are the Hearing Loss Association of America (HLAA) in the USA and the Canadian Hard of Hearing Association (CHHA) in Canada. (See "Sources of Help for Tinnitus" in Part IV of this book for further details.)

## Reduce Your Stress

There is often a direct relationship between the severity of your tinnitus and your ability (or inability) to cope with stress. Stress can cause tinnitus or aggravate your existing tinnitus.[27]

Too many people think that stress is all the bad things that life throws at you in quick succession. This is not exactly true. Increased tinnitus from stress can happen from good things too. For example, one lady's tinnitus shot up from a 3 (out of 10) to an 8 on her wedding day, even though she thoroughly enjoyed that day.[28]

Stress is how you **respond** to those situations. If you respond badly to those situations, you create harmful stress.

Your body has a built-in will to stay alive and will take action to protect itself from perceived threats to its well-being. It views things that upset you as threats. Therefore, if your tinnitus annoys you, your limbic (emotional) system will view this as a threat and will activate your body's emergency survival system—its "fight or flight" response.

When your body goes into "fight or flight" mode, it increases the blood flow to the big motor muscles in your legs and arms, which results in reduced blood flow going to your internal organs. Your heart rate, blood pressure and blood sugar all go up as your body pumps adrenaline into your system. Your endocrine glands change the level of various hormones in your body. At the same time your muscles tighten (especially the muscles in your abdomen and neck). In short, your body has revved itself up to deal with this threat—but there is nothing physical to ward off. Only a phantom threat exists.

Dr. Greenspan, the founder of the Centre for Stress and Pain-Related Disorders in New York, explains that in humans our internal alarm systems, unlike those of animals, can be activated not only by physical, but also by emotional and psychological threats. Also, unlike animals, when the threat has passed our bodies may not quickly return to normal. This is because our survival no longer actually depends on fight or flight. These perceived dangers are not clear-cut. As a result, our bodies don't always know when it is safe to return to normal again.[29]

You can reduce your stress by making every attempt to avoid nervous anxiety that only stimulates your already tense auditory system. Avoid over-fatigue. Make sure you get adequate rest and relaxation. Many people take their problems to bed with them. They worry about them before they go to sleep. Is it any wonder they wake up the next morning tired, tense and with their tinnitus roaring?

The long-term results of such stress include muscle spasms and a tight back, neck and head. Because tinnitus may disturb your sleep or break your concentration, you may react by becoming anxious, worried and depressed. In this state of mind you may take your feelings out on others. Thus begins a vicious cycle. This tension makes your tinnitus worse, which makes you tense up even more, which exacerbates your tinnitus yet again.

You learned to react to your tinnitus, which caused the problem in the first place. Fortunately, you can also break this vicious cycle and be a part of the solution.[30] Here are three qualities that will make you resistant to stress. Put into action, they will help you bring your tinnitus under control.

First, you need to look at change (in this case your tinnitus) as a challenge and opportunity rather than as a threat. If you view your tinnitus (change) as a threat, the above "fight or flight" changes occur in your body. However, if you see change as a challenge and an opportunity for growth, you body responds entirely differently. Your attitude makes all the difference. If you view your tinnitus-reducing strategies as a challenge and opportunity for growth and healing, you will do well. However, if you feel that you are a victim of tinnitus who has to undergo all this treatment—your tinnitus will not go away. It likely will get even worse.

Second, to be resistant to stress, you need to be an active participant rather than just letting things happen to you. When you are an active participant, you can choose to resolve a situation rather than looking at it as something inflicted on you.

Third, you need to feel that you are in control. You need to involve yourself in planning and actively doing something about your tinnitus. This will put you in charge. This way you and your body will work together against your tinnitus.[31]

What can you do? Since a lot of tinnitus can be traced to excess stress in your life, you need to get your life in order and reduce this stress. This may involve significant changes in your lifestyle. If you don't alter your lifestyle, your brain can return to its bad habits and the resulting horrible tinnitus. Therefore, put into practice what you have learned here about stress and about the other tinnitus-reducing strategies explained in this book. It is crucial that you reduce the stressful elements in your life, create solutions to your depression, and make the necessary major changes that impact your emotions.

Focus on learning to relax. I've found that teaching people to curb their stress and anxiety and to "hang loose" is one of the best tinnitus coping strategies. Read some books on relaxation techniques and practice those that work best for you. You will feel better as you help alleviate your tinnitus. You might want to try biofeedback (see the next section). You might also try relaxation therapy or take advantage of specialized types of massage to relax you. Do whatever works for you.

## Biofeedback

Biofeedback is a relaxation technique that teaches you to control certain autonomic body functions, such as pulse, muscle tension, and brain wave activity. You do biofeedback under the guidance of a psychologist.

If you have tinnitus, the goal of biofeedback is to help you manage the stress in your life by decreasing the stress and anxiety levels that may be contributing to your tinnitus. Even if you can't reduce your stress, at least you can try to change your body's reaction to this stress.

Using biofeedback therapy, you are taught to relax and are encouraged to relate your state of relaxation to the stress of living and the gradual reduction of your tinnitus. Many people notice a reduction in their tinnitus as they modify their reactions to stress.[32]

In one biofeedback study, 43.5% people with tinnitus experienced improvement while resting, and 24% experienced improvement in their tinnitus when using biofeedback during activity.[33] In fact, up to 80% of people taking biofeedback for tinnitus may find some relief from their tinnitus, and 20% may find total relief.[34]

## Increase Your Exercise

An excellent way to help reduce your anxiety and stress concerning your tinnitus is to exercise. Not only will exercise help improve your overall health, it also can directly and indirectly affect your tinnitus.[35] Here are four things exercise can do for you.

1. Vigorous exercise improves your blood flow—and that includes increasing blood flow to your ears. If your tinnitus is related to lack of adequate oxygen reaching your ears, you may find exercise is just the thing you need.

2. Exercise is a great way to help reduce your anxiety and lift your depression. People who exercise regularly generally suffer far less from anxiety and depression than those who quietly sit in a corner and worry about their tinnitus. Exercise helps burn up all the excess nervous energy you would otherwise use to fuel your fears over your tinnitus.

3. Exercise boosts your endorphin levels—and this makes you feel good. When you feel good you don't worry or obsess about your tinnitus like you otherwise would.

4. Exercise helps you to fall asleep more quickly because you are healthily tired and may fall asleep as soon as your head touches your pillow. That's good news if your tinnitus tends to bother you in the quietness as you try to fall asleep.

## Caution: Beware of Professionals That ...

When treating the common kind of neurophysiologic tinnitus, there are a number of misconceptions of which you need to be aware. For example, too many tinnitus practitioners focus on the conscious level—the cognitive part of your brain and at the same time ignore the crucial role your subconscious plays. They also typically ignore the fundamental role of conditioned reflexes.

Furthermore, they often focus only on your tinnitus without concurrently treating any associated conditions such as hyperacusis and misophonia. They may even fail to alleviate the effects of hearing loss.

Because time is money, some tinnitus practitioners believe that sound generators and/or hearing aids are sufficient to achieve improvement. Thus, they ignore the critically-important need for specific counseling regarding your tinnitus and teaching you how to deal with it.

If they do counsel you, the counsel they give is often too general or too abbreviated, and not tailored to your educational level, specific needs and background. Your counselor may even give false promises about your tinnitus going away forever.

Some tinnitus practitioners may use shortcuts, prescribe too much medication, run loud audiological tests when you have decreased sound tolerance, and fail to schedule follow-up visits.[36] Therefore, to get the best results, you need to seek out the best and most experienced tinnitus practitioner you can find.

## Making Good Tinnitus Treatment Choices

You are reading this because you want to get rid of your tinnitus. You probably have the following goals in mind, in descending order of importance.

1. Get rid of your tinnitus. Make it completely disappear.
2. Reduce the volume of your tinnitus, or at least reduce your perception of the volume of your tinnitus so it does not bother you.
3. Reduce the level of suffering/annoyance your tinnitus causes you.

In the pages that follow, there are a number of tinnitus treatments that can help you achieve your tinnitus goals. Sometimes it is possible to achieve goal No. 1. Unfortunately, often this is not a realistic goal. That is why most of the following treatments focus on goals 2 and 3—some focus more on either Goal 2 or Goal 3, while a few focus on both goals equally.

Since few if any tinnitus treatment therapies are mutually exclusive, you can try several of the tinnitus treatments mentioned in this book at a time if you so wish. Focus on those therapies that most closely match your goals.

As we have already seen, tinnitus is basically a psychosomatic condition. It has a physiological (physical) component and a psychological (mental/emotional) component. Consequently, you might expect therapies that treat both components should have the best results, and indeed, that is exactly what researchers have found.

For example, sound therapy, while good, is not best when used alone for reducing tinnitus. Studies have shown that using sound exclusively is only effective in 20% of cases.[37] To be really effective, you also need to treat the psychological component of your tinnitus.

Therefore, choose a treatment that contains both of these components (i.e. Tinnitus Retraining Therapy, Neuromonics, BeyondTinnitus) or choose two (or more) therapies at once—one or more from the physiological camp (i.e. Sound Therapy, myofascial therapy, hyperbaric oxygen therapy, etc.) and one or more from the psychological camp (i.e. Cognitive Behavior Therapy, counseling, Mindfulness, etc.) By doing this, you will give yourself the best chance to more quickly and more effectively gain control over your tinnitus.

The following chapters fit into one of three groups—(A) psychological therapies, (AB) combined psychological and physiological therapies, and (B) physiological therapies. In addition, a fourth group contains various natural and medical remedies that may be either (A) psychological or (B) physiological depending on the specific remedy.

This arrangement makes it easy to choose at least one "A" therapy and at least one "B" therapy (or a combined AB therapy) at the same time.

"A" Psychological Therapies
- Chapter 16 Take Control of Your Tinnitus
- Chapter 17 Change Your Attitude
- Chapter 18 Cognitive Behavior Therapy
- Chapter 19 Mindfulness-Based Tinnitus Reduction

"B" Physiological Therapies
- Chapter 20 Treating Somatosensory Tinnitus
- Chapter 21 Sound Therapies

"AB" Combined Psychological/Physiological Therapies
- Chapter 22 Tinnitus Retraining Therapy
- Chapter 23 Neuromonics Tinnitus Treatment
- Chapter 24 BeyondTinnitus Therapy

"A" or "B" Some are Psychological and Some are Physiological
- Chapter 25 Natural Remedies
- Chapter 26 Medical Remedies

---

**Chapter 14 Endnotes**

1 "'We Cannot Do Anything About Your Tinnitus.' This Is Simply Not True", 2016. p. 6.

2 Robb, 2015. pp. 18-19.

3 Tunkel, 2014. p. S1.

4 Tunkel, 2014. p. S6.
5 Tunkel, 2014. p. S6.
6 Tunkel, 2014. p. S1.
7 Henry, 2010a. pp. 2-3.
8 Tunkel, 2014. p. S11.
9 Info-Tinnitus, The Holistic Approach, 1990.
10 Hazell, 1997b. p. 3.
11 Hogan, 1998. p. 47.
12 Forstag, 2014. p. 21.
13 Forstag, 2014. p. 20.
14 Mayes, 2010. p. 165.
15 Forstag, 2014. p. 21.
16 Olsson, 1997a, p.2.
17 Info-Tinnitus, Solutions, 1990.
18 Results from ATA's Membership Survey, 2014. p. 9.
19 Mayes, 2010. p. 147.
20 Mayes, 2010. p. 147.
21 Mayes, 2010. p. 148.
22 Mayes, 2010. p. 149.
23 Mayes, 2010. p. 146.
24 Hazell, 1997c. p. 5.
25 Hazell, 1997a. pp. 3-4.
26 Walsh, 1997. pp. 1-3.
27 Rezen, 1985. p. 124.
28 Craggs-Hinton, 2007. p. 30.
29 Greenspan, 1998. p. 18.
30 Info-Tinnitus, Relaxation, 1990.
31 Greenspan, 1998. p. 19.
32 Tinnitus Treatment Options, 2002. pp. 1-2.
33 Hogan, 1998. p. 27.
34 Rizer, 2004. p. 6.
35 Craggs-Hinton, 2997. p. 68.
36 Robb, 2015. p. 17.
37 "'We Cannot Do Anything About Your Tinnitus.' This Is Simply Not True", 2016. p. 5.

Chapter 15

# Progressive Tinnitus Management

Progressive Tinnitus Management (PTM) isn't some new tinnitus treatment. Rather, it is a new delivery system concept, developed for the US military, in order to efficiently treat people (mostly military personnel) with tinnitus using two proven tinnitus treatments—namely, Sound Therapy (see Chapter 21) and Cognitive Behavior Therapy (CBT) (see Chapter 18). PTM teaches many different ways for you to use sound therapy to manage your reactions to your tinnitus. In conjunction with sound therapy, PTM uses Cognitive Behavior Therapy to help you change your thoughts and feelings towards your tinnitus. [1]

Note: The Progressive Tinnitus Management program avoids using the word "treatment", which you might interpret to mean that a specific course of treatment will permanently quiet or eliminate your tinnitus.[2]

This is because the basic premise of Progressive Tinnitus Management is that reducing or eliminating tinnitus is not normally an option since most military-related tinnitus results from loud noise and explosions. Therefore, the next best thing is to help those with military-related tinnitus learn to live more comfortably with their tinnitus.

Thus, intervention with PTM involves activities specifically designed to teach you how to reduce your reactions to your tinnitus (while no attempt is made to alter the tinnitus itself—which is in contrast to a number of other tinnitus treatments explained in this book).[3]

By learning to self-manage your reactions to your tinnitus, you gain the ability to know how to address any situation in which your tinnitus becomes bothersome or intrusive.[4] This, alone, can make a positive change in the quality of your life.[5] Therefore, any reference to "managing tinnitus" in the PTM program really means "managing your **reactions** to your tinnitus".[6]

The National Center for Rehabilitative Auditory Research developed the Progressive Tinnitus Management program for the US Department of Veterans Affairs to efficiently treat the enormous number of veterans with tinnitus.

**Progressive Tinnitus Management Resource Books**

The PTM program includes three supporting resource books. You can get the 3-book set on Amazon.com. Just search for *Progressive Tinnitus Management* and look for the 3-book set. It's not cheap at around $250.00.

The first book, the 160-page *Progressive Tinnitus Management: Clinical Handbook for Audiologists* explains the PTM program and gives audiologists the information they need about tinnitus in order to successfully conduct the program. You can also download and print a free copy of this book from http://www.ncrar.research.va.gov/Education/Documents/TinnitusDocuments/ClinicalHandbookAndSupplements.asp. (Note: You have to download and print each chapter and appendix separately.)

The second book, the 300-page *Progressive Tinnitus Management: Counseling Guide* is a spiral-bound flip-book designed and formatted to be used directly in the counseling process by both the audiologist and the person with tinnitus. The audiologist sees her page while the person with tinnitus sees his corresponding page at the same time. This book is only available in printed form. You can get a copy from Amazon.com for $90.00. Just search for *Progressive Tinnitus Management Counseling Guide*.

The third book, the 126-page *How to Manage Your Tinnitus: A Step-by Step Workbook* (3rd edition) is a self-help workbook for a person with tinnitus.[7] You can download and print this most useful book for free from http://www.ncrar.research.va.gov/Education/Documents/TinnitusDocuments/HowToManageYourTinnitus.pdf.

PTM provides a hierarchical way of prioritizing and progressively providing various clinical services for each person with tinnitus. As a result, each person with tinnitus receives services that progress to higher levels as needed. This is because people with tinnitus need varying levels of support and guidance in order to become self-sufficient in dealing with their tinnitus. Therefore, proper evaluation and the provision of appropriate education/counseling are the basic keys to the success of the PTM program.[8]

The beauty of the PTM system is that each person gets just the amount of treatment he needs in order to successfully manage his tinnitus. Some people with tinnitus only need their basic questions answered. Other people need basic education on tinnitus. Still others need a great deal of help. Thus, the system is set up to identify the levels of audiological and psychological help each person needs.

Fortunately, the majority of people with tinnitus either are not bothered by their tinnitus, or require only some basic education, and thus do not require extensive (and expensive) clinical intervention to learn how to manage their reactions to their tinnitus (Fig. 15-1).[9]

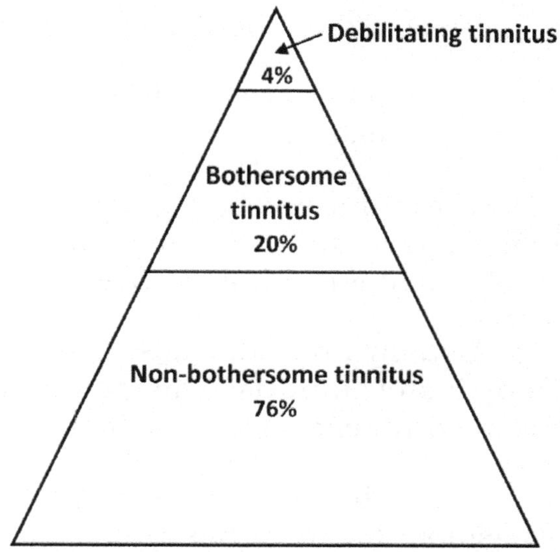


Fig. 15-1. This tinnitus pyramid represents all people who experience chronic tinnitus (about 15% of all adults). Only the people in the top two levels need help. The rest are not particularly bothered by their tinnitus.[10] Furthermore, many of the people in the middle section only want assurance that their tinnitus does not reflect some serious medical condition.

There are five levels in the PTM program. They are:

1. Triage.
2. Audiological evaluation.
3. Group education.
4. Tinnitus evaluation.
5. Individualized management.

Let's look at each of these levels in turn.

## Level 1: Triage

The first step in the Progressive Tinnitus Management program is determining the condition of your physical and mental health, and then scheduling/referring you for appropriate services.

When you complain of tinnitus, the primary concerns are to determine (in order of decreasing priority) if you:

1. Have a serious medical condition (physical or mental) requiring immediate medical attention.
2. Are experiencing symptoms of a non-urgent medical condition indicating the need for a medical examination.

3. Are experiencing symptoms of a non-urgent psychological condition indicating the need for mental health screening.

4. Have already been referred, or don't have any of the symptoms listed above, indicating you now need an audiologic examination.[11]

The tinnitus triage guidelines answer the question for any health care professionals that might encounter people with tinnitus, namely, "My patient complains about tinnitus. What should I do now?"[12]

Usually an audiologist conducts the initial evaluation of a person who complains of tinnitus. This audiological assessment and possibly fitting the person with hearing aids is often the only service the person needs.[13]

If you have tinnitus that is bothering you, you need an audiological assessment for three basic reasons.

1. The audiologist needs to evaluate your problem to determine if you should be referred to a medical doctor, ENT (ear specialist) or other health care professional for resolving any related medical or mental health issues.

2. Since tinnitus usually is associated with some degree of hearing loss, have your hearing evaluated, and if required, get hearing aids. This may be all that you need in order to bring your tinnitus under control so it no longer bothers you.

3. Your audiologist needs to evaluate whether specific tinnitus treatments can help you.[14]

If your tinnitus really bothers you (is clinically significant) you will typically answer "yes" to all four of the following statements.

- My tinnitus disrupts at least one of my important life activities.
- The degree of this disruption is more than trivial.
- This disruption causes a noticeable reduction in the quality of my life.
- The benefits from seeking tinnitus treatments would outweigh the cost, time and effort involved in taking them (i.e., overall it would be worthwhile).[15]

## Level 2: Audiological Evaluation

Once you have been triaged, you go on to Level 2. The main focus of Level 2 is to evaluate and manage your hearing problems, along with a brief assessment of how your tinnitus impacts your life. Consequently, you will receive a comprehensive hearing evaluation as well as written questionnaires to assess your perception of the relative impact of any hearing and tinnitus problems.[16]

This is because it is common for people with tinnitus to falsely attribute hearing problems to their tinnitus, when just the opposite is true. Hearing loss typically results in tinnitus. Therefore, your audiologist needs to determine how much of your complaint is due to a hearing problem, and how much is specifically due to your tinnitus.[17]

Level 2 is where your audiologist not only addresses your hearing loss and tinnitus, but also evaluates you for reduced tolerance to normal sounds.[19] Your audiologist will screen you for sound tolerance problems, hyperacusis and/ or misophonia by using the Tinnitus and Hearing Survey.[20] If you have any sound tolerance problems, your audiologist will suspend your progress through the PTM program while you undergo treatment for sound intolerance—what they call the Sound Tolerance Evaluation and Management (STEM) program.[21]

### Hearing Testing and Tinnitus

Numbers of people have mentioned that when taking a pure tone hearing test, they cannot separate or distinguish their constant, tonal kind of tinnitus from the test tones when the test tones are at or near the frequency of their tinnitus.

If this is your experience, there is a simple solution. Just ask your audiologist to switch her audiometer from using continuous tones to using pulsed tones (beep beep) or better yet, warble tones. I find warble tones are very easy to distinguish from my constant tinnitus sounds. If using pulsed tones, I listen for the gap between the two pulses to know I am hearing the audiometer's tone and not my tinnitus.

Most audiologists think they have to use the continuous tones, but it is acceptable to use pulsed, warbled, or continuous tones for threshold testing.[18]

If you have a hearing loss and require amplification you will need to get hearing aids. One benefit of wearing hearing aids is that wearing them can result in satisfactory management of your reactions to your tinnitus with minimal education and support.

Tinnitus treatment at Level 2 is ancillary, such as answering questions and providing you with educational materials.[22] If your audiologist determines that you still have tinnitus issues and need further help, she will advise you to go on to Level 3 and participate in the Level 3 group education workshops.[23]

## Level 3: Group Education

Level 3 group education workshops are for you if you require more help in directly addressing those situations where your tinnitus is affecting your life. The group education sessions are classroom-style sessions of PTM counseling. You will often find you are more motivated to attend group sessions rather than individual sessions because of the encouragement and support you receive from the other participants. Also, when you participate in group sessions, you tend to form a sense of camaraderie that further motivates you to continue to attend the sessions.[24]

The Level 3 program consists of five weekly group sessions. An audiologist leads two sessions and a mental health professional, typically a psychologist, leads three sessions. The audiologist will present information on how you can use sound therapy to help yourself deal with your reactions to your tinnitus. During the first session, you will receive the workbook, *How to Manage Your Tinnitus: A Step-by-Step Workbook.* This workbook contains step-by-step instructions for you to learn how to manage your tinnitus on your own.[25] You will use the Sound Plan worksheet[26] in your workbook to develop an individualized sound plan to help you manage your most bothersome tinnitus situation.[27]

The psychologist will lead three sessions on using the Cognitive Behavior Therapy (CBT) program. These three sessions focus on teaching the three CBT coping techniques: relaxation, cognitive restructuring (changing thoughts), and attention diversion (planning pleasant activities).[28]

By the time you have completed Level 3, you will have learned how to develop and implement individualized plans for using therapeutic sound and how to apply the principles of Cognitive Behavior Therapy to manage your tinnitus.[29]

### PTM Workbook

The self-help workbook you receive in Level 3 provides a description of key information that will be covered during the group education sessions. This workbook was designed for you to learn on your own, but many people find they benefit more with a "teacher" to provide some guidance and support.[30]

This workbook will help you come up with a personal sound plan—one that will work the best for you with your tinnitus.

There are three basic ways to manage your reactions to your tinnitus. First is through education and counseling, which is what this workbook and Level 3 sessions give you. Second is by using sound for tinnitus therapy. Third is by changing your thoughts and feelings towards your tinnitus (Cognitive Behavior Therapy). You can do these things on your own as you work through the various sections in your PTM workbook.[31]

This workbook is divided into four parts.

1. Introduction to tinnitus.
2. Step-by-step guide to using sound to help you manage your tinnitus.
3. Step by step guide to changing your thoughts and feelings in order to manage your reactions to your tinnitus (the Cognitive Behavior Therapy program).
4. Guide to protecting your ears from loud sounds.[32]

In Part 1 you will learn how to set goals in managing your tinnitus. For example, your goals might include: feel less stressed about your tinnitus; have fewer emotional reactions to your tinnitus; almost never think about your tinnitus; feel like tinnitus has little effect on your daily activities such as concentration, work, sleep, etc.; feel like your tinnitus is not much of a problem; and ultimately, feel that you have no need for further help.[33]

When you reach this stage you are now habituated to your tinnitus. Yes, you still have your tinnitus, but no, it is not a problem anymore—i.e. it does not bother you, nor does it affect your quality of life.

In Part 2 you will learn the details of using sound to help yourself deal with your tinnitus. You will come up with a sound plan tailored specifically to your needs.

In Part 3 you will learn how behaviors (other than sound therapy) can help you manage your reactions to your tinnitus, including:

1. Practicing relaxation exercises.
2. Increasing pleasant activities.
3. Learning how to change your thoughts about your tinnitus.[34]

Finally, Part 4 teaches you how to protect your ears. If you already have tinnitus and expose your ears to loud sounds, you can make your tinnitus worse. That is something you don't want to do if you're already having trouble dealing with your tinnitus. Therefore, you should always wear hearing protection when you are around loud noise.[35]

In addition, there are ten appendices that describe in more detail various aspects of tinnitus and hearing loss, and how you can manage your tinnitus.

For example, Appendix C explains that there are two basic approaches to tinnitus management. The first one is to eliminate your tinnitus completely—which would be wonderful—or at least to reduce the loudness of your tinnitus. The second one is to reduce your reaction to your tinnitus. In other words, become habituated to your tinnitus, so it no longer bothers you, which is the aim of the PTM program.[36]

## Level 4: Tinnitus Evaluation

If you think you still need more support and education in order to successfully deal with your tinnitus, you move on to Level 4: Tinnitus Evaluation. The main purpose of Level 4 is to determine whether you do, in fact, need personal one-to-one services by an audiologist and/or psychologist in order to successfully address your tinnitus problems. Therefore, at Level 4 an audiologist and psychologist will conduct in-depth assessments of your tinnitus and how it affects you.

The audiological evaluation involves a structured interview and filling out the Tinnitus and Hearing survey.[37] The various questionnaires and interview are the key to determining how your tinnitus impacts your life and if you need individualized support from an audiologist. In addition, the audiologist will evaluate various sound generating devices that may be appropriate for your tinnitus management using therapeutic sound, including ear level noise generators and combination hearing aid/noise generations, and personal listening devices.[38].

The psychologist will screen you for various mental health issues such as anxiety, depression, post-traumatic stress disorder, sleep disorders, etc. to determine whether you need additional one-to-one support to help you successfully deal with these issues in relation to your tinnitus.

## Level 5: Individualized Management

Level 5 primarily involves one-to-one counseling from an audiologist (using the counseling book *Progressive Tinnitus Management: Counseling Guide*) or a psychologist.

A psychologist or other mental health provider helps you further enhance your tinnitus-coping skills in areas such as relaxation techniques, attention control and planning for "flare-ups".[39]

Although the Progressive Tinnitus Management program is mostly being used by the Department of Veterans Affairs for military personnel, I hope it catches on in the private sector so **all** people with tinnitus have access to this program.

---

**Chapter 15 Endnotes**

1 Henry, 2010a. p. 5.
2 Henry, 2010b. p. 21.
3 Henry, 2010b. p. 22.
4 Henry, 2010b. p. 22.
5 Henry, 2010b. p. 21.
6 Henry, 2010b. p. 21.
7 Beck, 2014. pp. 30-31.
8 Henry, 2010a. p. vii.
9 Henry, 2010b. p. 22.
10 Henry, 2010b. p. 23.
11 Henry, 2010b. p. 15.
12 Henry, 2010b. p. 97.
13 Henry, 2010b. p. 24.
14 Henry, 2010b. p. 25.
15 Henry, 2010b. p. 22.
16 Henry, 2010b. p. 41.
17 Henry, 2010b. p. 25.
18 Tunkel, 2014. p. S14.
19 Henry, 2010b. p. 27.
20 Henry, 2010b. p. 101.
21 Henry, 2010b. p. 28.
22 Henry, 2010b. p. 57.
23 Henry, 2010b. p. 41.
24 Henry, 2010b. pp. 28-29.
25 Henry, 2010b. p. 25.
26 Henry, 2010a. p. 30.

27 Henry, 2010b. p. 29.
28 Henry, 2010b. p. 29.
29 Henry, 2010b. p. 25.
30 Henry, 2010b. p. 28.
31 Henry, 2010a. p. 6.
32 Henry, 2010a. pp. v- vi.
33 Henry, 2010a. p. 7.
34 Henry, 2010a. p. 37.
35 Henry, 2010a. p. 61.
36 Henry, 2010a. p. 72.
37 Henry, 2010b. p. 101.
38 Henry, 2010b. p. 30.
39 Henry, 2010b. p. 67.

# Chapter 16

# Take Control of Your Tinnitus

## Tinnitus and Your Emotions

Too often we think of tinnitus as a condition over which we have absolutely no control. Therefore, we put our trust in doctors to do something **to** us to fix our tinnitus.

Yet our doctors typically tell us, "There is nothing I can do. You just need to go home and learn to live with your tinnitus." Typically, they don't offer any hope, or any advice on how we might accomplish this. The result is that we are devastated, give up hope and often sink into deep depression.

That's the bad news—that's the typical medical model of tinnitus. However, it doesn't have to be this way.

Now here's the good news—**you can** do things to gain a measure of control over your tinnitus. And it is imperative that you do so, because if you don't, then by default, you have given control over to your tinnitus, and your tinnitus will run (and ruin) your life and drive you buggy in the process.

Tinnitus research has more and more revealed that tinnitus **suffering** is an **emotional** brain phenomenon. It is becoming clear that a person's state of mind is inextricably linked to the **distress** they experience from their tinnitus. In turn, the distress they experience reflects back to whether the person perceives tinnitus as a threat to their well-being or not.

## Tinnitus Is a Psychosomatic Condition

Although tinnitus is not commonly considered a psychosomatic condition, in actual fact, tinnitus basically is psychosomatic in nature. Psychosomatic is just a fancy word that comes from two Greek words—psychic—mind, and soma—body. Thus, it has both a physiological (somatic or body) component and a significant psychological (mental/emotional) component. To put it another way, tinnitus is always both a medical and a psychological phenomenon.[1]

Consequently, you might expect therapies that treat both components should have the best results, and indeed, that is exactly what researchers have found. Trying to treat the somatic part of tinnitus, which is what doctors typically try to do, without also helping the person improve their state of mind, typically does not work well, if at all.

Conversely, if you treat the person's emotional state of mind, you can typically help the person **more** than by trying to treat the somatic part of tinnitus alone. Research has shown the tinnitus therapies work best when they address your emotional and cognitive reactions to your tinnitus rather than just trying to treat your tinnitus as a physical condition of your body.[2] Of course, the best way is to treat both at the same time.

## Perception and Reaction: Your Limbic System in Action

Tinnitus, as currently understood, has two components: perception and reaction. Whereas a person may complain of the perception (sound) of tinnitus, the audiologist or psychologist treating the person with tinnitus must also appreciate the significance of the person's negative reaction (e.g. anxiety and depression) to tinnitus. Thus, it is important for health care professionals to recognize and attempt to manage both components.[3]

I'm amazed at the differences between people and their tinnitus. Some people hear tinnitus so faintly that they can only hear it when it is quiet, and yet they are totally overwhelmed by their tinnitus. Other people have screaming tinnitus, and they tell me, "It's no big deal."

You see, is not the volume that you perceive your tinnitus at that makes the difference. It is your emotional makeup.

At this point you may be wondering, "Why is it that 25% of the people with tinnitus **suffer** from it?" And the equally important question is, "Why do 75% of the people with tinnitus **not suffer** from it?"

In order to answer these questions, we need to delve into the subconscious mind. The part of your subconscious mind that is associated with your emotions is your limbic system.

Your limbic system has a number of different functions. At this point, I am specifically just talking about your limbic system and emotions that arise from real or perceived threats to your physical or emotional well-being.

One of the vital duties of your limbic system is to "listen" to every sound you hear and record in its "database" your emotional response to each sound.

Conceptually think of this database as a table with two columns. The first column contains the sound or word including the tone of voice or its context, and the second column contains a colored flag that denotes your emotional response to that sound.

Again, conceptually think of these flags as colored green for no emotional response, yellow for a mild response, orange for a moderate response, red for a strong response, and a double red flag denoting an extreme response.

Let's look at two scenarios that illustrate the two extremes of emotional response and learn how your limbic system deals with each.

In the first scenario, let's imagine you are a "sweet young thing". You live in a ground floor apartment. In fact, your apartment is actually built half into the ground. Thus your bedroom window is right at ground level. It's a warm summer night so you have your bedroom window open. It's 2 o'clock in the morning, and you are sound asleep in bed. That's the setting.

There is a faint, furtive footfall outside your open bedroom window. A "boogeyman" is lurking right outside your window. The almost imperceptibly-faint footfall sounds he makes wakes you out of a dead sleep. You bolt upright in bed. Your heart is pounding as a shot of adrenaline surges through your body. You are now in "fight or flight" mode—ready for action—whether to fight off the boogeyman or flee for your life.

What woke you up? It certainly wasn't the volume of the sound because the sound was so faint you could just barely hear it. What really woke you up was your limbic system doing its job to help protect your life.

Perhaps you didn't realize this, but your ears never sleep. They are always on duty. They listen to every sound around you and send those messages to your brain. There, at the subconscious level, your limbic system intercepts them and checks its database for any emotional response they have evoked in the past. It sees "furtive footfall at night" and beside it a double-red flag.

Your limbic system springs into action, cranks up its internal volume control to the max and shoots the message to the conscious part of your brain. Your conscious brain can't ignore that loud signal. Immediately your brain jolts you awake and primes you for action.

That's your limbic system doing its job.

Now let's look at another scenario. This time it will be one with no emotional response. Let's see how your limbic system responds.

In this example, let's consider the sounds your refrigerator makes. Assume you've had your fridge for a few years, and you are totally used to its sounds as it cycles on and off—doing its job of keeping your food cold. The normal sounds your fridge makes are totally lacking in any emotional content—there is no threat involved. Thus, your limbic system flags them with green flags.

The result is that you so totally ignore the sounds your fridge makes that if I asked you, "Is your fridge running right now?" you'd have to stop and specifically listen for that sound.

You need to do this—not because you can't hear the sound of your fridge, but because your limbic system is filtering them out. It doesn't bother you with sounds to which you have no emotional attachment, thus freeing you to concentrate on meaningful sounds. Again, this is your limbic system doing its job.

In the first scenario, your limbic system turned a very faint sound into an enormously loud perception of sound in order to get your attention, while in the second scenario, it took a much louder sound and turned the volume down so much you are not even aware of this sound most of the time because it is not important to you.

Let's carry this analogy a bit further and see how you and your limbic system interact.

Conceptually think of yourself as a two-floor house. You—the conscious you—live on the main floor while your limbic system lives in your subconscious—the basement. Furthermore, the floor separating you from your subconscious is so well insulated that no sounds from the basement—no matter how loud they are—can ever penetrate this sound barrier. Thus, what goes on in the basement never bothers you. As a result, you don't care if there is loud tinnitus downstairs because it doesn't bother you since you can't hear it. The only way you can hear what goes on down there is if you or your limbic system opens the basement door.

In our first scenario, when your limbic system processed the "furtive footfall" sounds, it immediately cranked its internal volume control wide open and opened the basement door. The combined effects of this bolted you out of a dead sleep ready for action.

In our second scenario, when I asked you if your fridge was running, conceptually, you opened the basement door and hollered: "Hey, limbic system is the fridge running?" In response, your limbic sends the fridge noise upstairs, and you hear it. Satisfied, you shut the basement door, at which point you no longer hear it anymore.

## What You Can Do to Gain Control of Your Tinnitus and Break Its Hold on You

Now you're probably wondering what all this has to do with controlling your tinnitus. Without explicitly saying so, I've just taught you how to gain control over your tinnitus.

The secret is to treat your tinnitus sounds exactly the same as you do fridge noise, **not** the way you treat furtive footfall sounds in the night. It's that simple.

You see, whenever you hear a new sound, whether it is a real sound or a phantom sound like tinnitus, it grabs your attention, at least momentarily. You wonder, "What is that sound?" Once you determine that the sound is not a threat to you in any way—and thus you have no emotional involvement, you basically forget all about it. Your limbic system observes your response and flags it with a green flag. Consequently, you are not even going to be aware of this sound most of the time even though you can hear it if you listen for it. Essentially, the basement door is shut.

However, if you **perceive** the sound (remember, this is **your perception**, whether it is true or not) as being threatening to you in any way—whether affecting your physical or mental well-being, your limbic system observes this and flags it with the appropriate flag depending on how strong your emotional response is. The stronger your emotional response, the higher the flag color from yellow right up to double red for things that are life-threatening.

### Having Tinnitus vs. Suffering from Tinnitus

Now let's look at the two different classes of people with tinnitus.

The first group—comprised of the 75% who are not bothered by their tinnitus—essentially treat their tinnitus as "fridge noise". They do not see their tinnitus as a threat to their well-being, but just as another meaningless environmental sound they are aware of hearing from time to time. In their minds, they see it as no big deal.

However, the second group—comprised of the 25% that suffer from their tinnitus—treat their tinnitus as a threat to their well-being. In effect, they treat their tinnitus sounds as though they were "furtive footfalls in the night", and their limbic systems do their jobs and flag the sound with higher-level colored flags.

If you are anxious and "high-strung", you cause yourself needless problems with your tinnitus. Since you are already anxious, you worry about every little change pertaining to your body. One day you notice this new faint sound. Maybe you can only hear it in quiet. However, you get upset and worry about it. Your thoughts go something like this. "What have I done now? Have I caused permanent damage to my ears? Is there something dreadfully wrong with my brain?"

These thoughts are all related to threats to your well-being. Your limbic system notices you worrying and appropriately flags this new tinnitus sound with a yellow flag and at the same time turns up the volume a bit and opens the basement door a crack. The result is that you hear your tinnitus louder, and it is more intrusive.

This causes you to worry even more, and your limbic system "cooperates", upgrades the flag to orange, turns the volume up more and opens the basement door wider. Now your tinnitus is really bothering you and you start to panic, "How can I ever live with this for the rest of my life?" and get totally overwhelmed. In turn, your limbic system again "cooperates" and upgrades the flag to red and finally double-red.

The result is that you now are consumed by your tinnitus. You can't think of anything else. You have trouble living in society so you withdraw to your own little world filled with tinnitus. You say to yourself, "I just can't live with this. I want to die."

Now, no matter how much you wish you could, you can't tell your limbic system anything. You can't just open the basement door and yell down, "Hey limbic system, turn down that racket right now if you know what's good for you!"

It just doesn't work like that. Your limbic system is an independent observer of your emotional responses. It simply observes how **you** respond to a given sound and then flags that sound in its database accordingly.

This is why **you need** to take control of your emotional res need counseling to help you realize that tinnitus is **not** a threat being; that there **is** hope for you; that you **can** take control of y responses; and thus, you **can successfully deal** with your tinnitus.

## Gaining Control of Your Tinnitus

You got yourself into this tinnitus mess by worrying about your tinnitus and thereby causing your limbic system to double-red flag it. That's the bad news.

Now, for the good news. Your limbic system's database is not written in stone. It is dynamic. That is why you can gain control over your tinnitus. You see, just as your limbic system flagged emotionally-charged sounds and made them louder and more intrusive as it observed your emotional response increasing, it will also do the opposite if it observes you decreasing your emotional responses.

Since you can't **tell** your limbic system anything, you have to **demonstrate** to it that you do not consider your tinnitus a threat to your well-being anymore. This is not easy, but it is essential that you begin to do it if you ever want to be free from the tyranny of your tinnitus.

In order to bring your tinnitus under your control, you need to do the opposite of what you have been doing. Instead of allowing yourself to be overwhelmed by your tinnitus, you need to learn how to ignore your tinnitus. You need to work on reducing your emotional response to your tinnitus until you have no emotional response to it whatsoever, and you now treat it just like fridge noise.

Here's how you can do it.

First, seek out someone who can build hope in you that you can succeed in controlling your tinnitus. You need hope so you will persevere with your tinnitus treatment. This is not a quick fix, but a long term project that can take up to 3 years. You need hope so you don't quit when the going is tough.

Second, learn as much as you can about your tinnitus. Knowledge takes away fear. When you clearly understand that tinnitus is not a threat to your well-being, you can begin to get your emotions under control.

Note, whenever you think about your tinnitus, read about it, study various tinnitus treatments, or talk about your tinnitus, it will typically make your tinnitus temporarily worse. Don't let that bother you. It happens to me all the time.

Third, once you understand tinnitus and realize it is not a threat to your life, totally and completely ignore your tinnitus by focusing on the loves of your life.

When your limbic system sees that you don't go ballistic any more over your tinnitus, it cooperates and reduces the double-red flag to a single red flag. The result is that your tinnitus reduces in perceived volume and is less intrusive. Now you are better able to deal with your life. You are able to sleep better. This makes dealing with your tinnitus even easier.

Continue to work on your emotional status towards your tinnitus. As you perceive the threat as less and less, your limbic system will continue to reduce the flag color to orange and then yellow and hopefully, finally to green. Treat each step as success. You **are** getting your tinnitus under control.

When you finally reach the green-flag stage, you have become habituated to your tinnitus. This is just a fancy word that means that your tinnitus no longer bothers you (or at least not very much).

After that, as long as you leave the basement door closed, hours may go by without your even being aware of your tinnitus. And when unbidden, you do hear your tinnitus, you now treat it just like fridge noise and soon forget about it for some more hours. The result is, your tinnitus no longer bothers you, even though it is there.

Does this really work? You bet it does. Over the years, I've helped many people successfully deal with their tinnitus. I've had numbers of people phone me, almost hysterical. Some want to commit suicide because their tinnitus is bothering them so much. A lot of people figuratively cry on my shoulder. But as I build hope in them, and teach them the secret of gaining control over their tinnitus, their mood lightens. By the end of the phone call, they are laughing and joking with me.

That shows what hope can do. The hard part is still ahead for them—actually putting into practice what they have learned. But they are on their way. You see, they **are** bringing their tinnitus under control. **You** can do the same!

---

**Chapter 16 Endnotes**

1 Moller, 2011. pp. 223-228.
2 Rabau, 2014. p. 19.
3 Tunkel, 2014. p. S16.

## Chapter 17

# Focus on Things Other Than Your Tinnitus

If your tinnitus is bothering you, you need to do two things. First, as we explain throughout this book, you need to change your attitudes towards your tinnitus. When you understand at the conscious level that your tinnitus is not a life threatening problem, you can gain a great deal of control over it at the subconscious level. Thus, you need to work on reprogramming your mind to quickly accept the reality of your tinnitus.[1]

Second, when you have accepted the reality of your tinnitus, and you have done your research and learned as much as you can about your tinnitus, you need to stop focusing on your tinnitus.

Did you know that one of the best ways to change your attitudes towards your tinnitus is to quit thinking about your tinnitus? You do not have to focus your attention on your tinnitus just because you can hear it.

For example, have you ever nearly fallen asleep when you heard (or more correctly, consciously became aware of) some repetitive sound that disturbed you—perhaps a dripping tap. You had not "heard" it at all until your mind fixed on it. And once your mind fixed on it, you could not put your attention on anything else. Your brain was truly hearing the sound all along, but since you weren't paying attention to it, you weren't aware of it.

In like manner, if you train yourself to no longer pay any attention to your tinnitus, you will actually not even "hear" your tinnitus. The solution is simple, but putting it into practice is another matter, especially if you have severe tinnitus.[2]

The truth is, tinnitus distress is strongly related to the amount of time you spend listening to your tinnitus and thinking about it. If you rarely think about your tinnitus, likely your tinnitus is not a problem. However, it becomes a definite problem when you find it difficult to focus on anything else because you are always thinking about your tinnitus. This just leads to increased stress, anxiety and depression. Thus, it is essential that you do all you can to spend less time checking up on, and worrying about, your tinnitus.[3]

Constantly and repetitiously mulling over your tinnitus will only make your tinnitus worse. That is why you need to consciously choose **not** to dwell on your tinnitus. Instead, you need to promptly and completely put your tinnitus out of your mind as much as possible. In short, totally and completely ignore your tinnitus.

However, my telling you to, "Ignore your tinnitus" is not the most helpful advice **unless**, at the same time, I give you practical tips on how you can carry this out. You see, it is impossible to just ignore something since you first have to bring the subject into your mind so you know what you are supposed to be ignoring—and this is exactly the opposite of what you are supposed to be doing!

The proper way to ignore something is not to tell yourself to ignore it, but simply totally and completely focus your mind on other things instead. For example, as I have said numerous times when I am helping people with tinnitus, "Did you ever notice that when you are passionately kissing/embracing your girlfriend/boyfriend/spouse, you don't hear your tinnitus?" You're not even aware of it. At that point, the last thing on your mind is your tinnitus! They all get a surprised look on their faces, followed by a knowing look as they realize this is true.

Only one person ever said that he could still hear his tinnitus, to which I retorted, "Obviously you weren't **passionately** kissing your wife!"

When you are completely focused on, and are thoroughly wrapped up in, something that is exciting or enticing to you, your tinnitus will not be important enough for your brain to even bother decoding it.[4]

Therefore, instead of worrying about your tinnitus, focus on living a happy productive life. Get involved in fun activities, productive projects, and the loves of your life. Keep busy with enjoyable activities and hobbies.

When you do this, your tinnitus will normally fade into the background and you will only really notice it when you are under extra stress, when you are overly tired, or when it is extremely quiet around you.[5] Refuse to dwell on the meaningless noise in your head. Instead of thinking how awful tinnitus is, think of more positive and productive things. If you do this you will ultimately adapt to the noise in your head. The result will be long periods when you will not notice your tinnitus, no matter how loud it is.[6] This works for me. This will work for you too if you refuse to let your tinnitus annoy you.

One of the worst things you can do is to opt out of life and quit doing the things you enjoy. Sitting around doing nothing just leaves you with a lot of time to think about your tinnitus. Whenever your tinnitus is particularly bothersome, keep yourself busy with pleasant, meaningful activities, especially activities where you need to use your mind.[7]

One man noted, "My tinnitus comes on whenever I think of it". I pointed out to him that it is not strange at all, but a good thing because it shows that he is habituated to his tinnitus. Thus, the only times he really notices his tinnitus is when he thinks about it.

Most of the time, I'm the same way. I can go for hours without even realizing I have tinnitus (although it is always there), but then the phone rings. Someone wants help with their tinnitus. Almost immediately my tinnitus "appears"—much louder and more intrusive than it was just a minute before. In fact, I now hear my tinnitus louder than I hear my own voice over the phone and that's pretty loud because of the enormous amplification I need in order to hear on the phone. This louder tinnitus lasts as long as I am on the phone—typically an hour or two.

Nor is this unique to me. One audiologist I know has a tinnitus clinic. He also has tinnitus himself. He told me he has the same experiences as I do. Those of us who spend time helping people deal with their tinnitus find our tinnitus (if we have tinnitus) becomes considerably louder when we are helping people because we are focusing on tinnitus by talking, writing and thinking about it. (My tinnitus is ringing away pretty loudly right now as I write this.) You might say that louder tinnitus is an occupational hazard for tinnitus counselors.

This illustrates just how important it is not to focus or think about your tinnitus if you want to bring your tinnitus under your control. If this happens to tinnitus professionals who understand, and are thoroughly habituated to their tinnitus, think how much more it affects people who do not understand tinnitus and are actively worrying about their tinnitus?

Now here's some good news. Once I get off the phone and quit talking/thinking about tinnitus and instead refocus on what I was doing before the phone rang, my tinnitus drops back to its old level and within a few minutes I may no longer be aware of it anymore because I am so habituated to my tinnitus.

This can happen to you too. That is why I tell people to focus on the loves of their lives and forget about their tinnitus. When you do this, your tinnitus can seem to disappear, but this only happens if you become truly habituated to your tinnitus. And that only happens if you totally ignore your tinnitus. And that only happens if you do not attach any emotional significance to your tinnitus. And that only happens if you do not see your tinnitus as a threat to your well-being. See how it all ties together? You have to begin working on your tinnitus at the most basic level if you want to successfully deal with your tinnitus.

If you are bothered by your tinnitus, you already know that focusing on your tinnitus can be a most difficult habit to break. This is where mind distraction/enrichment techniques come in. While Cognitive Behavior Therapy (see the next chapter) uses strategies to help you think differently about your tinnitus, mind distraction/enrichment strategies focus on helping you turn your thoughts away from your tinnitus.

This means that cognitive behavior techniques work best when you are having negative thoughts. Mind distraction/enrichment techniques work best when your tinnitus is grabbing your attention. Relaxation techniques work best when you are feeling tense or anxious.[8] At the same time, don't forget about sound enrichment techniques. They allow you to keep your ears busy with replacement sounds so that you are not so focused on your tinnitus.

Here's a simple formula—enriching your environment with real sound plus focusing on the loves of your life, not on your tinnitus equals reduced tinnitus distress.[9] and a happier life.

---

**Chapter 17 Endnotes**

1 Tinnitus Treatment Options, 2002. p. 2.
2 Tinnitus Resources, 2002. pp. 1-2.
3 Mayes, 2010. p. 91.
4 Hogan, 1998. pp. 133-134.
5 Vernick, 1993. p. 184.
6 Hazell, p. 41.
7 Mayes, 2010. p. 93.
8 Mayes, 2010. p. 98.

## Chapter 18

# Cognitive Behavior Therapy (CBT)

Cognitive Behavior Therapy (CBT) is a good "tool" for you to have in your tinnitus "toolbox". You can pull it out and use it to help yourself deal with your tinnitus. Although CBT can be used to treat a variety of conditions such as depression, anxiety, chronic pain and tinnitus,[1] it is most effective when used to treat a single, specific issue at a time—in this case, tinnitus.

Cognitive Behavior Therapy is not particularly new. It had its origins back in the 1950s and 1960s,[2] but health care professionals did not use it for treating tinnitus until around 1984.[3]

## What Is Cognitive Behavior Therapy?

Perhaps you are not clear exactly what the word "cognitive" means. According to the Merriam-Webster dictionary, cognitive means "of, relating to, or involving conscious mental activities (such as thinking, understanding, learning, and remembering)".

Thus, Cognitive Behavior Therapy focuses on correcting your thinking—that is, changing how you think about your tinnitus. It is just a fancy way of saying that how you think about something reflects in how you will react physically and emotionally to it.

Thousands of years ago, wise King Solomon wrote, "As a man **thinks** in his heart, so is he [or more accurately, so he becomes]" (Proverbs 23:7). This was true back in Solomon's time, and it is just as true today. Therefore, it should come as no surprise that it is also just as true in regards to how we think about our tinnitus.

Researchers more or less agree that "the larger part of tinnitus suffering is associated with negative psychological reactions to tinnitus, and these negative psychological reactions need to be addressed properly to effectively manage tinnitus."[4] Thus, the goal of CBT is to help you develop skills so you can identify and challenge your own irrational, negative thoughts that result in distress.[5] CBT also helps you change your negative cognitive, emotional and behavioral responses to your tinnitus, not to abolish the tinnitus sound itself.[6] In other words, CBT helps you restructure your negative thoughts so they are more accurate and helpful.[7]

Cognitive Behavior Therapy is a form of psychotherapy that is normally done by clinical psychologists. More correctly, we should say that when using the CBT program, the therapist and tinnitus sufferer collaborate together while working towards a positive outcome.

CBT presupposes that you are an **active** participant in your world, thus interpreting stimuli and using cognitive processes to view and/or perceive the world according to your interpretation. Consequently, you can change your thoughts and perceptions.[8]

Cognitive Behavior Therapy works on the emotional component of your tinnitus rather than on the loudness of your tinnitus. It aims to limit the attention you give to your tinnitus, rather than trying to eliminate your tinnitus. This, in turn, reduces your tinnitus-related distress and increases the quality of your life.

Researchers have not found any treatment to permanently eliminate tinnitus in most people. Thus, they have spent most of their time trying to eliminate or at least ameliorate psychological symptoms associated with tinnitus.[9] This is where CBT comes in.

The purpose of Cognitive Behavior Therapy is threefold:

- Change the way you perceive your tinnitus.
- Teach you ways to focus attention away from your tinnitus.
- Help you achieve control over your stress, anxiety and depression.

Several studies have confirmed that there is an association between psychological factors such as anxiety, depression and stress and severe tinnitus. Cognitive Behavior Therapy works because how you think about your tinnitus affects how badly you feel about your tinnitus. The more you pay attention to your tinnitus, the worse you feel regarding your tinnitus.

For most people with tinnitus, after an initial stress reaction, they simply stop reacting to the same boring tinnitus sound and become largely unaware of their tinnitus for most of the time. This process is called habituation. It occurs naturally as long as you regard your tinnitus as meaningless and not as a threat to your well-being.

In contrast, if you suffer from your tinnitus, you perceive it as a threat to your well-being—whether physical, mental, emotional, social or financial. Your thoughts reflect despair, persecution, hopelessness, loss of enjoyment, a desire for peace and quiet and a belief that no one understands what it is like. Other common themes include resentment about your persistent tinnitus, a wish to escape it and worries about your health and sanity.

Furthermore, if you suffer from your tinnitus, you will often complain of "feeling depressed, sad, irritated, anxious, frightened, panicky, agitated, angry or ashamed". In addition, you may become restless or withdrawn. You can't sleep and have difficulty functioning. You feel the need for antidepressants, sleeping pills or other tranquilizers.

Your emotions and behavioral reactions are the result of your assessment of an event and are not the result of the event itself. This is the A-B-C theory of cognitive behavior. "A" is the activating event. "B" is your beliefs (thoughts). "C" is the consequences (how you react, both physically and emotionally).[10]

The following table illustrates the association between tinnitus, specific beliefs and their emotional consequences.

| Activating Event "A" | Beliefs "B" | Emotional Consequences "C" |
|---|---|---|
| Ears ringing | "I cannot live with it." | desperate, hopeless |
| 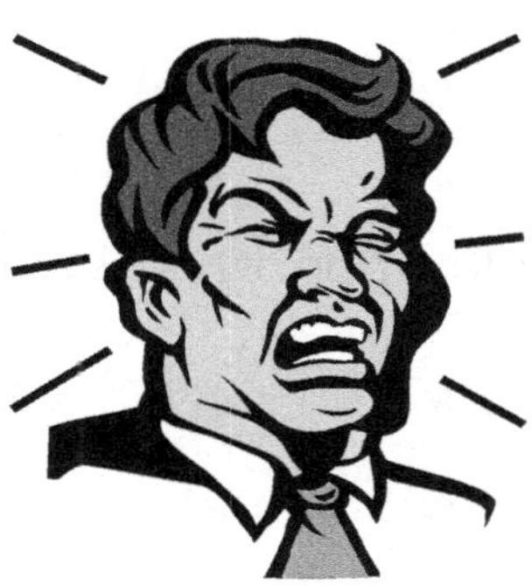 | "There is nothing I can do about it." | helpless, depressed |
| | "If I did not have to work in this noisy environment, I would not have gotten tinnitus." | anger, hostility[11] |

You see, it is the psychological processes, not just the audiological ones, that make the real difference in whether or not you habituate to your tinnitus or are distressed by it.

It is your thoughts, beliefs and expectations about tinnitus that create your problem in dealing with tinnitus. Tinnitus itself does not have the power to ruin your life. We can illustrate this by the fact that the majority of people permanently afflicted with tinnitus—even if they describe it as loud—do not feel distressed by it.[12]

For example, although about 50 million Americans have tinnitus (I'm one of them), only about 12 million are bothered by it. Why is it that roughly 75% of the people with tinnitus are **not** distressed by their tinnitus? Just as importantly, why is it that the other 25% **are** bothered by their tinnitus? This is the answer.

Distress due to tinnitus involves a lot of worry, or overly negative thinking, and a high level of stress, anxiety or tension. In fact, those that suffer from tinnitus often either get tinnitus, or notice their existing tinnitus getting worse, during or after a period of high stress.

Furthermore, people who suffer from tinnitus think about it **much** more than people who have tinnitus but do not complain about it. Therefore, if you are constantly worrying about your tinnitus with thoughts such as:

- I will have a nervous breakdown if this tinnitus keeps up.
- I will ruin my physical health.
- I won't get any peace and quiet ever again.
- I can't enjoy my life now.
- I can't do normal things anymore.
- I must avoid loud sounds and/or silence.
- My tinnitus is interfering with my job, so how will I support my family.

Don't be surprised if these thoughts become self-fulfilling prophecies.

All these negative thoughts increase your anxiety. This increased anxiety not only makes you tense, but also causes you to focus ever more narrowly on your tinnitus, which you perceive to be a threat to you. As a result, you begin to focus your attention on your tinnitus to the exclusion of other things. This makes your tinnitus seem much louder and more intrusive.

People with tinnitus are convinced that their tinnitus is making them depressed, anxious and worried. Furthermore, if they think that there is nothing they can do to alleviate their symptoms, they will likely become hopeless and depressed. Blaming a situation or person for the onset of tinnitus will create anger and hostility.

Cognitive responses to tinnitus can be very different between people. Regardless of the cause of tinnitus, "suffering" is a function of how you react to (or cope with) your tinnitus. You need to understand that your way of coping can be modified.[13]

Therefore, if you are distressed by your tinnitus, probably the largest key to reducing that distress is changing how you think about your tinnitus.

If you carefully examine your thoughts and beliefs about tinnitus, you will realize that the above thoughts are obviously **not** true since the vast majority of people with tinnitus are **not** distressed by their tinnitus.

Tinnitus is important—not because it exists, but because of what you believe it does, or will do, to you. As you have just learned, the ideas you harbor are seldom accurate. Thus, if you change your ideas about your tinnitus, at the same time, you will change your reactions to your tinnitus. The result will be that it becomes less intrusive in your life.[14]

Changing how you react to your tinnitus is not easy. In fact, it can be as difficult as learning to write with your left hand (assuming you are right-handed). However, the good news is that with the right techniques, you can alter the emotional meaning of your tinnitus so it becomes of little or no importance. Even though your tinnitus may remain just as loud, the distress connection between your hearing system and your limbic (emotional) system can be reset. The result is that when you change your reaction, you may experience dramatic improvement in how well you cope with your tinnitus.[15]

Bear in mind that the longer you have been distressed by your tinnitus, the longer it will take you to see positive changes. Change won't happen overnight, but it **will** happen if you continue with this therapy.

With Cognitive Behavior Therapy, you will learn effective coping techniques to deal with your negative feelings towards your tinnitus. As you alter the significance of tinnitus in your life, your tinnitus sounds will become more tolerable and eventually less noticeable.

## The Elements of Cognitive Behavior Therapy

There are a number of elements to the Cognitive Behavior Therapy program. Each addresses a different area related to how you feel about (and act) on your tinnitus. These various elements address either of the two main components of the CBT program—cognitive restructuring or behavioral modification. Typically, the following techniques are seldom used by themselves, but are incorporated into the overall CBT program where each element contributes to the overall success of the therapy.

### Cognitive Restructuring

Cognitive restructuring is where you identify any dysfunctional beliefs and negative thoughts you have towards your tinnitus. For example, you may think, "This noise is driving me crazy!" or "This is the worst thing that could ever happen to me." or "I can't live with all this racket! It's going to be the death of me."

Next, you challenge these negative thoughts and see them for what they are—catastrophic, unrealistic thoughts. Then you replace them with more constructive thoughts concerning your tinnitus such as, "My tinnitus doesn't actually hurt me. It is bad, but it generally gets better with time." or "I'm going to do something enjoyable, rather than focus on this noise in my head." or "Life is still good in spite of my tinnitus."

Thus, cognitive restructuring helps you think differently and adopt a different and more positive attitude towards your tinnitus. Together you and your therapist collaborate in identifying, testing, and challenging dysfunctional thoughts, beliefs and attitudes. Thus, you learn to recognize and abandon, rigid, unhelpful thinking patterns and replace them with constructive thoughts. You learn that the source of your distress is not the tinnitus sound itself, but the way you evaluate and interpret your tinnitus sounds.

By substituting new positive thoughts in place of your old negative thoughts regarding your tinnitus, you find that your tinnitus is now becoming less and less distressing.[16]

### Attention Control Techniques

Attention control techniques make you aware that you have control over where you focus your attention. You can **choose** to focus your attention on your tinnitus, or you can **choose** to focus your attention on other things apart from your tinnitus. When you totally focus on something apart from your tinnitus, you can make your tinnitus "disappear", at least for the moment.

It is empowering when you realize that you do have a measure of control over your tinnitus—that you **can** focus on your tinnitus, and you can focus **away from** your tinnitus.

In order to focus away from your tinnitus, you can use your other senses. For example, smell your coffee, taste your steak, feel the fabric of your sweater, and, of course, you can specifically listen to the various sounds around you and thereby ignore your tinnitus.[17]

## Imagery Techniques

You can use imagery techniques to change your negative associations related to your tinnitus either by masking the tinnitus sounds themselves, or by integrating them into positive scenes.

For example, you can imagine that your tinnitus is masked by the sound of a waterfall or the waves of the sea. You are not using real sounds to mask your tinnitus in this exercise, but are achieving tinnitus masking by your imagination alone.

You can also incorporate your tinnitus into pleasant scenes. For example, depending on your specific tinnitus sounds, you could imagine walking through a landscape by listening to the singing of the birds, or lying on a blooming field and hearing the noises of bumblebees and cicadas and other insects. Perhaps it is a cold and snowy winter day. Imagine yourself comfortably sitting in front of the fireplace hearing the sizzling of the teakettle and looking forward to enjoying a hot cup of tea.[18]

## Behavioral Techniques

If you are bothered by your tinnitus, you may tend to avoid certain social or work situations that cause you more stress. The CBT program encourages you to expose yourself to those situations in order to realize that, yes, you can cope in those situations without any major negative consequences.

However, sometimes you may choose to use your tinnitus as a "crutch" to allow you to avoid certain stressful situations that are totally unrelated to your tinnitus—for example, office work or participating in social events. You decide that your tinnitus is a legitimate excuse for avoiding those situations.

If you are doing this, you need to become aware of this underlying problem, and find ways to overcome this practice.[19]

### Relaxation Training

If you are bothered by your tinnitus, typically you are also tense. Therefore, relaxation techniques can help you to better cope with tension and anxiety related to your tinnitus. The most common form of relaxation training is called progressive muscle relaxation. In this technique, you learn how to decrease muscular tension and to quickly achieve a state of relaxation after detecting tension by sequentially tensing and relaxing various muscle groups.[20]

## How Well Does Cognitive Behavior Therapy Work?

One study showed that Cognitive Behavior Therapy was more beneficial than things such as tinnitus masking, for example. Another study revealed that Cognitive Behavior Therapy reduced the annoyance due to hearing tinnitus and that it improved a person's ability to cope with their tinnitus.[21] One researcher explained, "Those treated with CBT experienced less tinnitus severity and they experienced statistically significant improvements in their quality of life."[22]

Overall, after reviewing the extensive literature and clinical studies related to CBT, Korean researchers concluded that CBT is an effective and safe treatment for tinnitus.[23]

Therefore, if you cannot change your attitude towards your tinnitus on your own, perhaps you need to work with a CBT professional who can help you.

---

**Chapter 18 Endnotes**

1 Cognitive Behavioral Treatment of Tinnitus, ~2011. pp. 3-4.
2 Cognitive Behavioral Treatment of Tinnitus, ~2011. p. 3.
3 Cognitive Behavioral Treatment of Tinnitus, ~2011. p. 4.
4 Beck, 2014. p. 30
5 Beck, 2014. p. 30.
6 Cognitive Behavioral Treatment of Tinnitus, ~2011. p. 1.
7 Tunkel, 2014. p. 23.
8 Beck, 2014. p. 30
9 Cognitive Behavioral Treatment of Tinnitus, ~2011. p. 1.
10 Cognitive Behavioral Treatment of Tinnitus, ~2011. p. 2.

11 Cognitive Behavioral Treatment of Tinnitus, ~2011. p. 2.
12 Cognitive Behavioral Treatment of Tinnitus, ~2011. p. 2.
13 Cognitive Behavioral Treatment of Tinnitus, ~2011. p. 2.
14 McKenna, 2007. pp. 1-3.
15 Mayes, 2010. p. 19.
16 Cognitive Behavioral Treatment of Tinnitus, ~2011. pp. 4-5.
17 Cognitive Behavioral Treatment of Tinnitus, ~2011. p. 5.
18 Cognitive Behavioral Treatment of Tinnitus, ~2011. p. 5.
19 Cognitive Behavioral Treatment of Tinnitus, ~2011. pp. 5-6.
20 Cognitive Behavioral Treatment of Tinnitus, ~2011. p. 4.
21 Cognitive Therapy for Tinnitus, 2002. pp. 1-2.
22 Beck, 2015. p. 3.
23 Jun, H. J. 2013. p. 28.

Chapter 19

# Mindfulness-Based Tinnitus Stress Reduction

Another approach to helping bring your tinnitus under your control is a therapy called Mindfulness-Based Stress Reduction developed by Jon Kabat-Zinn. It basically uses Buddhist meditative practices, but without the Buddhism.[1]

As Jennifer Gans, Psy.D., the developer of the Mindfulness-Based Tinnitus Stress Reduction (MBTSR) program explains, "I am often asked if mindfulness has any religious significance, or if it is a Buddhist practice in conflict with other religions and beliefs. While mindfulness has been a part of the Buddhist culture and religion, as it is practiced in programs like MBTSR, it has no religious or even spiritual tenants."[2]

Mindfulness-based approaches are used in managing chronic pain, sleep disturbances, depression, anxiety, multiple sclerosis and other maladies. The good news is that it can also be particularly useful in managing tinnitus.[3]

## What Is Mindfulness?

Mindfulness is a therapeutic process—a mental state—achieved by focusing awareness on, and purposefully living in, the present as a way of relieving physical and emotional pain[4] while calmly acknowledging feelings and body sensations.[5] Mindfulness teaches that you can benefit by fully embracing your experience with tinnitus rather than pretending it is not there. You approach your Mindfulness experience with curiosity, acceptance, openness to whatever arises, and a gentle compassion towards yourself.[6]

The aim of Mindfulness is not specifically to make you relaxed and happy as such, but rather, to free you from the tendency to get drawn into automatic reactions to your thoughts, feelings, and sensations. Thus, Mindfulness enhances your awareness of your tinnitus so you are able to **respond** to it instead of **react** to it.[7] Furthermore, Mindfulness also helps relieve the anger and apathy that so many people with tinnitus experience.[8]

## Mindfulness vs. Cognitive Behavior Therapy

Mindfulness and Cognitive Behavior Therapy share a number of similarities, but have some important differences too. For example, Cognitive Behavior Therapy involves judging how rational, realistic, or logical your thoughts are with the goal of replacing thoughts that are irrational, unrealistic, or illogical. In contrast, Mindfulness accepts all thoughts, feelings and body sensations by simply observing them as they come and go. You do not judge them, nor do you make any effort to modify your thoughts, feelings or sensations.

While Cognitive Behavior Therapy aims to increase realistic, logical and rational thinking with the goal of relieving distress and reducing maladaptive behaviors, Mindfulness attempts to alter your perception of experiences in a kind, accepting and non-judgmental manner.[9]

Furthermore, rather than encouraging you to actively try to avoid distressing thoughts, sensations or feelings as you do with Cognitive Behavior Therapy, Mindfulness encourages you to do just the opposite—to move toward the distressing symptoms—thus unlocking your body's ability to habituate. Mindfulness teaches you to allow unpleasant thoughts, feelings or sensations about tinnitus to simply go in and out of your awareness without having to do battle with them.[10]

## How Mindfulness Works

If you have bothersome tinnitus, you have probably let your mind run, more or less, on autopilot. Your mind then falls into habitual ways of thinking about your tinnitus. Some of the habitual thoughts you develop around your tinnitus experience can prevent your mind from changing its habitual negative reactions towards the tinnitus sounds you hear into neutral or positive thoughts.

Furthermore, if you have chronic bothersome tinnitus, you rarely experience your unpleasant tinnitus sensations in isolation. You almost always will find your tinnitus sensations tightly wrapped "in a cascade of thoughts, judgments, memories, fears, emotions, sadness, regrets, beliefs, and feelings about past, present, and future experiences living with this chronic symptom".[11]

Thus, your tinnitus sounds may create a struggle between you and your tinnitus, leading to symptoms of anxiety, fatigue, sleep disturbance, difficulty with concentration and depression. You may also frequently report poor attention and focus, interference with work, and negative impacts on your personal relationships.[12]

The skills in the MBTSR program begin with making you aware of your habitual thoughts and beliefs about your tinnitus. It is common to hold on tightly to a narrow view of how bad your life will be if your tinnitus persists, or how you did something to cause your tinnitus fate. These thoughts keep you stuck in stories from the past and in predictions for a bleak future. However, with practice, you can train your mind, rewire old thinking habits, modify your behaviors and reactions, and ultimately, learn to more easily live with your tinnitus.[13]

Your brain has three basic parts. First, there is the brainstem that controls your subconscious bodily functions such as keeping your heart beating, keeping you breathing, etc.

Second, still at the subconscious level, is your limbic system. This is the seat of your emotions. One important part of your limbic system, the amygdala, has the specific task of taking information from internal and external sensations and determining whether these signals present a potential danger that requires immediate attention and monitoring, or if it can safely ignore these stimuli.[14]

Third, now at the conscious level, is your cortex. The thinking part of your brain—the medial pre-frontal cortex—sits directly behind your forehead. The pre-frontal cortex conducts your executive functioning tasks, including judgment, reasoning, emotional regulation, bringing awareness to certain things, and fear modulation. [15]

Your pre-frontal cortex plays a key role in correcting any misperceptions you may have regarding your tinnitus. This ability is called "response flexibility". Response flexibility allows you to stop, pause, think, and then choose a thoughtful response without falling back on your old knee-jerk habits. This is an important skill you need to develop if you have bothersome tinnitus. This is because your brain misperceives it as a threat, and then repeatedly reacts without conscious thought to these unfounded fears and frustrations.[16]

God designed your mind to be a "judging" machine. You constantly use your memories and what you have learned from the past to judge your present experiences, and to plan for the foreseeable future. This process can be life-saving when real danger is present. However, it can cause false alarms that cause unnecessary suffering when you continually anticipate threats that keep your mind and body overreacting and overworking.[17]

If you have bothersome tinnitus, it is important for you to remember that your brainstem and limbic system are just doing their jobs—constantly scanning the external and internal environment for potential threats to your survival. God hardwired these automatic systems into your brain in order to get your attention as soon as possible whenever they perceive any danger to your well-being. However, problems arise when these automatic, subconscious systems misperceive your tinnitus as a threat.[18]

So often, your alarming, yet often benign and meaningless, tinnitus sensations are misunderstood as a potential danger, requiring constant vigilance by the subconscious fear-determining centers in your brain. Thus, your brain constantly works overtime to determine whether the tinnitus stimulus is life-threatening, and requires a fight-or-flight reaction or not.[19]

When looking at how to alleviate your tinnitus, one important question to ask is, "What is the difference between the person who experiences bothersome tinnitus versus the person who experiences non-bothersome tinnitus?"

As you dig deeper into this question, you will probably find it is not what is happening **in** your ears, but rather what is happening **between** your ears—in other words, it's not what you are hearing, but what you are thinking and perceiving that makes all the difference.[20]

People with non-bothersome tinnitus generally hear the sounds associated with tinnitus, but they do not develop the frustration, depression, or anxiety associated with bothersome tinnitus.[21]

In people with bothersome tinnitus, researchers believe that the amygdala misinterprets the "level of threat" that the tinnitus sounds represent. Thus, it seems that the people who experience bothersome tinnitus remain on chronic alert to the sensation, while those who interpret the tinnitus sensation for what it is—a meaningless, benign perception of a sensation—are able (automatically and subconsciously) to allow the sensation to drop into the recesses of their awareness. This may be the reason some people experience bothersome tinnitus, while others do not.[22]

Your pre-frontal cortex is slightly slower in processing than your amygdala. This partly explains why your brain tends to place sounds in the "better-safe-than-sorry" danger category. However, you can enlist this conscious part of your brain to exert more control over bringing awareness to certain processes such as fear modulation and response flexibility.[23]

In order for your medial pre-frontal cortex to communicate with the subconscious regions of your brain, you need to develop a system of neuronal connections to unlearn your old fears of tinnitus. At the same time, your brain needs to build new communication wiring between your rational medial pre-frontal cortex and your automatic brainstem and limbic systems.

The good news is that, when directed, your pre-frontal cortex can send fibers to your overactive amygdala that serve to calm it down so that you can use reasoning to put tinnitus in the benign category where it belongs. To grow these additional neuronal fibers takes hard work, consistency and commitment.[24]

This is where meditation comes in. Meditation (a well-known Mindfulness practice) can lead to cortical growth in those parts of the brain associated with focal attention, fear, and emotional regulation.[25]

Thus, the central goal of mindfulness–based programs is to help you train your brain to convince your fast-acting and mis-appraising amygdala that keeping tinnitus in your awareness is a waste of both energy and resources. Instead, like it does with the sounds of fans and white-noise machine sounds, it can also let tinnitus sounds safely recede into the recesses of your mind.[26]

Since your brain is plastic, this means the actual structure in your brain can change with experience. In Mindfulness, practice is a way of influencing this change by positively creating new wiring in your brain circuitry. Using mindful awareness, you can shine a light on the inner workings of your mind. By doing so you can see an accurate picture of your habitual reaction to your tinnitus and see it for what it really is—a sensation that does not need to be monitored by your mind, poses no credible threat to your survival, and therefore, you can safely allow it to fade from your conscious awareness.[27] Thus, even though your tinnitus is still there, you will gain relief from the distress of your tinnitus.

## The Effectiveness of Mindfulness

Mindfulness works for numbers of people. For example, in a small study before taking the Mindfulness-based Tinnitus Stress Reduction Program, the participants self-reported an average tinnitus handicap inventory questionnaire score of 50.6. After taking the program, the average score dropped to 41.7 (a moderate level) and then further dropped to an average of 22.8 (a mild level) at the 12 month mark. As researcher Jennifer Gans reported, "We found the perceptions of chronic tinnitus changed, with participants noting that they felt an increased tolerance, acceptance and courage to live with it, even 12 months after completing the program. People commented that their tinnitus no longer seemed like a dreadful curse; it was just another sensation that could be annoying but was not insurmountable."[28] In addition to a decrease in tinnitus annoyance, depression and anxiety scores also went down, and quality of life scores went up after participants completed the program.[29]

Obviously, Mindfulness won't totally relieve you of the distress you feel towards your tinnitus, but even reducing your distress by one-third to one-half is certainly a step in the right direction.

Dr. Gans developed the eight week, skill-building Mindfulness-Based Tinnitus Stress Reduction program to teach you how to develop more healthful and positive ways of relating to the unpleasant sensations of your tinnitus. This program includes in-depth tinnitus education and mindfulness skill building.

It teaches you step-by-step the skills you need to help the thinking part of your brain to more accurately determine real threats, and to calm knee-jerk reactions to your bothersome tinnitus.[30] Each week's class integrates elements of deep breathing, gentle yoga, relaxation, and meditation to help you develop new, more effective ways to relate to your tinnitus experience and to the stress in your daily life.[31]

You can find more information on the Mindfulness-Based Tinnitus Stress Reduction program, and an online version of the Mindfulness course at Dr. Gans' website: http://www.mindfultinnitusrelief.com. The on-line course currently costs $335.00.

You may want to try Mindfulness therapy along with various other treatments mentioned in this book. If it works for you—great—use it. If it doesn't work for you, put it back in your "tinnitus toolbox" and try another "tool".

---

**Chapter 19 Endnotes**

1 Gans, 2010. p. 52.
2 Gans, 2014. p. 24.
3 Gans, 2014. p. 24.
4 Gans, 2014. p. 24.

5 Study Explores Mindfulness-based Tinnitus Relief, 2015. p. 36.
6 Gans, 2014. p. 24.
7 Mindfulness-Based Cognitive Therapy, 2011. p. 1.
8 Gans, 2014. p. 24.
9 Gans, 2010. pp. 52-53.
10 Gans, 2010. p. 56.
11 Gans, 2015. p. 28.
12 Gans, 2015. p. 28.
13 Gans, 2015. p. 28.
14 Gans, 2015. p. 29.
15 Gans, 2015. p. 30.
16 Gans, 2015. p. 29.
17 Gans, 2015. p. 29.
18 Gans, 2015. pp. 29-30.
19 Gans, 2015. p. 29.
20 Gans, 2015. p. 29.
21 Gans, 2015. p. 29.
22 Gans, 2015. p. 30.
23 Gans, 2015. p. 30.
24 Gans, 2015. p. 30.
25 Gans, 2015. p. 30.
26 Gans, 2015. p. 30.
27 Gans, 2014. p. 25.
28 Study Explores Mindfulness-based Tinnitus Relief, 2015. p. 36.
29 Gans, 2014. p. 24.
30 Gans, 2015. p. 30.
31 Gans, 2015. p. 28.

## Chapter 20

# Treating Somatosensory Tinnitus

If you have somatosensory tinnitus, there are a number of different treatments you can try to see which helps you. Note that tinnitus originating in the muscles of the head and neck is typically more difficult to effectively treat because there may be several causes at the same time.

As a result, you may find that you need to try some or all of the below treatments at the same time as each one helps a specific area of your body. Since these areas often interact and affect each other, when treated together, they will tend to "fix" all these problem areas.

The two main approaches for treating somatosensory tinnitus fall into one of two broad categories; either physiotherapy (including massage therapy) or chiropractic treatments. Sometimes a given condition can be treated using various techniques from both of these categories. A good example of this would be the various therapy techniques for treating temporomandibular joint problems. If you have somatosensory tinnitus, you need your temporomandibular joint and neck evaluated before your doctor/chiropractor/physiotherapist can select the best treatment option for you.[1]

In addition to the above two main categories, there are other less common treatments including transcutaneous electrical nerve stimulation (TENS) near the ear region and auriculotherapy (joint therapy).[2] (Note: TENS is explained in the "Transcutaneous Electrical Nerve Stimulation" section of Chapter 26.)

In many cases, improvement in somatosensory tinnitus is closely related to the duration of the symptoms. Therefore, it is essential that doctors and ENTs assess this type of tinnitus and refer the person to a physical therapist, massage therapist or chiropractor as soon as possible instead of wasting time by prescribing drugs. (Drugs do nothing to treat the underlying cause of somatosensory tinnitus caused by postural, vertebral or articular [joint] disorders).[3]

## Temporomandibular Dysfunction

If you have a temporomandibular disorder (TMD), you also most likely have muscle tension in both your jaw and neck, as well as tinnitus, vertigo/dizziness and a feeling of fullness in your ears. Therefore, the first step in treating your TMD should be reducing your muscle tension.[4]

If your tinnitus is caused by TMD, your dentist or chiropractor may be able to realign your jaw and thus not only cure your TMD pain, but also reduce or eliminate your tinnitus and other symptoms.

Susie found her tinnitus was dentally related. She says, "I was getting tinnitus so badly that I could not sleep at night without my hearing aids on and the TV on. My dentist rebuilt my bite because, in my case, the ringing in my ears was a result of my jawbone pushing on the vessels around the auditory canal. The bite adjustment has stopped my tinnitus completely."

Effectively treating TMD can really improve your tinnitus. (Note: If you are over 60 years of age, the success rate for eliminating tinnitus is not as high for some reason.) Recent research shows that TMD therapy improves tinnitus in 46 - 96% of patients who have TMD and coexisting tinnitus.[5] One TMD clinic reported that 84% of their last 1,200 TMD patients who also had tinnitus reported that their ear sounds were "gone" or "almost gone" after treatment.[6]

In another study of 93 people, "52 said that their tinnitus had resolved, 28 reported experiencing significant improvement, and 13 reported minimal or no improvement. No one reported experiencing a worsening of the condition."[7] That's good news if you suffer from tinnitus related to TMD.

## Physiotherapy and Massage Therapy

When treating somatosensory tinnitus, physiotherapy and massage therapy basically work to reduce muscle tension and consequent pain, which often reduces or eliminates somatosensory tinnitus.

In addition, a physiotherapist can indirectly help improve various psychological conditions. For example, in the case of tinnitus related to emotional factors, physical therapy can help improve anxiety and depression by teaching people deep diaphragmatic breathing techniques, the countdown technique (counting from 60 to 0), meditation (using images and words), Jacobson's progressive relaxation, or mindfulness (see Chapter 19).[8]

The two main techniques physiotherapists and massage therapists use to reduce muscle tension are trigger point therapy and myofascial release. Since these are closely-related techniques, we will look at them together.

## Trigger Point Therapy and Myofascial Release

Trigger point therapy (TPT) is a proven manual therapy where a practitioner uses her fingers to apply moderately deep pressure to the trigger points (knots) in your muscles in order to release those trigger points using a method called Trigger Point Pressure Release.[9]

The practitioner presses on your trigger points until you no longer perceive any sensory abnormality, referred pain or discomfort at the trigger point.[10] The pressure squishes the toxins out of your muscles and into the bloodstream, where they can be eliminated.[11] This reduces the chemical irritation of the muscle and nerve endings inside the muscle. In turn, this reduces the muscle tension, local pain and referred session sensations like pain, tingling, pressure and tinnitus elsewhere in your body.

If you want to do trigger point therapy on yourself, a good guideline for how hard to press is about as hard as you can and still be able to relax. You work on each muscle for 1 to 3 minutes. For very small muscles or muscles that have very few trigger points, 1 minute is usually enough. If you are interested, you can learn more about how to perform these techniques in the article *What is the Therapy to Remove Trigger Points of Tinnitus.*[12]

Myofascial therapy (MFR) follows right on the heels of the trigger point release therapy. Myofascial maneuvers are similar to stretching exercises.[13] The practitioner applies deep pressure to the muscle, and at the same time stretches it. The purpose is to stretch the fascia surrounding the muscle, and to reduce or stretch out adhesions between muscle and fascia or between separate fascial membranes.[14]

When treating somatosensory tinnitus, the focus of fascial release techniques and trigger point techniques is on the muscles at the base of the skull and neck, as well as the muscles on the side of the face. Stretching the fascia and reducing trigger points allows the ringing to diminish and possibly cease.

Note: Myofascial dysfunction (MFD) treatments only work on the portion of your tinnitus caused by myofascial dysfunction. Thus, you may need to use MFD treatments in conjunction with conventional or upper cervical chiropractic treatments (see the section on "Chiropractic Treatments" later in this chapter) for effective relief.

## Habits to Avoid to Prevent Tinnitus Trigger Points

There is a lot you can do to prevent trigger points from forming in the first place. Often, all you need to do is replace bad habits with good habits. These habits include proper posture, adequate movement, exercise, practicing relaxation and stretching certain muscles. By following these good habits, you will avoid or greatly reduce trigger point problems such as pain and tinnitus in the future.

### 1. Posture

"What is the correct posture for sitting at your desk for eight hours a day? Do you know? What does it look like? I'll give you a hint. This is a trick question. There is **no** correct posture for **sitting eight hours a day**! No one should be sitting all day long without getting up regularly."[15] Therefore:

**Habit #1.** Do not sit longer than 20 minutes without standing up. If you do nothing else, stand up, then squat down as low as you can, then stand or jump up and reach for the ceiling, then sit back down again. Better yet, walk around for a little bit before you sit down again. It only takes a few steps to benefit your body.

**Habit #2.** Hold you head/neck, shoulders, arms and back in a way that minimizes muscle tension. Here's how to do it.

If you are going to stay in a position longer than 5 minutes:

A. Center your head directly over the center of your shoulders and the center of your hips

B. The line between the center of your ears and your eyes should be angled slightly up (or horizontal), so that you are looking straight forward (or slightly downward).

C. Keep your elbows directly below your shoulders, right next to your side.

D. Keep your elbows bent to 90 degrees or slightly straighter.

E. Don't forget Habit #1.

### 2. Movement/Exercise

Your body was made for movement, so move it. Exercise regularly. Walk your dog for a mile or two every day, or go out at lunchtime and walk around the block a couple of times. Arrange your office so that everything is not all near you. For example, locate your printer on the other side of the room. Thus, every time you print something off, you will have to get up and walk over to retrieve your print out. This may be bad from an efficiency point of view, but it'll do wonders for your body in helping prevent trigger points forming (and other health problems).

**Habit #3.** Move around and exercise regularly.

### 3. Relaxation

Tight muscles in your head, jaw, neck and shoulders are almost always the result of stress. Furthermore, tight muscles can lead to somatosensory tinnitus. Therefore, if you fail to relax you can undo all the effects of good posture and cause trigger points in the process. So don't skip this step. Here are two relaxation techniques that you can practice.

**A. Progressive Relaxation:** Fully contract each muscle of your body. Be as selective as possible in contracting only individual muscles, but do the left and right at the same time. After fully contracted, breathe out and fully relax the muscle. Progress through your whole body, from toe to trunk, from fingers to head and face.

**B. Diaphragm Breathing:** Breathe in and out very slowly. Take approximately 4 to 6 seconds to breathe in through your nose and 8 to 12 seconds to slowly release the air through your mouth.

**Habit #4.** Fully relax occasionally throughout the day, even if for only 60 seconds at a time. Do it again for 15-30 minutes before you go to bed.

### 4. Stretching

**A. Jaw Stretch:** Place the tip of your tongue at the top of your mouth, directly behind your front teeth. Slowly open your mouth, keeping your tongue in place. Open as wide as you can without pain or popping your jaw.

**B. Neck Stretch:** Here are three neck stretching exercises.

1. **Forward—backward:** Start with your head tilted all the way forward. Put your hands on the back of your head and gently resist your head movement as you tilt your head all the way back to look straight up. Then put your hands on your forehead and resist the movement as you bend your head forward again. Repeat this two more times.

2. **Rotation:** In a similar manner, but this time with your hands on the sides of your head, turn your head all the way to one side. Use your hands to gently resist as you turn your head all the way to the other side. Repeat back to the first side. Do this two more times.

3. **Side-to-side:** With your hands on each side of your head, and starting with your head tilted all the way over to one shoulder, use your hands to gently resist the movement of your head as you bring your head up straight and then down to your opposite shoulder. Repeat back to the first side. Do this two more times.[16]

**Habit #5.** Carefully stretch your jaw and neck occasionally (at least twice) during the day.

When you regularly practice these 5 habits, this will go a long ways towards preventing myofascial trigger points from forming in the first place. If you already have had somatosensory tinnitus and have been treated for it, practicing these habits will probably prevent your somatosensory tinnitus from ever coming back.

## How Well Do Trigger Point and Myofascial Release Therapies Work?

Trigger point and myofascial release therapies can work well in reducing somatosensory tinnitus caused by tight muscles in your face and neck.

For example, in one double-blind, placebo-controlled, randomized trial, participants had a significant decrease in tinnitus loudness, and in pain intensity, a decrease in tinnitus handicap inventory scores and a decrease in the number of myofascial trigger points (MTPs).[17]

In the above study, 37 people from the experimental group and 34 people from the control group were analyzed blind by a researcher before treatment began and again after 10 weeks of treatment. Ultimately, 3 people with tinnitus in just one ear benefitted from complete tinnitus relief; 2 people with tinnitus in both ears felt complete relief in one of their ears; and 1 person reported an improvement in the number of tinnitus sounds they heard (a decrease from 7 to 3). All of these people still maintained their relief at their two-month revaluation.

Six out of 37 people is only 16% that had a positive change in their tinnitus, but if you were one of the 16%, you'd be glad you took this treatment.

Other studies have shown that the results for myofascial dysfunction treatment for tinnitus vary all over the place. Some people have no change in their tinnitus. For others, their tinnitus totally disappears. In one study of people with myofascial-related tinnitus, approximately 25% experienced total relief. Another 25% experienced significant improvement in their tinnitus. Unfortunately, the remaining 50% didn't see any improvement. [18]

Note: One recent study showed that people with normal pure tone audiograms and chronic pain had the best treatment results when their myofascial trigger points were deactivated, regardless of whether their tinnitus was constant or intermittent or unilateral or bilateral.[19]

Another interesting finding was that people whose tinnitus reduced in intensity when they moved their bodies a certain way had better results than those whose tinnitus got louder when they did the same thing.[20]

These results show that trigger point and myofascial release therapy often need other complementary therapies such as chiropractic treatment at the same time. Even so, if you think trigger points or myofascial dysfunction may have caused your tinnitus, you would be wise to seek out specific treatment for these conditions. Health care professionals trained in trigger point deactivation typically include chiropractors, physiotherapists, massage therapists, osteopathic physicians, occupational therapists and acupuncturists.

Trigger point and myofascial release therapies are important tools in your tinnitus toolbox to help you gain control of your tinnitus, so take advantage of them if you have somatosensory tinnitus. See if they will work for you.[21]

## Arlen's Atlas Therapy

A quasi-trigger-point therapy is called Arlen's atlas therapy. This therapy is applied to the top vertebra in your neck, commonly called the "atlas". If your tinnitus is caused by tension in the muscles of your neck, you might want to give Arlen's atlas therapy a try.

Here's how it all seems to tie together.

The short muscles in the back of your neck consist of two layers. The inner layer has 10 to 100 times more neural density than do other skeletal muscles. Furthermore, the nerves for proprioception (helping you keep your balance) comprise 90% of the nerve function as compared to 10% in most other skeletal muscles. This helps us regulate our posture in space.

When everything is working normally, a constant flow of neural impulses flows to the brain stem from the six senses (proprioception being number six) and from the cerebral cortex in your brain.

However, anything that irritates these inner cervical muscles or puts them under tension causes them to send a large number of nerve impulses to the balance center (vestibular nuclei) in the brainstem.

If the brainstem becomes overloaded with too much information from one or more of the senses, it can result in symptoms such as dizziness, nausea, vomiting, nystagmus, blurred vision, and tinnitus.

It is this enormous neuronal response that seems to cause this type of somatosensory tinnitus. The solution is to reduce the tension in these inner cervical muscles. When this happens, the cervical muscles reduce their balance and pain sensor output.

This is where Arlen's atlas therapy comes in. Arlen's upper cervical treatment lowers the proprioception (muscle/tendon signals) and nociception (pain signals) output, reducing the flow of information to the brain stem to normal.[22] This gets things back on track, and the result is your tinnitus begins to fade away.[23]

**Proprioception vs. Nociception**

**Proprioception** (pro-pree-oh-SEP-shen), from the Latin proprius, meaning "one's own", "individual," and capere, to take or grasp, is the sense of the relative position of neighboring parts of the body and the strength of effort employed in movement. The ability to sense stimuli arising within the body regarding position, motion, and equilibrium. Proprioception helps us keep our balance.

**Nociception** (noe-see-SEP-shen) is from the Latin word "nocere" "to harm or hurt". It is the encoding and processing of harmful stimuli in the nervous system, and, therefore, the ability of a body to sense potential harm. This process, called nociception, usually causes the perception of pain.

It is important to begin treating the neck muscles as soon as possible after any traumatic event that causes neck muscle tension. This is because any delay gives the brain time to form an internal tinnitus loop due to the plasticity of the neural system. You don't want this to happen, because breaking such a tinnitus loop is not easy. It is much better to prevent tinnitus from forming in the first place.

In cases of whiplash injury, the distorted or otherwise damaged muscles of the neck should be treated within several days by atlas therapy (or upper cervical chiropractic treatment or craniosacral osteopathy) in order to get the neck back to normal and thus prevent tinnitus and other symptoms forming as a result of this neck trauma.[24]

In contrast to conventional chiropractic treatment (see the following section), Arlen's atlas therapy is performed without traction, rotation or extension of the cervical spine. Rather, Arlen's atlas therapy involves a high amplitude, low velocity "impulse" to the "wing" of the atlas. "No repositioning of the atlas is involved, as is attempted by chiropractors, even though the impulse has to travel in the direction of the reposition."[25]

The good news is that Arlen's atlas therapy causes the muscles to relax and this seems to quiet down abnormal nerve impulses to the brainstem. For example, in one study of 11 people with whiplash injuries, 7 experienced a complete normalization of vestibular disturbances, 3 improved, and only one person remained unchanged.[26]

Atlas therapy does not eliminate tinnitus in people who have longstanding, painful tension in their necks, but this therapy can substantially reduce their tinnitus. However, when people with recent neck tension from whiplash were treated with several sessions of atlas therapy, typically their tinnitus totally went away as their muscles permanently relaxed.

Thus any treatments that permanently relax the muscles at the back of your neck have the potential to reduce tinnitus from this source. These include not only atlas therapy, but also acupuncture, craniosacral therapy and upper cervical chiropractic treatment (see following section).[27]

## Chiropractic Treatments

Chiropractic is a type of health care that deals with the nervous and musculoskeletal systems in your body. The influence of the musculoskeletal system upon certain types of tinnitus is well recognized.[28] Often, proper chiropractic treatment can successfully relieve tinnitus from this cause.

Tinnitus can be a symptom of an injury to your upper cervical spine (neck). Therefore, if you have somatosensory tinnitus, probably your best option for treatment is to have chiropractic adjustments to your head and neck. When your head is properly balanced or realigned with your neck, your tinnitus can improve or even disappear.

Chiropractors talk about subluxations. In medical terms, a "luxation" is a complete dislocation of two bones. In contrast, a subluxation is an incomplete luxation (some degree of dislocation). Thus, a subluxation occurs when the alignment between two bones is altered, yet at the same time, the two joint surfaces remain in contact with each other (Stedman's Medical Dictionary). I just say my neck is "out".

Subluxations may be quite small—only 1 or 2 mm—but this can be enough to cause problems. Medical doctors typically discount these slight subluxations as not being medically significant. Typically, when they read cervical X-rays, they say everything is normal because they can't see any broken bones or tumors. Furthermore, they think any misalignments will right themselves on their own. However, the truth is that many times this never happens, and you have to go to a skilled chiropractor for a spinal adjustment to get things restored to normal.[29]

Somatosensory tinnitus can result when various muscles are "tight" and out of balance as we saw in the previous section. This is because when the muscles are "tight" or unbalanced, they either pull the vertebrae "out", or the opposite occurs where the vertebrae get knocked out of place and cause the muscles to become unbalanced and "tight". Either way, the end result can be tinnitus.

Let's look at this in more detail.

Your head, which typically weighs around 10 or 11 pounds, rests on top of the two-ounce, doughnut-shaped atlas vertebra (C1). The atlas is also called the "yes" bone because your head rocks back and forth on its two articulations when you nod your head to indicate "yes".

Your second vertebra (C2) is called the "axis". This is the vertebra that allows you to turn your head left and right. You could call it the "no" bone because it allows your head to rotate left and right as you shake your head "no".[30]

Incidentally, your atlas and axis are your two most freely moveable vertebrae; and as a result, are the ones most commonly misaligned and also the easiest vertebrae to be misaligned.[31] Since your C1 and C2 vertebrae are intimately related, if one goes out, the other is probably out too. Furthermore, Dr. Michael Burcon, probably the world authority on using chiropractic to treat Meniere's Disease explained, "they both usually go out in the same direction".[32] However, they are not necessarily "out" by the same amount.

You might not realize this, but your brainstem actually extends down into the atlas and axis cavity so your spinal cord basically begins with the C3 vertebra. In fact, five of your twelve cranial nerves originate in your brainstem. The base of the brain controls many important bodily functions, such as breathing, blood pressure, the sleep center, and balance.[33]

Thus, if your top two vertebrae are out of alignment, they put pressure on the base of your brainstem. This can cause interference at the point where your head and neck join (the atlas) and interfere with the free flow of signals up and down your nervous system—sometimes with serious consequences.[34]

This is where specialized (upper cervical) chiropractic treatment comes in. Adjusting the atlas (and axis) can take this pressure off your brainstem, thus alleviating many problems by allowing your brain to send its healing messages throughout your body and allowing your spine to revert to its proper alignment.

"If the atlas is out of its proper position, it can irritate, constrict or disrupt vital nerve signals to any portion of your body. This can cause muscle or joint pain, organ dysfunction, lowered immune system and countless other conditions that you would not ordinarily relate to a problem originating in your neck"[35] including tinnitus.

Note that an atlas subluxation both posterior (behind) and inferior (below) on the right can irritate the 8th cranial nerve (the vestibulo-cochlear nerve that controls balance and hearing) on the left side and that can lead to symptoms such as tinnitus.[36]

Dr. Burcon explains, "When the **atlas** is the **major** subluxation, vertigo with vomiting is the major symptom. However, when the **axis** is the **major** subluxation, hearing loss, ear fullness and tinnitus are the major symptoms."[37]

Furthermore, when your vertebrae are not in correct alignment, this can also affect your autonomic nervous system, thereby influencing circulation to your head and inner ears.[38]

One fairly-common incident that can knock your atlas and axis out of proper alignment is whiplash caused by a vehicle accident.

If you've ever been in a car accident and had whiplash, you may have found that your ears started ringing. It probably never crossed your mind that tinnitus and whiplash might be related, but they can be.

There are primary as well as secondary causes that can give rise to tinnitus after whiplash. Primary causes include direct trauma to your head such as hitting the side window, the back of the seat, the steering wheel, mirror and/or windshield. Secondary causes often involve your temporomandibular joint (TMJ)—the hinge of your jaw—which is commonly injured as a result of whiplash. By itself, TMJ (now often referred to as TMD) can cause ear pain, tinnitus, vertigo (dizziness), hearing loss, and headaches.

As we have just seen, many nerves in your head and neck arise from your neck, as well as from the cranial nerves. Therefore, spinal adjustments to your neck as well as certain cranial adjustments can have a dramatic benefit in the treatment of whiplash-induced tinnitus.[39]

The good news is that adjustments to your upper cervical spine can restore balance to your nervous system and calm your nerves. That is why a number of people with tinnitus have reported improvement in their tinnitus after undergoing something as simple as a neck adjustment. As one chiropractor explained, "A number of our tinnitus patients' symptoms have improved following spinal corrections".[40]

For example, chiropractic treatment reduced tinnitus, vertigo and hearing loss in a person with a cervical subluxation (neck out of place) and temporomandibular disorder.

In a Swedish study of 1,504 people who went to chiropractors, as a surprising bonus, 23% of the patients reported improvements in non-musculoskeletal symptoms. Interestingly, the 7th most common unexpected benefit, affecting about 3% of these people, was less ringing in their ears (reduced tinnitus). This means that in people going to conventional chiropractors, neck problems are obviously causing increased tinnitus, and some of this tinnitus is alleviated by conventional chiropractic treatments.[41]

If your tinnitus is caused by the bones in your neck/jaw not being in the correct alignment, you may find that chiropractic treatment is quite effective in getting your tinnitus under control.[42] This doesn't work for everyone of course, but if your upper cervical spine is "out", it is definitely worth looking into.

## Conventional Chiropractors vs. Upper Cervical Chiropractors

Conventional chiropractors are the kind of chiropractors most people immediately think of when they think of chiropractic. He's the guy who grabs your head and twists your neck 'hoping' to unlock, some 'locked' vertebrae so it moves freely again. He's the one that uses force and cracks, crunches, rotates, or takes your neck to its full range of motion and moves it with high velocity in the other direction. In short, conventional chiropractors manipulate your back and neck. [43]

Conventional chiropractors have their place to be sure. If you have any vertebrae "locked", they are the people to go to. However, when it comes to your ears and things like tinnitus, a conventional chiropractor is **not** the best doctor to go to. For this, you want an upper cervical chiropractor.

Upper cervical chiropractors gently align those critical top two vertebrae in your neck—the "atlas" and the "axis"—so your body can begin to function normally again and hopefully get rid of your tinnitus.

You might ask, "What's the difference between the two? They're both chiropractors, aren't they? Can't I just go to any chiropractor for upper cervical treatment? Aren't all chiropractors trained in spinal adjustments?"

The answer is "yes", all chiropractors are trained in spinal adjustments, but their training does not prepare them to be **experts** in specifically adjusting the atlas and axis vertebrae!

Conventional chiropractors are people who have attended a recognized chiropractic school and received their Doctor of Chiropractic degree (DC). To obtain this degree they must first earn a 4-year bachelor level degree followed by a 4-year doctoral degree in chiropractic.[44]

All upper cervical chiropractors have also earned their Doctor of Chiropractic degrees, but in addition, they have also taken a 1-year post-doctoral specialty in upper cervical spine treatment techniques along with associated clinical training. Only about 2% of chiropractors go on to take the upper cervical post-doctoral training.[45]

There are a number of different approaches to upper cervical chiropractic adjustments—about 10 or so. All of them require extra training. Furthermore, all of them require extra time with each patient. Dr. Burcon is partial to the "hands-on" Blair method, but he is quick to point out that the other methods are all good too.

In addition to the Blair method for treating the upper cervical spine, some of other methods include the Atlas Orthogonal, the HIO (Hole-in-One) Toggle Recoil, the Kale Brainstem, the NUCCA, the Knee Chest, the Orthospinology/ Grostic, the Quantum Spinal Mechanics and the Palmer Specific to name some of the more common ones. You can learn more about these various upper cervical treatment methods at http://www.upcspine.com/tech.htm if you are interested.[46]

## Finding an Upper Cervical Spine Chiropractor

By now you probably are eager to find an upper cervical chiropractor and see what they can do to help you bring your tinnitus under control. Fortunately, upper cervical chiropractors are easy to find if you know where to look.

Greg Buchanan's website at http://www.upcspine.com/ gives a wealth of information on upper cervical chiropractic. Furthermore, he maintains a list of upper cervical chiropractors scattered all over the world so you (hopefully) can find one near you. Just go to the above link and click on the fifth button across the top "Practitioners". From the drop-down menu choose your area of the world. If you live in the USA or Canada, choose North America, then click on the "View" button (on the right) for your state (or province) and you will see an alphabetic listing (by chiropractor's last names—not business names) of the upper cervical chiropractors in that state/province. Each listing gives not only all the contact information you need, but also what method of upper cervical techniques they use, what instruments they use, whether they take X-rays or not, etc.[47]

You can also go to the main web page for each of the various upper cervical chiropractic associations (each organization is associated with one specific method) and look at the listing of chiropractors trained in their method. These listings may be more complete and up-to-date than those on Buchanan's website.

To find an upper cervical chiropractor that practices a specific method (such as the Blair method), go to http://www.upcspine.com/tech.htm and click on the name of the method you want to investigate (in the column on the left) or on the "Read More" link at the bottom of the paragraph describing the method on the main part of the page. Usually there is a listing of chiropractors using that method somewhere on that website.

I'd suggest you look for upper cervical chiropractors that have/do the following:

1. A good number of years of experience (a minimum of 15 or 20 years). This is because it takes years of practicing to become an expert upper cervical chiropractor.

2. A chiropractor that uses the Blair method (if you can find one reasonably near you).

3. A chiropractor that has a proven track record in successfully treating people with somatosensory tinnitus.

4. A chiropractor that uses at least two methods to tell if you are in adjustment (X-rays and thermography, for example).

5. A chiropractor that takes X-rays so he won't miss tiny subluxations.[48]

---

**Chapter 20 Endnotes**

1 Sanchez, 2011. p. 1091.
2 Rocha, 2015. p. 3.
3 Rocha, 2015. p. 3.
4 Sanchez, 2011. p. 1091.
5 Klemons, 2010. p. 1.
6 Klemons, 2010. p. 2.
7 Klemons, 2010. p. 2.
8 Rocha, 2015. p. 3.
9 Teachey, 2012. p. 2.
10 Sanchez, 2011. p. 1091.
11 Hobbs, 2014. p. 2.
12 Tinnitus Synergy, 2014. pp. 1-6.
13 Rocha, 2015. p. 3.
14 Hobbs, 2014. p. 5.
15 Hobbs, 2014. p. 2.
16 Hobbs, 2014. pp. 3-4.
17 Sanchez, 2011. p. 1091.
18 Teachey, 2012. p. 3.
19 Sanchez, 2011. p. 1092.
20 Sanchez, 2011. p. 1092.
21 Teachey, 2012. p. 3.
22 Sanchez, 2011. p. 1091.
23 Kaute, 1998. pp. 165-166.
24 Kaute, 1998. p. 166.
25 Koren, 2004. p. 2.
26 Kaute, 1998. p. 165.
27 Kaute, 1998. p. 166.
28 Teachey, 2012. p. 2.
29 Bauman, 2015. p. 11.
30 Bauman, 2015. p. 8.
31 Blair Upper Cervical, 2002. p. 1.
32 Dr. Michael Burcon, 2015. Personal communication.
33 Bauman, 2015. p. 8.
34 Bauman, 2015. p. 8.
35 FAQ, 2002. p. 1.

36 Bauman, 2015. p. 10.
37 Burcon, 2014. p. 35.
38 Whittaker, 2013. p. 1.
39 AdvancedWellness, 2012. p. 1.
40 Tanase, 2015. p. 1.
41 Koren, 2004. p. 1.
42 Tinnitus 1-2-3, 2012. p. 1.
43 Buchanan, 2002. p. 1.
44 Bauman, 2015. p. 19.
45 Bauman, 2015. p. 20.
46 Bauman, 2015. p. 20.
47 Bauman, 2015. pp. 24-25.
48 Bauman, 2015. p. 25.

## Chapter 21

# Sound Therapy

Sound therapy is one of the two proven ways to mitigate the effects of the common forms of subjective tinnitus. (The other is various forms of counseling mentioned in previous chapters.) Sound therapy got its start back in the 1970s when researchers began using it to mask a person's tinnitus.[1]

When talking about tinnitus, sound therapy is using sound intended either to change in a positive way how you feel about your tinnitus and/or how you react to your tinnitus.[2] Thus, in practical terms, if you have tinnitus, sound therapy helps to:

1. Habituate you to your tinnitus by inducing a sense of relief from the stress of your tinnitus.

2. Reduce the contrast between background environmental sounds and your perception of tinnitus.

3. Distract your attention away from your tinnitus.[3]

In order to habituate to your tinnitus, you want to avoid silence so your ears have real sounds to focus on. Fortunately, there are a number of ways you can use sound therapy to do this. For example, you can use amplification (hearing aids), tinnitus maskers (using white noise), background environmental sounds, notched music, fractal music and so on.

It is important to realize that neither you nor your audiologist can predict how your tinnitus will respond to sound therapy prior to your trying it out. People differ; the causes of tinnitus are complex and varied, and your stress response to tinnitus plays a very significant role in how bothersome your tinnitus is to you and how well you will respond.[4]

Sound therapy can take time. For some people it provides almost instantaneous relief. However, to habituate to your tinnitus so you no longer need sound therapy can take between 6 and 18 months. As a result, if the change seems too slow, you may return to your audiologist feeling discouraged, frustrated and desperate.

This is why it is essential that you receive appropriate counseling **at the same time** you are taking tinnitus sound therapy. You first need to understand what tinnitus is in order to overcome or avoid the negative associations that prevent you from habituating to your tinnitus.[5]

The key is to stick with your sound therapy program. Don't give up.

> The benefit of sound therapy may come sooner or later, may be dramatic or subtle, may be influenced by other factors related to your overall health and stress management, and may result in good days and bad days, even within the context of an overall positive trend.[6]

## Which Tinnitus Sound Therapy Is Right for Me?

The majority of tinnitus management protocols emphasize that, since tinnitus is a perception of sound, sound therapy should be an essential part of any tinnitus treatment. There are several non-amplified sound therapy options, which include narrowband noise (for masking purposes), broadband noise (for habituation), modulated noises and/or filtered music.[7]

Furthermore, how people perceive their tinnitus influences how they feel, and in turn, react to their tinnitus. We all perceive our tinnitus differently, and our perceptions

**Broadband vs. Narrowband sounds**

"Broadband sound is white noise, or a 'shhh' sound. Many people with tinnitus find this soothing. The term 'white noise' refers to a sound which encompasses all possible sound frequencies at once, much as white light includes all color frequencies of the visual color spectrum.

Narrowband sound is similar to broadband sound, but instead of including all possible sound frequencies it includes only those within a certain range, or band (hence a 'narrower band' of frequencies.) To the user, it also has a 'shhh' sound, though at a different pitch than white noise. It may be at a higher pitch and sound more like a sizzle or at a lower pitch and sound more like wind in a cove."[8]

can vary greatly from one person to another. As a result, it should be no surprise that we also vary in the sounds we prefer to use in sound therapy.[9]

Thus, it is important to determine not only what sounds you like, but what sounds are most effective in reducing your perception of tinnitus.[10] That is why choosing the correct sound to use in tinnitus sound therapy often has a significant impact on whether sound therapy works well or not.[11]

Not only do the sounds we prefer vary from person to person, they can even vary from time to time with the same person. For example, your preferred sounds can vary with your mood, time of day, or current activities.

In general, there are three types of sound you can use to help you deal with your tinnitus.

1. **Soothing sounds**: These sounds make you feel better as soon as you hear them. They help reduce the stress and tension you feel from your tinnitus.
2. **Background sounds**: These sounds reduce the contrast between your tinnitus and quiet environments. Thus, they make it easier for you to ignore your tinnitus.
3. **Interesting sounds**: These sounds keep your attention. They help you shift your attention away from your tinnitus and focus on the interesting sounds you are hearing.[12]

You don't necessarily need three different kinds of sounds. Some sounds can have all three characteristics. For example, certain kinds of music can sooth you, provide background sound so that you don't hear your tinnitus as well, and also be interesting—such as music you love.[13]

Note: The Progressive Tinnitus Management program (see Chapter 15) classifies sounds into the three above categories. Other tinnitus management programs talk about calming, therapeutic, and distracting sounds.[14] However you name them, these sounds do the same things.

Based on these categories, some sound devices are designed to produce relaxing or soothing sounds in order to reduce the stress that can exacerbate your tinnitus. These sound therapy devices, targeting your relaxation response, can be an important part of your tinnitus sound therapy.[15]

Other devices are tinnitus maskers. These devices are designed to cover up your tinnitus with another more pleasant sound. Yet other sound therapy devices target your tinnitus on a neurological level by interrupting the perception of your tinnitus sound and giving your brain something more interesting to focus on.[16]

The sounds used for sound therapy can vary in their timing (beat), frequency spectrum and emotion-evoking characteristics. In addition, individual differences can influence how effective a given sound is over another sound.[17]

For example, the hearing aid manufacturer, ReSound, has incorporated their tinnitus sound generator—Nature Sounds—in some of their hearing aids. These hearing aids generate alternative sounds to standard white noise. At the time of wring this, your audiologist can activate these Nature sounds when fitting you with ReSound Aventa hearing aids.[18]

ReSound has also developed the ReSound Relief app for tinnitus. This app gives even more sound therapy options. Thus, there should be some sounds that work for you. Nature Sounds are synthesized versions of natural water sounds and can also include environmental sounds, music and personal imported sounds.[19]

Sounds used in tinnitus therapy should not being irritating or annoying. Broadband sounds, such as white noise, have proven to be effective for managing tinnitus and many people habituate to their tinnitus after listening to broadband noise.[20]

However, some people find white noise particularly irritating to them and therefore it is not a good choice for their tinnitus therapy. That is why we need a variety of tinnitus sound therapy options. Having sounds that we prefer and accept is one of the keys of successful sound therapy.[21]

Some people prefer to listen to computer-generated, dynamic sounds that enhance short-term variations in amplitude over traditional broadband noise. For example, one study showed that modulated sounds—particularly low-frequency amplitude tones with a higher frequency in the tinnitus pitch range—were the most effective in reducing tinnitus loudness.[22]

ReSound has determined that most people prefer air and water sounds for tinnitus sound therapy. These sounds cause the least amount of annoyance when compared to narrowband and broadband white noise as well as other nature-inspired sounds.[23]

Other hearing aid manufacturers have developed other tinnitus sound therapy sounds such as fractal music and S-Tones. (We'll discuss these later in this chapter.)

## Which Tinnitus Sound Therapy Device Is the Best?

Just as there are a number of sound therapies, there are also a number of sound therapy devices from hearing aids to sound generators to white noise machines. When asked, "Which sound therapy devices do you favor and why?" Dr. Jastreboff replied,

> Sound is more important than any particular device. Consequently, the optimal device depends on the specific patient. Since the majority of tinnitus patients have hearing loss, the combination devices (hearing aid plus sound generator in one shell) are optimal. For misophonic patients, who typically have normal hearing, sound generators are recommended. The stress should be placed on sound and not on the particular instrument.[24]

## Enrich Your Environment with Sound

You do not need to go to an audiologist and purchase a fancy sound device in order to help yourself deal with your tinnitus. You can enrich your environment with sound yourself. This gives your brain real sounds to listen to and hopefully your brain will "let go" of the tinnitus to which it is locked on.

Sound enrichment benefits many forms of tinnitus by activating neural plasticity (in the good way). It takes time to grow new neural connections. Thus it may take 6 to 8 months or longer to reduce your tinnitus to an acceptable level.[25]

When using sound enrichment, you should never use loud sound. Sound enrichment always uses soft to moderate sound.[26] In general, the length of time you use sound enrichment daily likely will vary depending on how severe your tinnitus is. If you have more severe tinnitus (or sound sensitivity) you will find that you need longer sessions of sound enrichment—the longer you use sound enrichment each day the better. Remember, sound therapy takes several months to produce noticeable results, so don't give up before it has had time to work.[27]

There are two main kinds of sound enrichment you can employ depending on your goal at the time—relaxation sound enrichment and distraction sound enrichment.

The goal of **relaxation sound enrichment** is obviously to help you relax. When you are relaxed, you will find that your tinnitus will not bother you as much as if you are anxious and tense.

In order to use sound enrichment for relaxing, the sounds you choose need to soothe you. For some people, this means listening to soothing music. For others, it means listening to the sounds of nature. Nature sounds include sounds such as the sound of water (ocean waves lapping on the beach; rushing water in streams and rivers; and waterfalls); the sounds of wildlife, particularly the sounds of birds chirping and singing; and weather sounds such as wind, rain or thunderstorms. You can hear these sounds outdoors while communing with nature, or you can purchase CDs with these nature sounds on them so you can bring the sounds of nature into your bedroom in the city.

You may already have soothing sounds in your home. For example, you may find the hum of your refrigerator, fan or furnace soothing, or it may be the bubbling sounds from your fish tank. Obviously, hearing these latter sounds depends on your degree of hearing loss.

The goal of **distraction sound enrichment** is to distract you from focusing on your tinnitus. Distraction sounds are many and varied. They include listening to people talking, watching the TV, listening to the radio or to the various sounds made during the course of your work or hobbies.

## Sound Therapy at Night

If your tinnitus prevents you from falling asleep at night, or if you wake up in the middle of the night and can't get back to sleep because of your tinnitus, you may question, "Should I use sound therapy at night to help me go to sleep and stay asleep?"

The good news is that even while you are sleeping, sound therapy continues to help you habituate to your tinnitus. As Dr. Jastreboff explains,

> Since habituation of tinnitus-evoked reactions can take place during sleep as well, it is important to take advantage of sound therapy **all** night long. This strategy can help reduce the relative strength of tinnitus and improve sleep while facilitating the process of habituation. Ear-level devices are not optimal for use during the night. Typically, patients use table-top sound machines and/or sound pillows. Using sound therapy all night long is an effective method for improving sleep quality, which is disrupted in the majority of tinnitus patients.[28]

The most commonly-recommended type of sound to use for sleeping is white noise, although if you are sensitive to sound, you may find that pink noise works better for you.[29]

Set the sound to run constantly throughout the night—not just until you fall asleep again. This is because your ears never sleep so your brain is getting the benefit of sound enrichment even while you sleep. Set the sound level to whichever level works best for you—whether at the non-masking, mixing, partial masking or complete masking level.[30] (See the section on "Tinnitus Masking" later in this chapter for more on this.)

### Stream Soothing Sounds to Your Hearing Aids

Here's another sound therapy approach you can use to enrich your listening experience if your hearing aids have a streamer. Since modern streaming devices can connect to virtually any audio device, they can wirelessly turn your hearing aids into a personal headset.

If you have a smart phone, iPod, tablet or computer, search for apps for tinnitus. At the time of writing this (Feb, 2016), a minimum of 100 apps in the Apple iTunes store pop up when you type in the search term "tinnitus" and choose "iPhone". Many of these apps produce various tinnitus therapy sounds. You will probably find a good number of similar apps in the Android store.

All you need to do is download one or more of these apps to your smart phone, iPod, tablet or computer and then stream the relaxing sound files to your hearing aids. And if you search for "relaxation music" and choose "iPhone Apps" you will get at least another 100 relaxation music apps. The variety of sound apps you can find to help you deal with your tinnitus is almost endless.

**Tinnitus Apps**

There are a number of apps that may help complement your tinnitus therapy program. For iPhone users there are Whist, Tinnitus Pro: Music Therapy, Sleep Pillow, White Noise, ReSound Relief, Tinnitus, Phonak Tinnitus Balance, Sleep Bug White Noise, Beltone Tinnitus Calmer, Oticon Tinnitus Sound, myNoise, Soothing Sounds Lite, SimplyNoise, Tinnitus Therapy Lite, Free Sleep Sounds, Tinnitus Help, Link Tinnitus Sound, EQ HearAid + Tinnitus Masker, Noisli and many others, but these are more than enough to get you started. Try them and see which ones work best for you.

## Tinnitus Masking

If you spend a lot of time in quiet places, or if you are hard of hearing like I am and do not regularly wear your hearing aids, your brain automatically turns up its internal volume. One result is that typically you now perceive your tinnitus as louder.

The obvious way to overcome this is to add in some background sounds that your subconscious can listen to. Then your brain will turn your internal volume back down to where it should be.

When you listen to background sounds, these real sounds, at least to some extent, mask your tinnitus. This gave rise to the tinnitus treatment called "Tinnitus Masking". In fact, this was the earliest way people used sound therapy for dealing with their tinnitus. Tinnitus masking, as its name implies, uses another sound to cover up or mask your tinnitus sound. Thus, masking helps reduce the distress you feel from your tinnitus.

The objective of tinnitus masking therapy is to use sound to induce tinnitus relief and promote habituation.[31] You can mask tinnitus in one of two ways.[32]

1. **Total masking**: Total masking is using another **louder** sound to completely cover up (mask) your perceived tinnitus.
2. **Partial masking**: Partial masking is using another **softer** sound to reduce your focus on your tinnitus because you hear this other sound in addition to your tinnitus. Partial masking works on both your conscious (psychological) level and on your subconscious (central auditory perception) level.[33]

When you add sound to your environment, you are helping to mask your tinnitus with other sounds. Using partial or complete masking to change or hide your tinnitus can give you a sense of being in control,[34] and that alone can help reduce the distress you feel towards your tinnitus.

There are actually four degrees of sound enrichment that sometimes go under the general term of "tinnitus masking". J. L. Mayes, in her excellent book, *Tinnitus Treatment Toolbox* explains:

> The term "masking" is sometimes used to describe the effect of covering up the sound of tinnitus with another sound. At a **non-masking** loudness level, the outside sound and tinnitus can both be heard clearly. As the loudness of the outside sound is increased, eventually the tinnitus and the outside sound will start **mixing** or blending together without changing or masking the tinnitus sound. As the loudness continues to increase, **partial masking** can begin to happen. With partial masking, the tinnitus and outside sound blend together and the tinnitus starts to change (e.g. sound softer or different). As the loudness of the outside sound increases more, some people's tinnitus can be **completely masked** or covered up to the point that they can't hear their tinnitus any more.[35]

The purpose of each of these levels of masking is different. For example, in order to get quick relief from your tinnitus, you may want to completely mask it. Traditional sound therapy treatments did just that by masking your tinnitus with a background sound such as broadband noise. Note that, in most cases, the masking noise must be at least as loud as your perceived tinnitus in order to provide you with sufficient relief from your tinnitus.[36]

Therefore, complete masking usually works best for people who have tinnitus that is easily covered up. By setting the volume a bit louder than you hear your tinnitus, it masks your tinnitus and can bring you almost immediate relief while you are listening to it. This is not true of everyone with tinnitus. For example, I can still easily hear my tinnitus over loud sounds, so it would be difficult to completely mask my tinnitus.

Now that you understand the basics of tinnitus masking, here are some ways you can use sound enrichment to mask or partially mask your tinnitus. When using sound therapy the idea is to build up sound in the space around you so you always have some real sounds to hear instead of just your tinnitus.

**Masking with External Sounds:** You can mask your tinnitus with normal external sounds. One way to do this is by listening to good music, or having the radio, television or stereo playing in the background or listen to your MP3 player, iPod or iPhone or similar device. To be effective, set the sound level so it partially or completely masks your tinnitus. I am listening to a piece by Mozart as I write this. It effectively masks my tinnitus, or at least it distracts me from consciously hearing my tinnitus. Incidentally, listening to good classical music has two other benefits. It stimulates your brain (makes you smarter) and it relaxes you (reduces your stress). Others buy recordings or CDs of naturally-soothing sounds such as waterfalls, ocean waves, rain fall, jungle sounds or whales that also tend to mask your tinnitus. These can be remarkably valuable to you if your tinnitus bothers you while you are "up and around".

At night if your tinnitus is more noticeable because your surroundings are quiet, add some sound to your bedroom. Any sounds such as a ticking clock, fan, an automatic radio that turns off after you are asleep, or some relaxing sounds on CDs or MP3 players will help mask the irritating noises in your head.

**Masking with Hearing Aids:** If you have both hearing loss and tinnitus, an effective way to mask your tinnitus is just to get and wear hearing aids. Thus, your first step could be to get your audiologist to fit you with hearing aids. If you are like many people, simply wearing hearing aids can mitigate the effects of your tinnitus because hearing real sounds again will partially mask your tinnitus sounds, not to mention help take your mind off these sounds.

Some new hearing aids have sound generators built in so you get a double benefit of hearing more real sounds plus listening to various tinnitus therapy sounds. (See the section "Hearing Aids with Built-In Sound Generators" later in this chapter for more on these hearing aids.)

**Masking with Special Tinnitus Maskers:** Alternately, you could try wearing an actual tinnitus masker. These devices are designed to cover up your tinnitus with another more pleasant sound.

Depending on the device, it may look like a behind-the-ear hearing aid or a pocket pager. They produce "white noise" (or hopefully "pink noise" even if they still colloquially call it "white noise") or some other sounds or music at a sufficient level to hide your tinnitus, or at least make it less noticeable.

Since the goal of sound therapy is to create a real external sound that will induce your brain to stop its excessive spontaneous neuronal hyperactivity in the damaged area of the cochlea, another approach can also work.

In this approach, rather than using broadband white noise for tinnitus relief, you use sounds near the frequency of your tinnitus. The more closely the masking sound corresponds with the tinnitus frequency, the more effectively it will suppress your tinnitus.[37]

Some people find it is much easier to cope with the external noise produced by a tinnitus masker than with their constant tinnitus. In one study, 16% reported relief from tinnitus just by wearing their hearing aids, 21% reported relief using a tinnitus masker, while 63% found some relief using a combination hearing aid/tinnitus masker.

Tinnitus masking has some downsides to it. First, although masking may provide tinnitus relief by making it inaudible, once you remove your tinnitus masker, your tinnitus will eventually return. Second, the level of sound required to mask your tinnitus may annoy you.

Third, for most people, tinnitus masking is not the real answer. This is because tinnitus masking and tinnitus habituation are complete opposites. In one study, people who used tinnitus-maskers for 10 to 15 years were still annoyed by their tinnitus after all those years. Why? When they wore their maskers, they couldn't hear their tinnitus, so they never learned how to ignore it and become habituated to their tinnitus. However, when these same people switched to tinnitus habituation therapy, they achieved this goal in only one year! Masking or suppressing tinnitus by white noise is only possible about 30% of the time anyway. Although masking can provide symptom relief, it cannot produce habituation.[38]

### White Noise vs. Pink Noise

What's with the "color" of noise—white noise, pink noise, red noise, etc.? As audiologist Theresa Cullen, Au.D. explains, "This rainbow of masking sounds contain all the frequencies that are audible to humans—20 – 20,000 Hertz—but the way power is distributed among those frequencies differs".[39]

In case you are interested, white noise is a sound containing a blend of all audible frequencies distributed over the various audible frequencies with **equal energy per hertz** (frequency). Thus the sound energy is the same between say 50 and 60 Hz as it is between 4,000 and 4010 Hz. Putting it another way, white noise has equal power distribution throughout all frequencies, so both low and high frequencies are presented at the same volume. Most people hear white noise as a hissing sound or much like the static you heard in years gone by when an FM radio was not tuned to any station.

In contrast, the energy in red (or Brownian) noise is inversely proportional to frequency, so higher frequencies are softer than lower frequencies. That is, red noise has most energy in the lower frequencies and less and less energy as you go up the frequency spectrum. The energy per frequency decreases by 6 dB per octave.

About 1996, researchers defined "pink" noise. Why pink noise? Because its half way between white noise and red noise. In pink noise, the power per hertz decreases as the frequency increases so the lower frequencies are louder than the higher frequencies. This is because pink noise has **equal energy per octave**. However, because lower octaves contain fewer frequencies than higher octaves, the energy per frequency reduces by 3 dB per octave as you go up the frequency spectrum. For example, there are just 125 frequencies in the octave from 125 Hz to 250 Hz, but a whopping 8,000 frequencies in the octave between 8000 Hz and 16000 Hz!

Cutting through the technical jargon, for all practical purposes, pink noise is really just natural-sounding "white noise" (as your ears perceive it), with louder lows and softer high frequencies. Consequently it is more pleasant to listen to. In contrast, true white noise sounds harsher and tends to grate on your nerves as it has much more power in the high frequencies. As a result, pink noise can be a better choice for masking tinnitus sounds.

Dr. Cullen continues, "Each color of masking noise has its own suggested uses. Most habituation therapies start with white noise because it presents the widest range of frequencies. Pink noise is often recommended for sleeping. However, there is no harm in trying out different masking sounds to find what best works for you. You may find that one sound is consistently useful, or that different sounds work better for specific situations."[40]

Therefore, for long term control of your tinnitus you may want to try Tinnitus Retraining Therapy (TRT) and a white-noise sound generator (see Chapter 22). TRT uses noise generators set to a low volume. The white noise is set to the "mixing point" where the masking noise and your tinnitus blend together (non-masking mixing level).[41]

The idea is not to make your tinnitus inaudible, but to bring about changes in your subconscious hearing system. At the same time, the noise generators reduce the contrast between your tinnitus and complete silence (when tinnitus naturally emerges). Studies indicate that up to 80% of people are helped by TRT with devices set at or below the mixing loudness level.[42]

## Residual Inhibition-Inducing Therapies

### Tinnitus Masking for Residual Inhibition

When you mask your tinnitus for a period of time with a louder sound and then turn off the masking sound, you may find that you no longer hear your tinnitus at all, or it is now at a reduced volume. The "fancy" term for this is "residual inhibition."

Residual inhibition can be one positive side effect of masking your tinnitus. This resulting residual inhibition may last from a few minutes, to a few hours, weeks, months or years.[43] If this works for you, great! Then you'd only have to wear a tinnitus masker long enough to produce another stretch of residual inhibition. If you were lucky, you might only have to wear a tinnitus masker for say half an hour or so at a time in order to produce a week's worth of residual inhibition. Unfortunately, for most people residual inhibition is measured in seconds or minutes, not in days or weeks.

Residual inhibition is the natural process of the nervous system becoming desensitized to external stimuli over time. You can also invoke residual inhibition, albeit briefly, by overwhelming the auditory system with a very loud noise—a power saw, for example. One man found this was effective in temporarily stopping his tinnitus sounds.[44] (Note: I don't recommend this as the loud sounds from a "screaming" power saw are much more likely to make your tinnitus worse than to cause residual inhibition to occur!)

Residual inhibition can also occur when you mask your tinnitus with a frequency of sound that closely matches the pitch of your tinnitus and then turn the sound off. At this point, for numbers of people, their tinnitus either disappears, or is greatly reduced in volume.

One man discovered this for himself. He reported, "I have tinnitus. Tonight I was surfing the web and found a site that played pure tones at various frequencies when you clicked on the corresponding buttons. To my surprise, most of my high-pitched tinnitus went away for a while after listening to the higher-frequency sounds!"

The closer you match the pitch of the external sound to your tinnitus, typically the more your tinnitus is reduced, and the longer the residual inhibition lasts. Obviously, this works best for people whose tinnitus consists of a single, constant frequency of sound.

Thus, if your tinnitus is a constant tone, and you listen to a pure tone sound of the same frequency for 30 seconds or a minute, often you will find that your tinnitus disappears (or is greatly reduced) for several seconds (typically 30 to 60) immediately after you turn the tone off.

The sound does not need to be loud for residual inhibition to occur. In fact, you can cause residual inhibition with sounds just 10 dB louder than your tinnitus. (Note: You perceive a 10 dB increase as a sound that is twice as loud as before.) Also note that making the masking sound louder does not increase the length of time of the resulting residual inhibition.

Incidentally, the length of time you mask your tinnitus is no indication of how long your resulting residual inhibition will be. For example, if masking it for 60 seconds results in 1 minute of residual inhibition, it does not follow that masking it for 60 minutes will result in 1 hour of residual inhibition.[45]

A number of different tinnitus treatments cause residual inhibition for varying lengths of time afterwards—ranging from just seconds, to hours, to days, to several weeks or even months. In a few cases, the tinnitus may permanently disappear. I wish we were all so lucky!

There have been several commercial attempts to use residual inhibition to help people that suffer from their tinnitus. One product that showed early initial promise was the *Quiescence* tinnitus management software, but unfortunately, it seems to have fallen by the wayside. Even so, researchers are still studying the residual inhibition phenomenon, trying to understand more of how it works. Perhaps, in the future, they will discover a way to make the effect last long enough that it becomes a useful treatment for tinnitus.

Following are two tinnitus treatments that may produce significant residual inhibition. Unfortunately, in spite of their initial promise, neither one seems to be commercially viable for whatever reason. However, I've listed them here for your information as they really did work for some test subjects, and may yet provide the basis for future residual inhibition treatments.

## "Phase-Out" Phase Shift Tinnitus Reduction

If you have subjective tinnitus at a constant pitch (single frequency), you may be able to reduce your tinnitus. Fortunately, about 76% of people with subjective tinnitus do have mono-frequency tinnitus. Drs. Daniel Choy and Ivan Kaminow pioneered this unique treatment in 2000. It was granted FDA approval in the USA in 2003.

This treatment, called "Phase-Out" or the "Padden-Choy procedure" is now available via apps for the iPhone and iPad and Google mobile platforms, so you can treat yourself any time you feel the need to. (The iPhone app is called *Phase-Out*.)

In order to use this program, first you need to determine the exact frequency and loudness of your tinnitus. Then you listen to a special phase-shifted signal that matches your tinnitus in frequency and volume.

This sound signal is sequentially shifted out of phase by 6° at a time. You listen to this phase-shifted signal for 30 seconds, then it shifts another 6° out of phase for 30 seconds and so on until it has stepped sequentially though 6°, 12°, 18°, 24° and so on in 6° increments until it comes the full circle at 360°. This whole process takes 30 minutes.[46]

Treatment consists of listening to this phase-shifted sound several times a week. How often you need to do this varies from person to person.

After listening to the phase-shifted sounds, you may discover your tinnitus either partially or completely disappears. This residual inhibition may last from a few minutes, to a few hours and up to several weeks. The average is for this residual inhibition to last about one week.

When your residual inhibition wears off, you simply listen to your smart phone for 30 minutes a few times, then put it away until the next time you need it.

At present, there are no known negative side effects to this treatment.

How well does this "Phase-Out" phase shift tinnitus reduction program work? For people that meet the tinnitus criteria, between 83% and 91% of them experience a significant reduction (defined as 6 dB or greater) or a complete cessation of their tinnitus for a period of time.

The "Phase-Out" website reports,

> From 2000 to 2007, with a three decibel reduction (50% on a linear scale) as the success level and a treatment schedule of once a week, for three weeks, the success rate for the procedure world-wide was 61% with an average fall of 8.5 decibels.

> From 2007 to 2010, with the treatment schedule compressed to three times per week, the success rate increased to 81%, with an average fall of 7.6 decibels.
>
> In 2011, when the treatment schedule was further compressed to three consecutive days, 67 of 67 patients dropped their volumes by 8.4 decibels (86% on the linear scale). At this level, no tinnitus is audible.

Note that although this system shows some promise, the Phase-Out app has a serious drawback such that you may not want to use it. The big problem is that the set-up process is tedious and when you get it all set up, you cannot save your settings. Thus, you have to go through this whole process each time you want to use it.

Probably, you should wait until they update this app to make it more user-friendly. However, this may not happen as the last time they updated this app was May, 2012, which was 4 years ago at the time I wrote this.

You can learn more about the "Phase-Out" program at http://phaseoutapp.com/. The *Phase-Out* app for the iPhone is available on iTunes for $9.99.

## UltraQuiet Therapy

Another promising treatment for tinnitus, based on residual inhibition, is *UltraQuiet* therapy. Instead of masking your tinnitus with a sound at or near your tinnitus frequency, *UltraQuiet* therapy uses the frequencies well above human speech (10,000 Hz to 20,000 Hz) so the masking sound does not interfere with your hearing speech.

During this therapy, you listen to music (which has been processed and shifted in pitch) through a special bone-conduction transducer placed on the mastoid bone behind your ear. *UltraQuiet* therapy uses music rather than white noise since music has been found to be a better tinnitus-masking sound than white noise. The volume is set quite low—only about 6 dB above the softest sound you can hear—so it is not loud and intrusive.

You listen to this processed music for between 30 minutes and an hour twice a week for 4 weeks. The goal is to effect changes in your brain's tinnitus-generating circuits, resulting in long-term inhibition.

The interesting thing about this therapy is that it seems to produce relatively long term residual inhibition. Of eight people in one study, two had residual inhibition lasting 4 weeks, one for 1 week and four had residual inhibition lasting for 3 to 5 days. Two reported no residual inhibition.[47]

If you want to learn more about this therapy and learn whether it might benefit you, you can contact one of the pioneers in this therapy—Dr. Abraham Shulman, MD, Martha Entenmann Tinnitus Research Center, Health Science Center, State University of New York, 450 Clarkson Avenue, Brooklyn, NY 11203.

## Amplification (Hearing Aids, Cochlear Implants & Other Devices)

Since tinnitus and hearing loss often go together, it is no surprise that a majority of the tinnitus patients seen by audiologists require treatment for both hearing loss and tinnitus. Therefore, if you have both hearing loss and tinnitus, your audiologist could first try fitting you with hearing aids.

You see, when you strain to hear because of your hearing loss, you can actually make your tinnitus worse.[48] In such cases, wearing hearing aids or cochlear implants can be beneficial in helping get your tinnitus under control as your ears focus on real sounds. Furthermore, wearing hearing aids can help reset your brain's hearing system and reduce the over-activity associated with silence resulting in tinnitus.[49]

As Dr. Baguley, the head of Audiology/Hearing Implants at Cambridge University Hospitals in Cambridge, England explains, "Hearing aids are an enormous help for most tinnitus patients most of the time, even when their hearing loss is mild".[50]

That is why many people find that when they put on their hearing aids or cochlear implants in the morning, they soon forget about their tinnitus. Hearing real sounds again partially masks their tinnitus sounds, not to mention taking their minds off these sounds. Thus, their tinnitus simply fades into the background for the rest of the day.

Note that hearing aids by themselves, although helpful, do not give the good results that wearing them while combining them with other tinnitus treatments such as Tinnitus Retraining Therapy do. When asked what percentage of patients experience tinnitus relief from the use of hearing aids only, Dr. Jastreboff explained, "In my experience, if hearing aids are used alone, the success rate is about 15%; when hearing aids are used as part of TRT, their effectiveness is over 80%".[51]

In addition, by masking your tinnitus with hearing aids—and since 80% of people with tinnitus have hearing loss—this will typically help you reduce your stress and allow you to communicate more easily and engage in pleasant social situations, which your untreated hearing loss may prevent you from enjoying.[52].

Here's something else of which you should be aware. Modern hearing aids can cut out a lot of background noise. Normally this is a blessing. However if you have tinnitus, you need to avoid silence. Therefore, your audiologist should adjust your hearing aids so they do not remove all the typical lower-frequency background sounds. You may even want your audiologist to program another program with the noise reduction turned off so your ears can take full advantage of any background sounds to help mask your tinnitus.[53]

Your reaction to the configuration of a particular hearing aid or sound generating device is subjective. Thus, there is no right or wrong combination of features for you to use when it comes to tinnitus treatment. As a result, your audiologist should try different combinations of features at various settings to find out what's right for you.[54]

One question that people ask is, "If I have tinnitus in only one ear, should I get two hearing aids?" This is a good question. Since the vast majority of people with tinnitus already have some hearing loss in both ears, you should go with two hearing aids. This is because "if you fit one ear only, you're very likely to replace your tinnitus with an even more annoying sense of imbalance—everything being louder in the one ear".[55]

## Middle Ear Implants

Middle ear implants such as MedEl's *Vibrant Soundbridge* are alternatives to conventional hearing aids. One advantage is that middle ear implants allow more power to be delivered to the cochlea, especially in the higher frequencies. For example, using the *Vibrant Soundbridge,* people with severe tinnitus and high-frequency hearing loss achieved relief of their tinnitus after being implanted. People with significant residual inhibition (residual inhibition was explained earlier in this chapter) of their tinnitus and high-frequency hearing loss seem to be the best candidates for this implant.[56]

## Cochlear Implants

If you are deaf, or nearly deaf, and have tinnitus, quite often getting a cochlear implant will cause your tinnitus to reduce significantly or go away. Cochlear implants may help to reduce your tinnitus in two ways. First, as with hearing aids and middle ear implants, your cochlear implant may increase ambient normal sounds and thus mask your tinnitus. Second, the electrical stimulation of your auditory nerve by your cochlear implant may suppress your tinnitus.[57]

In one study, half of those who had tinnitus before they received their cochlear implants experienced tinnitus relief soon after they were "turned on".[58] For those with **severe** tinnitus before their cochlear implants, the good news is that up to 90% received relief from their tinnitus.

Unfortunately, 5–7% of the people getting cochlear implants experience a worsening of their tinnitus. That is why in the USA, it is forbidden to implant CIs in people who have normal hearing in both ears, yet suffer from tinnitus.[59]

Although you are not eligible for cochlear implants if you still have significant useable hearing in your better ear, there is one exception. If you have incapacitating tinnitus in your deaf ear, even though you have normal hearing in your good ear, you may be approved for a cochlear implant in your deaf ear in hopes that this will alleviate your tinnitus.[60]

However, getting a cochlear implant in your deaf ear, if you have normal hearing in your other ear, isn't the only option you have. Dr. Jastreboff explains,

> I have a number of patients with unilateral deafness who improved very well. I do not use or recommend cochlear implants on these patients but rather suggest CROS or BiCROS hearing aid systems. The method is based on combining information from the visual and auditory systems and is very effective. When using cochlear implants in patients with total deafness and tinnitus, it is necessary to remember that while it is helpful for about 40% of patients, some patients may experience a worsening of tinnitus after cochlear implantation.[61]

## Hearing Aids with Built-In Sound Generators

If wearing hearing aids by themselves isn't enough, or don't work for you, then your audiologist may try hearing aids specifically designed for people with tinnitus. These hearing aids offer the benefit of amplification along with supplemental tinnitus therapy sounds built in.[62]

When using hearing aids that have tinnitus therapy options built in, such hearing aids should be flexible enough to work:

- In one or both ears
- In just one or in multiple programs
- At different intensities in each ear
- At different intensities in the various programs
- With different noise types in each program and/or in each ear.

In addition, such hearing aids should also have a volume control designed such that the wearer can adjust the volume of the tinnitus therapy signal independently from the volume level of the hearing aid's microphones.[63]

When setting the level of the tinnitus therapy signal, follow the Tinnitus Retraining Therapy (TRT) protocol. That is, look for the mixing point where the tinnitus therapy sounds generated by the hearing aid mix with the person's tinnitus without masking it. This is because, in order to achieve habituation, the tinnitus therapy sounds must not completely mask the tinnitus. Instead, the person needs to hear both sounds.[64]

A typical setup would give you one program with regular microphone input and another program with the therapy sound mixed in.

Note: If you have normal hearing and have tinnitus, one approach would be for your audiologist to fit you with hearing aids and set the hearing aids to "noise only" mode without any microphone input.[65]

Some hearing aids offer built-in nature sounds as a tinnitus therapy option. Such sounds provide a positive, soothing and stress relieving listening experience. These hearing aids are ideal if you prefer a more natural therapy signal.[66]

## Hearing Aids with Built-In Fractal Tones

Another way of enriching your environment with real sound and at the same time gaining some relief from your tinnitus is wearing hearing aids that have fractal tones built in. For many people, fractal tones are much more pleasant to listen to than white noise.

Fractal tones use harmonic, but semi-random, musical relationships that are generated by a recursive process where the algorithm is applied multiple times to process its previous output. The resulting pleasant, ever-changing, harmonic but unpredictable relaxing tones—which sound much the same as wind chimes—follow the rules governing relaxing music, but are not associated with any music you may remember.[67]

The aim of this unpredictable fractal "music" is that you will listen to these tones passively, rather than actively.[68] This is by design because a "limitation of real music is its familiarity, which can produce active, rather than passive listening. Moreover, you can potentially retain repetitive music passages in your memory. This can either cause boredom, or unwanted memory repetitions, known as earworms."[69]

This is why they use fractal tones. Such tones achieve the benefits, but avoid the potential drawbacks of music. The result is that it is easier for you to habituate to your tinnitus because when you are passively listening, you are neither focusing on the fractal tones nor on your tinnitus.

In addition, the fractal tones these hearing aids generate can give you some degree of relief from your tinnitus. The theory is that the fractal tones help you relax and thus reduce the annoyance you feel towards your tinnitus.[70]

Note: You want to set the volume of the fractal tones so that you can hear them, but they should be relatively soft. Furthermore, the tones should not interfere with normal conversational speech. The idea is to set the volume so that the annoyance level of your tinnitus just begins to decrease.[71]

The manufacturer of Widex hearing aids has been the push behind using fractal tones for tinnitus therapy. Some Widex hearing aids include fractal tone generators for tinnitus sound therapy, which they call Zen music, rather than just producing white noise.

When given the choice between listening to sound therapy containing fractal tones versus programs containing broadband (white) noise, tinnitus sufferers overwhelmingly chose fractal tones—probably because of the inherent relaxing qualities of the Zen tones.[72]

In 2012, Widex introduced their integrated tinnitus management program, which they called Zen therapy (WZT). The objective of Zen therapy is ensuring that tinnitus does not negatively impact a person's quality of life.[73]

There are four key components to Zen therapy:

1. **Counseling** to educate the person and to assist the limbic system to modify its negative interpretation of tinnitus.

2. **Amplification** to stimulate the ears and brain.

3. **Zen fractal tones** (generated by hearing aids) designed to both relax and provide acoustic stimulation.

4. **Relaxation** strategy program including relaxation exercises and sleep management strategies.[74]

Widex advises people to use the Zen programs as much as they need to in order to control their tinnitus, let them relax and to avoid silence whenever possible.[75]

In one study, even though the participants had habituated to their tinnitus to an acceptable level, they recognized and in some cases achieved, an even greater appreciation for the benefits received from amplification—either by assisting their hearing or by continuing to minimize their tinnitus distress. This is particularly relevant considering that 17 of the 19 subjects originally complained about their tinnitus, not difficulty hearing.[76]

Thus, the good news is that as you begin to habituate to your tinnitus, you have less and less need for sound therapy, but you will find that your use of hearing aids alone or hearing aids plus fractal tones increases even after you have successfully resolved your tinnitus distress.

Furthermore, the Zen program is effective in reducing tinnitus handicap scores in a short period of time.[77] A survey of patients who had been fitted with hearing aids containing fractal tones indicated that 69% had reductions in their tinnitus reaction questionnaire's scores greater than 20 points.[78] The majority of the reduction occurred fairly rapidly—within the first two months of treatment.[79]

In case you are interested, Widex currently has a couple of hearing aids with built-in Zen (fractal) tones—the Clear 440 and the Mind 440.

## S-Tone Sound Therapy

Traditional sound therapy devices, including hearing aids, provide relief by masking a person's tinnitus with a background sound such as broadband noise. However, in most cases, the masking noise must be at least as loud as the perceived tinnitus in order to provide sufficient relief for the person with tinnitus.[80] In contrast, S-Tones are designed to provide relief at volumes 50% softer than the person's tinnitus, thus reducing the sound burden.

SoundCure developed the proprietary S-Tones. S-Tones occur when the carrier frequency is matched to the pitch (frequency) of your tinnitus and are modulated at 40 Hz. The result of listening to S-Tones is that the S-Tones produce synchronized, robust neural activity in your auditory cortex. In turn, modifying the activity of your auditory cortex interrupts tinnitus generation.[81]

S-Tones are effective at low volumes. Furthermore, they are more effective than broadband noise in reducing tinnitus. The S-Tones from SoundCure showed a greater reduction in tinnitus perception, even at soft volume levels, when compared with broadband noise.[82] Thus, S-Tones may be a good alternative to broadband white noise if you find white noise does not work for you.

The S-Tones are generated by SoundCure's Serenade device. You can learn more about S-Tones and SoundCure's tinnitus program at http://www.soundcure.com.

## "Notched" Music Therapy

Another version of sound therapy for tinnitus sufferers that shows promise consists of listening to a specially-modified version of your favorite music for about 2 hours a day for a year.[83, 84] How hard can that be when one of the benefits is reducing the volume of your tinnitus?

In order for this to work, there are two conditions you must meet. First, your tinnitus must be a tonal kind of tinnitus that stays at a constant frequency. Second, the music you listen to must be digitally modified to take out the frequency of your tinnitus—hence the term "notched music"—as you have a notch where there is no sound at your tinnitus frequency.

The way the researchers created this "notch" was to filter out a whole octave of sound centered on the frequency of your tinnitus. Then, you just listen to your music for about 2 hours a day for the next year. By the end of 6 months, you'll likely notice that the volume of your tinnitus has dropped significantly.

After 12 months, the people in the above study found their tinnitus had dropped in volume by about 28%, and their annoyance at their tinnitus had dropped around 22%. In contrast, those in the placebo group (who listened to their favorite music without the notch) actually had their tinnitus increase about 9% and their annoyance at their tinnitus increase about 7%. (There was no indication in this study as to what kind of music people listened to, nor at what volume.)

In another study, researchers studied 26 people who listened to notched music over a two-month period. "Their results found that attentively listening to notched music (without other sensory distractions) significantly reduced tinnitus-related activity in the brain"[85] thereby making their tinnitus quieter and less intrusive.

The reason this notched music therapy appears to work is neural plasticity. Apparently our brains are more amenable to change based on listening to sounds we like rather than to ones we dislike—hence the need to choose music you particularly like.

It appears that notched-music therapy may prove to be an enjoyable, low-cost and casual (relaxed) treatment for reducing tinnitus a significant amount.

One source of notched music customized to your specific tinnitus is available on-line at AudioNotch: Tailor-made Notched Sound Therapy at http://www.audionotch.com/. Subscription is $39.95 for 2 months, $79.95 for 6 months and $99.95 for 12 months. You listen to their customized notched-music on any MP3 player or your computer. They produce MPEG-3 files so any device that can play those files will work, including presumably many smart phones.

Another source of notched music, again customized to your exact tinnitus pitch, is produced by ProMedical Audio at http://promedicalaudio.com/. They have an app for the Apple iPhone so you can listen to your customized notched-music via your iPhone. The app, "Tinnitus Pro: Music Therapy" is available on the iTunes store for $19.99.

## Biomental Therapy

Dr. Hans Greuel in Germany has come up with yet another form of sound therapy called Biomental Therapy. His program also consists of two parts—learning about tinnitus and listening to special sounds. (Note: This is somewhat similar to Tinnitus Retraining Therapy and Neuromonics in some ways, yet, at the same time, is very different.)

Dr. Greuel's theory is that tinnitus (and some other ear disorders such as sudden deafness and Meniere's disease) are simply natural protective reflexes fighting against too many burdens. Basically, he feels that excess tension or stress hinders the blood circulation in your ears. This ultimately results in a noticeable disturbance in your ears, which is manifested in your brain as tinnitus.

He believes that tinnitus occurs mainly when you are under stress. After three to six months of constant stress, tinnitus impresses itself on your mind. You are now conditioned to it. This is why it seldom disappears on its own. Like Dr. Jastreboff, he believes that just as you became conditioned to your tinnitus, you can undergo treatment to de-condition (heal) yourself of tinnitus.

The first step of his program is to become informed about tinnitus and how it develops. Also, you need to read about people who have been successfully treated for their tinnitus. This gives you understanding and hope that it will work for you too. He gives much of this information in his book, *Up To The Ears—Sudden Deafness, Vertigo, Tinnitus*. He discusses the reasons behind tinnitus. You will then understand the close connection between stress and tinnitus. It is most important that you understand, and know as much as possible about, tinnitus and the conditions that trigger it. These triggers include such things as muscle tension in your jaw and neck, grinding your teeth, back tension resulting in back problems, high blood pressure, etc.

(Note that the symptoms of stress he mentions are basically the same as the symptoms we saw in Chapter 20 on Somatosensory Tinnitus. Thus, if you fit this profile, you would probably do well to seek out one or more of the somatosensory tinnitus treatments and use it in conjunction with Biomental Therapy.)

The second step is watching some video therapy, and listening to some audio therapy, files. These sounds will help cover up your tinnitus, and also help you relax. As you relax, the blood flow to your ears (and the rest of your body) will improve.

Concentrate on relaxing several times a day. When you have learned to relax with these sounds, it is possible that these sounds alone will stimulate healing. Therefore, listening to the tapes regularly is a prerequisite for successful healing.

The success rate is impressive. Tinnitus sufferers had a success rate of 88%. One lady who had suffered with tinnitus for 10 years and had tried many things without success wrote, "I have a typical tinnitus-personality. I recognized six qualities of myself in the book *Up To The Ears*. In only one week (of listening to the tapes) I was able to feel the pleasant sensation of warmness in both ears and a feeling of complete relaxation." After four months of listening to the tapes, she told how she now sleeps through the night, and gets up feeling refreshed and calmer. Her tinnitus is not as loud as it once was. She concludes, "Life is simply much nicer for me now".[86]

Since I wrote the above some years ago, Dr. Gruel has changed his program significantly. You can learn the details of his program on his "Tinnitus-Help Teletherapy Center" website at http://www.ohrfrei.de/eta1.html. This is now an on-line program that you can access for a very reasonable 85 Euros (about $92.00 USD).

## Healing Your Ears with Sound

Healing your ears with sound is yet another development in treating tinnitus. Actually, there are several versions of it used under different names. Note that these treatments are typically not specifically designed just for tinnitus, but are also used for other auditory-related problems such as hyperacusis (extreme sensitivity to sound), Meniere's disease and hearing loss, as well as for unrelated conditions such as autism.

No one really knows why these treatments seem to work but several theories have been proposed (more than 20 and counting).[87] It may be that the stimulation of the middle ear acts as physical therapy for the inner ear since each frequency stimulates a different area of the cochlea.[88] It may be that neural inhibition kicks in. This is where some neurons, when stimulated, inhibit the activity of other neurons.

Consider the information about the following two sound therapies in light of what you now know about tinnitus as revealed in Chapters 2 & 3, and also the information explained in Chapter 22 "Tinnitus Retraining Therapy".

## Dr. Tomatis' Sound Therapy

Dr. Tomatis' Sound Therapy consists of listening to special tapes/CDs/iPods of classical music that has been especially electronically altered to give your ears a "workout". You can listen while you are working or relaxing.

Dr. Alfred Tomatis, an ENT in France (now in Luxembourg), pioneered this version of sound therapy back in the early 1970s. Since then it has been modified several times.

For example, another doctor, Guy Berard made some modifications to the sound therapy program and called it "Auditory Integration Training". (See the next section.)

In addition, the mother and daughter team of Patricia and Rafaele Joudry made yet another variation to this sound therapy program and explain it in their book, *Sound Therapy: Music to Recharge Your Brain*. It explains how to listen, and what benefits you can expect for conditions such as tinnitus, fatigue, insomnia, stress and anxiety, hearing loss, sound sensitivity (hyperacusis), dizziness, Meniere's syndrome, jet lag and learning, memory and concentration problems.

Rafaele also authored, *Triumph over Tinnitus*. This book explains sound therapy's role in helping people with tinnitus. If you are interested, you can get these books through her Sound Therapy International website at http://www.soundtherapyinternational.com/v3/.

Sound therapy practitioners use Dr. Tomatis' Sound Therapy in treating various disorders such as hearing loss, tinnitus, Meniere's disease, hyperacusis, ADD, ADHD, autism, sleep disorders and a number of other conditions.

Dr. Tomatis' Sound Therapy doesn't work equally well for all these conditions. Thus, you have to understand what this version of Sound Therapy **realistically** can and cannot do for you.

This sound therapy is indeed a valid treatment for certain conditions, especially for children with learning disabilities, ADD, autism and related conditions. In fact, this is where sound therapy excels.

One Sound Therapy Practitioner explained, "I have seen incredible results in all 3 of my children with special needs from listening [to sound therapy music using an] iPod with bone conduction headphones".

However, when I asked her specifically what sound therapy had done for her ears, she told me that although she had been using sound therapy on herself for the past 9 months, she hadn't seen any difference in her tinnitus. This shows that this sound therapy does not work for everyone, not even for some firm believers in the program. On the other hand, it does work wonders for some people. Thus, like other tinnitus treatments, you really can't know if it will work for you unless you try it.

In general, for the **average** person with conditions such as hearing loss, hyperacusis, tinnitus and Meniere's disease, I don't think Dr. Tomatis' Sound Therapy is the best "starting choice". However, if you have tried other treatments and nothing is working for you, then by all means, give it a try. You may be surprised.

Dr. Tomatis' Sound Therapy sets out to rejuvenate both the middle ear and the inner ear. Its object is to keep your ears functioning at maximum efficiency, your inner ear fluids balanced, your middle ear muscles well toned, and the sensory cells in your cochlea stimulated. The idea is that when this is done, you should hear better, not suffer from vertigo so much, and find that your tinnitus is gone or much reduced.

Here is the theory behind Dr. Tomatis' Sound Therapy. (I'm not sure I agree with his theory.) Sensorineural hearing loss results from damage to the inner ear where the hair cells transmit sound signals to the auditory nerve. Loud or prolonged noise "flattens" these fine, hair-like appendages, called cilia, in the cochlea. "Flattened" cilia no longer pick up sound vibrations, so the sound does not reach your auditory nerve. A diagnosis of nerve deafness does not necessarily mean that the nerve is damaged, it may just be that the cilia have been "flattened".

Furthermore, Dr. Tomatis feels that a certain amount of hearing loss results when the two tiny muscles in the middle ear, the tensor tympani (attached to the anvil) and the stapedius (attached to the stirrup) lack proper tone. Good muscle tone and flexibility are essential if the middle ear mechanism is to accurately conduct sound to the inner ear. Lack of muscle tone means that the ear loses its ability to recognize certain frequencies of sound. Thus, these sounds never reach the inner ear.

When you listen to the sound therapy music, you exercise these two tiny muscles. Basically, Dr. Tomatis' Sound Therapy involves listening to music that has been altered such that the high frequencies and low frequencies are randomly shifted in and out. This challenges your ears with constantly alternating sounds of high and low tones, which causes your ear muscles to repeatedly tense and relax. This exercise restores the muscle tone and improves the functioning of the whole ear mechanism.

At the same time, you stimulate the hair cells in your cochlea. In Dr. Tomatis' Sound Therapy, the low-frequency (low tone) sounds are progressively removed and the high frequencies are augmented. Although quiet, the high-frequency sounds are raised in pitch until the only sounds you hear are between 8,000 Hz and 16,000 Hz. These high-frequency sounds stimulate the cilia. When the cilia have been "flattened" by too much noise the high-frequency sound stimulates them to return to their upright position. This restores the person's hearing in high frequencies to some degree.[89]

Dr. Tomatis' Sound Therapy gives you an opportunity to listen to these healing, high-frequency sounds even in the midst of a busy, noisy environment. Listening to this Sound Therapy music for three hours per day compensates for, and counteracts, the draining, stressful effect of much low frequency noise.[90]

According to Dr. Tomatis, his Sound Therapy has succeeded where tinnitus maskers have failed because it soothes the whole body, calms the mind and revitalizes the run-down brain cells.

Dr. Tomatis' Sound Therapy does not work for every person with tinnitus by any means. However, a number of people have reported that this sound therapy stopped their tinnitus when nothing else would work. Other people have noticed a significant reduction in their tinnitus. It has worked for people in their teens and in their eighties. It has worked for people who have had tinnitus for more than thirty years, and also for those who are just beginning to have tinnitus.

As with most tinnitus treatments, success takes time. It may only take twenty-four hours; but then again, you may not notice any results for fourteen months! Usually more severe cases take longer, so you should persist with the therapy for at least six months. The initial results of a listener survey showed that 20% found their tinnitus stopped completely. Another 36% reported their tinnitus was not as loud. An additional 44% experienced other benefits such as improved sleep and reduced stress, which made their tinnitus easier to cope with.[91] As Dr. Tomatis' Sound Therapy is a self-help program, its success depends very much on your motivation and commitment.[92]

If you want to investigate this therapy further, visit Dr. Tomatis' website at http://www.tomatis-group.com. From there you can find the official centers that practice this therapy throughout the world. Just click on the "Tomatis Network" button.

## Auditory Integration Training

Auditory Integration Training is another offshoot of the sound therapy originally developed by Dr. Alfred Tomatis. Dr. Guy Berard modified this treatment and brought it to the United States in 1992, calling it Auditory Integration Training.

Like Dr. Tomatis' Sound Therapy, the purpose of Auditory Integration Training is to recondition and normalize auditory responses in the middle ear and cochlea.[93] As a side benefit, this often reduces or eliminates tinnitus. Note that Auditory Integration Training is used in treating autism and other sensory disorders as well.

Auditory Integration Training consists of three detailed tests for hearing and a series of 20 half-hour listening sessions. These sessions are held twice a day for 10 days. The two sessions each day are held at least three hours apart. You listen to music that has specific frequencies filtered out, as determined by your initial assessment. The music is altered to randomly shift in and out the high and low frequencies. As well, the volume also shifts randomly. This makes the music sound distorted.

During each session, you will listen to this processed music through earphones. The music is played at a moderately loud, but not uncomfortable level.[94] As you listen, your ears receive a workout since the music is constantly changing from low to high frequency and from soft to loud.

For more information on Auditory Integration Training, visit http://www.auditoryintegration.net.

**Chapter 21 Endnotes**

1 Powers, 2015. p. 22.
2 Powers, 2015. p. 22.
3 Tunkel, 2014. p. S21.
4 O'Dell, 2015. p. 21.
5 Powers, 2015. p. 24.
6 O'Dell, 2015. p. 21.
7 Sweetow, 2015b. p. 30.
8 SoundCure, 2015. p. 1.
9 Piskosz, 2015. p. 26.
10 O'Dell, 2015. p. 20.
11 Piskosz, 2015. p. 28.
12 Henry, 2010a. p. 12.
13 Henry, 2010a. p. 12.
14 Piskosz, 2015. p. 26.
15 Sweetow, 2015a. p. 34.
16 O'Dell, 2015. p. 21.
17 Piskosz, 2015. p. 26.
18 Piskosz, 2015. p. 27.
19 Piskosz, 2015. p. 27.
20 Piskosz, 2015. p. 26.
21 Piskosz, 2015. pp. 26-27.
22 Piskosz, 2015. p. 26.
23 Piskosz, 2015. p. 27.
24 Robb, 2015. p. 17.
25 Moller, 2011. pp. 597-604.
26 Mayes, 2010. p. 78.
27 Mayes, 2010. p. 80.
28 Robb, 2015. p. 18.
29 Mayes, 2010. p. 77.
30 Mayes, 2010. p. 76.
31 Tunkel, 2014. p. S22.
32 Powers, 2015. p. 22.
33 Powers, 2015. p. 22.
34 Mayes, 2010. p. 79.
35 Mayes, 2010. p. 72.
36 Multicenter Study Finds S-Tones Beat Broadband Noise in Tinnitus Relief, 2014. p. 52.
37 BeyondTinnitus, 2011b. pp. 2-3.
38 Hazell, 1997b. p. 3.
39 Cullen, 2014, p. 22.
40 Cullen, 2014, p. 22.
41 Tunkel, 2014. p. S22.
42 Mayes, 2010. p. 74.
43 Coexisting with Tinnitus by Masking, 1997. pp. 1-2.
44 UB study finds that "crossed wires" in brain pathways controlling vision and hearing play a role in tinnitus, 2002. p. 2.

45 How is Tinnitus Diagnosed, 2004. p. 3.
46 Johnson, 2007. p. 2.
47 Goldstein, 2001. pp. 6-8.
48 Mayes, 2010. p. 42.
49 Mayes, 2010. p. 45.
50 Beck, 2015. p. 2.
51 Robb, 2015. p. 17.
52 Beck, 2015. p. 3.
53 Powers, 2015. p. 23.
54 Powers, 2015. p. 24.
55 Beck, 2015. p. 2.
56 Moller, 2011. pp 613-618.
57 Tinnitus Treatment Options, 2002. p. 2.
58 Tinnitus Treatment Options, 2002. p. 2.
59 "'We Cannot Do Anything About Your Tinnitus.' This Is Simply Not True", 2016. p. 6.
60 Moller, 2011. pp. 619-624.
61 Robb, 2015. p. 18.
62 O'Dell, 2015. p. 21.
63 Powers, 2015. p. 22.
64 Powers, 2015. pp. 22-23.
65 Powers, 2015. p. 23.
66 Powers, 2015. p. 24.
67 Sweetow, 2015b. p. 30.
68 Sweetow, 2015a. p. 34.
69 Sweetow, 2015b. p. 30.
70 Fractal Tones via Amplification for Tinnitus Relief, 2010. p. 1.
71 Sweetow, 2015a. p. 35.
72 Sweetow, 2015a. p. 39.
73 Sweetow, 2015b. p. 31.
74 Herzfeld, 2014. p. 24.
75 Herzfeld, 2014. p. 26.
76 Sweetow, 2015a. p. 38.
77 Herzfeld, 2014. p. 29.
78 Sweetow, 2015b. p. 30.
79 Sweetow, 2015a. p. 39.
80 Multicenter Study Finds S-Tones Beat Broadband Noise in Tinnitus Relief, 2014. p. 52.
81 SoundCure, 2015. p. 1.
82 Multicenter Study Finds S-Tones Beat Broadband Noise in Tinnitus Relief, 2014. p. 52.
83 Stracke, 2010. pp. 1-4.
84 Okamoto, 2010. p. 1.
85 Pape, 2014. p. 29.
86 Greuel, 1997.
87 Some Theories of AIT, 1997.
88 Treatment Possibilities, 1997. pp. 23-25.
89 Steele & Steele, 1997a. pp. 1-2.
90 Lacerte Marketing, 1997. pp. 1-2.
91 Treatment Possibilities, 1997. pp. 25-26.
92 Steele & Steele, 1997b. pp. 2-3.
93 McCarthy, 1997. p. 4.
94 Basic Information About Auditory Integration Training, 1997. p. 1.

Chapter 22

# Tinnitus Retraining Therapy (TRT)

Tinnitus Retraining Therapy (TRT) (also called auditory habituation or habituation therapy) is becoming increasingly popular as more and more medical professionals use it to effectively treat tinnitus. Dr. Pawel Jastreboff originally developed this therapy in 1988, and it has withstood the test of time.

When asked how TRT had changed over the past 25 years, Dr. Jastreboff replied,

> The model did not change over that time; however, its clinical implementation changed quite a lot. For example, we introduced the concept and treatment of misophonia, put more stress on retraining the subconscious part of the brain, and substantially changed the sound portion of the therapy. As a result of all of these changes, the time required for seeing improvement shortened substantially. In the early days, it took on average one year of TRT before patients saw some improvement. Nowadays, they may begin to see improvement in one month.[1]

If you have severe subjective tinnitus, this is one method you might want to try. Tinnitus Retraining Therapy has proven to work on many cases of previously intractable tinnitus. TRT has been used with great success by Dr. Jastreboff in the United States and Dr. Hazell (and since his retirement by Jacqueline Sheldrake) in Britain.

As Dr. Jastreboff explains,

> There are many treatments for tinnitus available now, but no method is as effective as TRT. For example, Cognitive Behavior Therapy (CBT) does

nothing for decreased sound tolerance and hearing loss, and published results show that it is not as effective as TRT. TRT can help save the quality of life of patients with tinnitus, decreased sound tolerance and misophonia.[2]

Tinnitus Retraining Therapy retrains the subconscious parts of your brain to ignore the sound of your tinnitus so that you are not aware of it, or, at least, are not annoyed by it any more. This is done in two stages. First you learn to remove your emotional response to your tinnitus. Second, you retrain your brain so you no longer pay attention to your tinnitus.[3]

Dr. Jastreboff based Tinnitus Retraining Therapy on the following principles.

- Your ears (and other sensory organs) process information at several different levels, and each level contributes to the final message that your brain processes.
- Your auditory (hearing) system is closely connected to the parts of your brain that control your emotions and your automatic response to danger signals.
- Your nervous system is like a giant filter, and continually modifies itself. Therefore, it enhances significant signals, and decreases its response to irrelevant signals.
- Your brain treats new sounds, and sounds associated with negative experiences, as significant. Such sounds elicit an emotional response that prepares your body for action. When these sounds are repeated, they are enhanced in your perception and are not buried under other signals. Repeated sounds that have neither a positive nor negative association evoke no response, and thus result in their habituation. Eventually you do not notice such sounds.[4]

Tinnitus Retraining Therapy involves an extensive audiological evaluation. You need a proper examination by an ear specialist to determine if you have any hearing problems or tinnitus triggers that need to be addressed. Next, you attend several directive counseling sessions where you learn all you can about tinnitus. You need this full explanation and understanding of what is going on in your ears, auditory pathways and brain to remove your emotional response to your tinnitus. Tinnitus Retraining Therapy also uses external sound, and for most people, external sound generators. It does not involve either surgery or drugs. The two major parts of TRT are directive counseling and wearing low-level, broadband noise generators.

When you successfully complete this treatment you will no longer be bothered or annoyed by your tinnitus. However, if you concentrate on and want to hear your tinnitus, you will. This is why it is a treatment, not a cure.[5]

## Caution—Find a Skilled TRT Practitioner

Tinnitus Retraining Therapy works very well when it is conducted properly. Unfortunately, not everyone that practices TRT does it properly. Therefore, Dr. Jastreboff cautions:

> Common misconceptions include: focusing on the conscious, cognitive part of the brain and ignoring the crucial role of subconscious centers; ignoring the fundamental role of conditioned reflexes; treating only tinnitus without concurrently treating hyperacusis and misophonia and without alleviating the effects of hearing loss; belief that use of ear-level instruments (i.e., sound generators, combination devices, hearing aids) are sufficient to achieve improvement; and ignoring the importance of specific counseling based on the neurophysiological model.
>
> Common errors are: counseling that is too general or too abbreviated and not tailored to the patient's educational level, specific needs and background; inconsistent counseling from a team treating the patient; false promises about the perception of tinnitus going away forever; use of shortcuts in the treatment without sufficient experience and understanding of TRT; inappropriate diagnosis (categorization) of patients; improper use of sound generators; too much medication that inhibits neural plasticity; running loud audiological tests when patients have decreased sound tolerance; and lack of follow-up visits.[6]

## Directive Counseling

By far the most important aspect of Tinnitus Retraining Therapy is the directive counseling. This is where you lay your fears concerning tinnitus to rest. This is where you demystify your tinnitus and discover how and why tinnitus affects you like it does. And most importantly, this is where you gain hope that leads to success! This is why you can even help yourself just by regularly reading this and other chapters in this book![7] For some people, this is all they need to habituate their brains to their tinnitus. They do not need to wear noise generators! You may find this so in your case.

The fundamental goal of directive counseling is to help you eliminate, or at least decrease, the negative feelings you associate with your tinnitus. In these sessions you will learn how your auditory system and brain work together and how this is relevant to your tinnitus. As you learn more, your fear and anxiety about your tinnitus will decrease.

The reason this works is because a known danger does not create as strong a reaction in your autonomic nervous system as an unknown danger does. It is this reaction of your autonomic nervous system that causes you to be annoyed by your tinnitus. Through directive counseling you work to decrease your autonomic nervous system's response to your tinnitus. And yes, this really works! One person said that he was pleasantly surprised with the immediate feeling of relief he felt after his directive counseling sessions although his tinnitus had not yet changed.

Following are some of the basic things you need to know about your tinnitus. We've covered some of this in previous chapters but it is summarized here as it is important to really know this. This knowledge will reduce your fears and anxieties.

## We Can All Hear Tinnitus

First, you need to understand that tinnitus is very common. You are not alone. In fact—surprise—everyone can "hear" tinnitus because tinnitus is a natural phenomenon.

Yes, given the right conditions we can **all** hear tinnitus. Here is the surprising proof. In an experiment, 80 young people without any signs of tinnitus were put in a soundproof room (one at a time) for just five minutes. Guess what? Ninety-four percent reported hearing buzzing or whistling sounds in their head or ears. The sounds they heard are identical to the kinds of tinnitus sounds we hear!

Our brains are so sensitive that they can detect the minute random background electrical activity continuously present in the myriads of nerve cells (neurons) in our auditory systems. Not only can our brains detect this neuronal activity, but under the right conditions, we can also hear this as sound. Every one of our neurons contributes, to some extent, to our tinnitus.[8]

What happened in the above experiment was this. The brains of these students, not hearing their usual background sounds any more, cranked up their internal hearing sensitivity until they could hear something—even if it was only the normal, random, meaningless, neuronal activity in their auditory systems.[9] Their tinnitus was temporary. When they came out of the soundproof room, their tinnitus disappeared as their brains turned the internal volume down again.

Even under normal conditions most people hear tinnitus from time to time. For example, after going to a loud disco or nightclub you've probably found your ears rang for a while after that. This is normal, and generally only lasts a short time (even though the loud music that caused it in the first place can leave you with a permanent hearing loss).

About 10% of the general population experience constant tinnitus. This happens because their brains focus on the meaningless weak background neuronal activity. Their brains do this because these people hold negative emotions relating to their tinnitus.

We need to distinguish between temporary tinnitus without any negative emotions associated with it, and the persistent tinnitus that causes distress. Note, too, that unrelated emotional events often trigger persistent tinnitus or make it worse. Such events could be things like bereavement, work or family stress, accidents or sickness, retirement, or moving to a much quieter place. Persistent tinnitus may also start while you are depressed or anxious. Quite often, tinnitus becomes permanent when you feel hopeless—when you despair that nothing can be done to stop it.

**Transient Ear Noise**

Almost everyone seems to experience transient ear noise a few times in their lifetimes. It typically occurs as a sudden whistling sound and may be accompanied by the perception of hearing loss.

This transient auditory event occurs only in one ear. Furthermore, it seems to occur completely at random without anything precipitating it. Often the ear feels blocked during the episode. The symptoms generally dissipate within a minute or so.[10]

For example, occasionally I will experience a sudden piercing whistle. The volume builds up to a peak in a matter of milliseconds and then rapidly reduces to nothing in maybe 5 to 10 seconds.

Some people have described these brief episodes of ear noise as "brief spontaneous tinnitus", but tinnitus experts do not consider them to be true tinnitus. In order to be considered true tinnitus, according to these experts, such episodes must last for at least 5 minutes and occur at least twice a week.[11]

If you have an untreated hearing loss—for example, you do not wear appropriate hearing aids—you have about twice the chance of having troublesome tinnitus. Here is why.

If you are hard of hearing, you often strain to hear. By constantly straining to hear, you are telling the lower levels of your brain to crank up the internal volume so you can hear better. Unfortunately, when your brain does this, it also picks up the random background neuronal activity. If you are old enough to remember tape recorders, you could think of this as similar to listening to a tape recorder with a tape in it—but you do not know the tape is blank. What do you do? You keep turning up the volume until you hear the background hiss of the blank tape.

How loud you hear tinnitus (or whether you even hear it) depends on whether your brain suppresses these sounds as meaningless, or whether it amplifies them because it thinks they are important and indicates a real or potential threat to your well-being.[12] If your brain perceives your tinnitus as random and meaningless, then it is easier for it to find other things to occupy its time. However, as soon as meaning is attached to a sound stimulus, it becomes "important" and thus your brain makes sure you "hear" it.[13]

## Most People Are Not Bothered by Tinnitus

Fortunately, these internal "sounds" seldom bother us. Most people (83% of the general population) are not normally aware of these sounds. In fact, they cannot even hear them except under unusual conditions. Why? They treat their tinnitus like any other sound they want to ignore. They have trained their brains to ignore (habituate to) these meaningless sounds. They can usually hear their tinnitus (when they listen for it), but they typically ignore it and their tinnitus is lost in the many meaningful sounds vying for their attention. The same principle holds true for other meaningless sounds. Think of the noise your fridge makes. You can hear it if you listen for it, but normally you don't hear it as your brain filters it out as meaningless background noise.

This should give you hope. You could be among this vast majority (97%) of the population that copes so well with tinnitus that it is not a factor in their lives. For those of you who find your tinnitus bothersome, annoying or debilitating, there is help for you. Keep reading.

## Here's How Tinnitus Develops

You likely first noticed your tinnitus when it was quiet around you. Maybe you had been to a concert where loud music was played, or perhaps you worked around loud noise. Now it is quiet, and you notice a ringing sound in your ears. Possibly you took a prescription drug. Maybe you were straining to hear in a quiet place and some random stray signals within your inner ear or in the lower part of your brain got past your lower level neuronal filters and now penetrate your consciousness.

Regardless of the source, when your tinnitus first emerges, it is a new signal. Because it is new, you notice this novel, unknown sound. It sounds like your ears are ringing. Since you do not have any pre-existing memory patterns of this sound, you have no means of categorizing it. Furthermore, new experiences tend to make you anxious. That is why your brain, until it properly evaluates what your tinnitus means, regards it with understandable suspicion.[14]

So, because it is a new sound, you focus on it. How annoying it is. You think, "I'll never be able to sleep with all this racket inside my head". You begin thinking, "I must have damaged my ears". Or you wonder, "Will it ever go away?" or even, "Do I have a brain tumor?" You want to know, "Just what's going on?" All your thoughts are centered on negative emotions—annoyance (that you can't sleep), fear (that you have damaged your ears or have a brain tumor), anxiety (what's happening to me?) and depression (it's never going to go away).

The conscious parts of your brain constantly communicate with the sub-conscious parts such as your limbic and autonomic nervous systems. Thus your emotions are involved. As well, your body is prepared for action. When these systems react to any sound, they keep your entire brain (both conscious and sub-conscious) focused on that sound. As a result, it is now impossible to ignore your tinnitus.

So guess what will happen? It's exactly the same thing that happens to every signal that your brain "hears". Because you are worrying about these sounds (a negative emotion), your limbic system—instead of filtering out these meaningless sounds—assumes they must be important, and cranks up your internal volume! Now you hear your tinnitus even louder. This upsets you even more. So what does your limbic system do? It thinks, "Boy, this must be a very important sound—look how upset master is getting! I'd better crank up the volume some more because he really needs to hear this!" And thus begins the vicious cycle that can drive tinnitus sufferers batty.

If your tinnitus troubles you, obviously you perceive it as a threat, or at the very least, something annoying rather than something that is of little or no consequence. The lower levels of your brain, including your autonomic nervous system, quickly react to perceived threats and immediately bring them to your consciousness. In the same way that an animal, alerted to danger by the sound of a predator, focuses on that sound in order to survive, you too consider that tinnitus is threatening or warning you. Consequently, you focus on it. Unfortunately, in this case, your built-in self-preservation system is working against you!

About 85% of those with tinnitus do not find their tinnitus intrusive, disturbing or anxiety provoking. This is something that tinnitus sufferers find very hard to believe! You must accept that it is your **reaction** to hearing your tinnitus that creates your distress, **not** the tinnitus itself. In truth, the loudness and pitch of your tinnitus does not play a significant role in how much your tinnitus annoys you.[15]

Whether your tinnitus annoys you or not is determined exclusively by the degree to which you experience negative feelings about your tinnitus (from your limbic system) and the increased tension you feel (from your autonomic nervous system). It has nothing to do with your auditory (hearing) system! This is just the opposite of the conventional wisdom regarding tinnitus.

## Retraining Your Brain

You now know that what triggers your tinnitus in the first place is an entirely separate factor from habituating yourself to your tinnitus once you have it. Also, you now know that how you react to your tinnitus determines whether it will persist and annoy you.

You have learned that tinnitus results from a conditioned reflex at the subconscious levels in your brain. As such, it is beyond your control. However, it is still accessible to behavioral retraining techniques. Herein lies the key to success. Tinnitus retraining is not just an abstract learning exercise in which you learn that your tinnitus is not a threat to you and your well-being. You also need to re-program your subconscious neuronal networks to pick up such signals on a "need to hear" basis. Because your neural networks have trained themselves to focus on certain signals in your auditory pathways, you must now retrain these same filters to ignore them.

In order for you to do this, you must discard the traditional concepts that tinnitus is caused by ear damage, dead hair cells, or the like. At the same time, you need to thoroughly understand that you perceive tinnitus because your neuronal networks have modified the way they filter the signals in your auditory pathways. You must understand (and believe) that these filters can be reset so they will no longer transmit tinnitus messages to the conscious part of your brain. This can happen because the presence of any continuous stimulus usually results in a process called habituation, whereby you respond less and less to the stimulus as long as it does not have any special negative meaning.[16]

If you have a hearing loss, you must be carefully fitted with hearing aids to remove any listening strain. Straining to hear can actually make your tinnitus worse by causing your neuronal networks to further amplify the sound signals in the sub-conscious parts of your brain. This makes it easier for them to pick up the tinnitus signals at the same time. Also, if you just wear one hearing aid when you have a hearing loss in both ears, you are likely making further trouble for yourself. This makes your hearing asymmetrical and is bad for your tinnitus.[17] This is why it is important to be fitted with appropriate hearing aids before you begin Tinnitus Retraining Therapy. Note that getting inappropriate hearing aids from someone who is not experienced in tinnitus management can actually make your tinnitus worse.[18]

The idea in Tinnitus Retraining Therapy is to block tinnitus-related neuronal activity from reaching the conscious level of your brain where you hear it. You also need to prevent tinnitus-related neuronal activity from activating your limbic and autonomic nervous systems. In order to make this happen, you must first train your brain to classify tinnitus-related neuronal activity as representing neutral, non-significant signals. Then, and only then, will your neuronal networks begin to filter out these sounds, and not bring them to your conscious attention.

You need to realize that your tinnitus does not spell a lifetime of anguish and despair. This may take several months or even years. If you also have other sources of anxiety or depression, it can take even longer. This process is not easy since firmly held beliefs are hard to change. However, be assured, you can change. With appropriate directive counseling from professionals, you can change even your strongly held views that tinnitus is a threatening and unpleasant experience that you cannot alter.

To habituate to your tinnitus, you first have to remove any negative associations attached to it. Signals that induce fear, indicate danger or are associated with unpleasant situations can never be habituated. This is because if you are to avoid danger and unpleasant situations, your brain must never ignore (or habituate to) sounds that warn you.

When we sleep the conscious parts of our brains shut down—we neither see, hear nor feel anything. However, even soft sounds can still awake us. When a sound has special meaning we learn to respond to it, like a baby waking in the night or the creaking of a floorboard when someone steps on it. This is because the subconscious filters in our auditory pathways will detect weak patterns of sounds if they are important to us. These conditioned responses also trigger activity outside our auditory systems because of the large number of connections to our limbic (emotional) systems and autonomic nervous systems (which turns on our body's "ignition key" to prepare us for action, whether it be flight or fight). This precludes sleep or concentration on less important things.

Each sound that we hear, and learn the meaning of, has an "emotional label" attached to it. This may change from time to time according to how we feel at that time, and depending on the context in which we hear it. So, once tinnitus loses its sinister meaning, no matter how loud or unpleasant it has been, it does begin to diminish. In many cases, we may not hear it for long periods of time.

This process takes a long time (often 2 years or so). During the initial stages your tinnitus gradually becomes less unpleasant (but you will still hear it as a loud sound). You are in the process of habituating your **reaction** to your tinnitus. You are not as annoyed as you used to be by your tinnitus.

Next, you will notice that your tinnitus is becoming quieter for longer periods of time. Eventually it disappears, or becomes a natural part of the background "sound of silence". You have now habituated to your **perception** of tinnitus. This is the final stage in Tinnitus Retraining Therapy. You no longer hear your tinnitus because your neuronal networks have filtered it out, and not sent it to the conscious part of your brain. In fact, you may no longer be able to hear your tinnitus, even when you listen for it.

How well does Tinnitus Retraining Therapy work? One study evaluated the efficacy of Tinnitus Retraining Therapy in 702 patients. "After an average of 33 months of treatment, 68% of patients described an improvement in their tinnitus. Of those reporting improvement, 80% described habituation of their perception of tinnitus. Success rates were strongly correlated to the total length of treatment and to adherence to the TRT recommendations."[19] Thus, the key to success in using TRT is to commit to following the entire program for as long as it takes to bring your tinnitus under control. If you do not do this, you are basically wasting your time and money taking the Tinnitus Retraining Therapy program.

## Low-Level Sound Generators

The second major part of Tinnitus Retraining Therapy uses low-level sound, often from special sound generators, to help habituate your brain to your tinnitus.

As you have learned, tinnitus often emerges when there is silence around you. In fact, most people first hear their tinnitus at night in a well-soundproofed bedroom or in a quiet living room. How long your tinnitus lasts depends on the negative emotions you attach to it, and also on the contrast it creates with your normal auditory environment. Thus, if you are in a quiet room, there is greater contrast between your tinnitus and the silence around you—so you more easily hear it. If you have tinnitus you should avoid silence as much as possible. That is why good tinnitus retraining programs include sound therapy (typically white noise). It reduces the contrast between your tinnitus and complete silence.

Incidentally, if you have a significant hearing loss, unless you wear your hearing aids all the time, you mostly live in a world of silence. This is especially true if you live alone. The house is silent even when there are environmental noises that hearing people readily hear. Therefore, you will be able to hear your tinnitus far more easily than people with normal hearing will. This is one reason you should wear hearing aids all the time.

However, if you don't—and I am one of these, since I only wear my hearing aids when I am specifically talking with people—you should surround yourself with some faint background sounds to reduce the contrast between your tinnitus and the silence. I don't often do this when I am writing since it breaks my concentration. As a result, I easily hear my tinnitus because all is so quiet—the only sound that intrudes into my silence is the faint clicking of my keyboard as I type. If my tinnitus begins to bother me, I play some classical music.

In Tinnitus Retraining Therapy, your counselor will advise you to avoid silence and immerse yourself in a low-level, emotionally-neutral sound environment. This sound can come from various sources. Its purpose is to increase the activity of your auditory filters. The preferred instruments are broadband noise generators that look much like behind the ear hearing aids. Using these special noise generators speeds up the process of retraining. However, if you use them, it is critical that you use them correctly, or your tinnitus may get worse.

About 60% to 70% of the people taking Tinnitus Retraining Therapy use these noise generators, but they are not absolutely essential. In fact, for many people with tinnitus, just enriching their sound environment according to specific directions, combined with specific counseling, is all that they need.

Note that the directive counseling is a crucial element of Tinnitus Retraining Therapy. Even the best noise generators in the world will not help you much without proper counseling. Also, although you can use white noise on its own to give yourself some temporary relief from tinnitus, unless you combine it with the retraining approach, you have little chance of permanent relief.

In contrast to tinnitus maskers, which produce sounds louder than your tinnitus, the white noise generators used in Tinnitus Retraining Therapy have an entirely different goal. Tinnitus masking was once thought to be useful because it made your tinnitus inaudible. This has proven to be largely counter-productive. You see, your brain needs to be able to detect your tinnitus in order for Tinnitus Retraining Therapy to work. This is because in order to retrain your neuronal networks to habituate to your tinnitus, you must be able to hear it. It is impossible to retrain your brain on something that it cannot detect!

Therefore, in Tinnitus Retraining Therapy you set your noise generators to a very soft level that blends and mixes with your tinnitus. It is very important that you set the volume low enough so it does not mask your tinnitus. White noise contains all frequencies, and therefore, very gently stimulates all the nerve cells in your subconscious networks, allowing them to be more easily programmed, or reset, so that you can no longer detect your tinnitus. The white noise also reduces the contrast between tinnitus and otherwise total silence.[20]

Incidentally, some people find their tinnitus gets louder soon after using white noise generators. This is temporary, and is actually a positive sign that their brains will habituate to their tinnitus.

The process of retraining your neuronal networks takes one to two years, although you can see results as early as one month.[21] Once your brain habituates to your tinnitus, you can discontinue this treatment.

## Tinnitus Retraining Therapy Works

Does Tinnitus Retraining Therapy really work? You bet it does—often simply reading about it without even getting professional help! In a letter to Dr. Hazell, one person wrote, "Just reading your advice on tinnitus seems to have reduced my ear noise by 50% and I am less worried about it". This is quite common. According to Dr. Hazell, many people have similar experiences. So by reading the information in this chapter (and indeed this whole book), you have involved yourself in a simple form of tinnitus retraining without knowing it.

More than 80% of the people who go through Tinnitus Retraining Therapy find significant relief. There is another plus to this treatment—there are no negative side effects! It does not create any harm to you or to your body.[22] You achieve success when you realize that tinnitus is no longer an issue in your life.[23]

Using Tinnitus Retraining Therapy, some doctors report that 65% of their patients have been helped in the first year of treatment.[24] Ultimately, about 15% of their patients no longer notice their tinnitus, while about 80% find that their tinnitus improves to the extent that they are no longer aware of it unless they focus their attention on it. Even then, their tinnitus is not annoying or bothersome.[25] But get this—20% of the people who had long-standing, distressing tinnitus can no longer even hear it at all now! Wow![26]

Here is some more good news. Studies show a trend of continuing tinnitus reduction, even after ending TRT.[27]

Most people have heard of actor William Shatner who played the intrepid Captain Kirk on Star Trek for so many years. What a lot of people don't know is that he developed a severe case of tinnitus as a result of an explosion on the Star Trek set when he was in the wrong place at the wrong time. His tinnitus was so severe that he even began contemplating suicide until he tried Tinnitus Retraining Therapy. Here is his story.

About 1989, Shatner began to notice a new sound in his ears. This noise increased and bothered him more and more. Like many others, Shatner discovered that his tinnitus was worse in quiet surroundings. He noticed it most in bed at night, and before getting up in the morning. The incessant noise in his head frightened him. As Shatner says, "My terror came from two things. One was the sound itself. The other was fearing that it was going to get worse and you're never going to be able to sleep or concentrate again." In his darkest moments, he thought, "Will it be this way for the rest of my life?" It was at this point that he began to think of suicide.

Then his son-in-law suggested that he see Dr. Jastreboff. In January 1996, under the direction of Dr. Jastreboff, Shatner began the Tinnitus Retraining Therapy treatments. He was fitted with white noise generators to habituate his brain into hearing, but not listening to, the sounds in his head. As he says, "There's something comforting about it (hearing the white noise), like hearing rain on the roof or traffic in the background but not listening to it". Slowly he retrained his brain to ignore his tinnitus.

What was the result? After just three months of treatment Shatner said, "I've become accustomed to the hissing. My anxiety has gone. 80% of the time I can deal with the noise I'm hearing now. I've got tinnitus, but it doesn't affect me in my general life. Certainly it doesn't affect my work."

This is in stark contrast to the horror stories Shatner had heard of people who wouldn't even come out of their houses anymore because of their tinnitus. Recently, he made a call to a man in California who had promised to support Dr. Jastreboff's research. When he called, the man's wife told Shatner that in his depression her husband had committed suicide because of his unrelenting tinnitus. As Shatner now knows, this is a needless tragedy. Help was available if only the man knew where to look.

Shatner is now speaking up. He reassures people that although there is no cure in sight, there is help for their tinnitus. He encourages tinnitus sufferers, "Do not despair!"[28] He should know. Tinnitus Retraining Therapy worked for him!

**Chapter 22 Endnotes**

1 Robb, 2015. p. 17.
2 Robb, 2015. p. 19.
3 Hazell, 1997b. p. 3.
4 Jastreboff, 1997b. p. 1.
5 Olsson, 1997b. pp. 1-3.
6 Robb, 2015. p. 17.
7 Hazell, 1997a. pp. 5-6.
8 Hazell, 1997a. pp. 2-3.
9 Jastreboff, 1997b. p. 2.
10 Henry, 2010b, pp. 1-2.
11 Henry, 2010b. p. 2.
12 Hazell, 1997b. p. 2.
13 Hogan, 1998. p. 60.
14 Hazell, 1997a. pp. 2-3.
15 Jastreboff, 1997b. p. 2.
16 Hazell, 1997b. p. 2.
17 Hazell, 1997c. p. 3.
18 Hazell, 1997a. pp. 4-5.
19 Thong, 2014. p. 19.
20 Olsson, 1997b. p. 2.
21 Robb, 2015. p. 17.
22 Jastreboff, 1997b. pp. 3-4.
23 California Tinnitus Assessment Center, News & Notes, 1997. pp. 1-2.
24 Wade, 1995. pp. 26-27.
25 Jastreboff, 1997a. p. 2.
26 Hazell, 1997c. p. 1.
27 Moller, 2011. pp. 575-596.
28 Shatner, 1997.

Chapter 23

# Neuromonics Tinnitus Treatment

Neuromonics Tinnitus Treatment is a relatively new treatment for tinnitus. Developed by audiologist, Paul Davis, Ph.D. of Australia to reduce the disturbing effects of tinnitus, Neuromonics opened for business in Australia in 2001. It came to the USA in late 2005. More and more tinnitus treatment centers are adding it to their arsenal of tinnitus treatments.

The goal of Neuromonics is to reduce the physical, mental and emotional disturbance you perceive as a result of your tinnitus. To that end, Neuromonics uses a number of the same concepts used in Tinnitus Retraining Therapy (explained in the previous chapter), including the importance of directive counseling and the use of sound generators (although how these two programs use sound is different).

## Determining Whether Neuromonics Is the Right Tinnitus Treatment for You

Some tinnitus treatment protocols work for some people and not for others depending on the kind and cause of their tinnitus. Neuromonics is no different—it works for many people but not for everyone.

Neuromonics seems to have a few advantages over standard Tinnitus Retraining Therapy. One apparent benefit is that in the initial treatment stages, Neuromonics often gives a greater reduction in tinnitus symptoms more quickly than TRT because, unlike with TRT, it uses tinnitus masking at this point. Another apparent benefit of Neuromonics is that it uses music. Since most people find music more pleasant to listen to than straight white noise, people ore likely to successfully complete the Neuromonics program because of the music. A third benefit is that with Neuromonics you don't need to wear a tinnitus masker all your waking hours like you would have to with TRT. Instead, you'd typically wear the Neuromonics sound generator between 2 and 4 hours a day.

Audiologist James (Jim) Shafer, Au.D., has used Neuromonics since early 2006, and has been using TRT even longer. When asked how these two tinnitus treatments compare to each other, and why a person would choose Neuromonics instead of TRT, he explained that when properly done, since both use directive counseling and sound generators, it largely boils down to a matter of personal preference, lifestyle and cost.[1]

Neuromonics is not for everyone. Here are some of the factors that might cause a person to choose Neuromonics versus TRT (or any other tinnitus treatment).

- Neuromonics is only a good choice for people who have normal hearing or who have mild to moderate hearing losses. With greater losses, TRT with its sound generators combined with hearing aids provides a better "fit".

- To get the most out of the Neuromonics program, a person should have 2 to 4 hours (preferably 4 hours) during each day when they are reasonably relaxed. This is because the Neuromonics music is designed to relax you and slow down your heart beat. This just doesn't happen if you are caught up in the frenetic morning rush hour, if you are jogging on your treadmill, or if you are frazzled with a high stress job and never have a moment to yourself. If this is you, then TRT may be a better choice.

- Neuromonics is not for you if you don't like listening to music in the first place. If you'd prefer just listening to white noise, then opt for TRT instead of Neuromonics.

- Another factor to consider is the size and placement of the sound generators. With TRT, you wear what looks like either in-the-ear or behind-the-ear hearing aids (and indeed they now often are dual purpose devices—both sound generators and hearing aids at the same time, if that is what you need). You wear them just like you would normal hearing aids. The Neuromonics sound generator is more like an MP3 player or iPod. You wear it on your belt or put it in your pocket and plug in the special ear buds. Because of the ear buds in your ears, you can't wear hearing aids at the same time.

- Cost may be a factor. For example the total cost of TRT begins around $2,500.00 to $3,000.00, whereas the total cost of the Neuromonics treatment is more in the range of $4,500.00 to $6,000.00.
- Neuromonics is likely not for you if you have a fluctuating hearing loss since the Neuromonics sound generator needs to be programmed to fit your specific level of hearing.
- To be successful with the Neuromonics treatment, you need the ability to organize your day to fit in treatment periods. You do not need to find one 4-hour block of time. Neuromonics works just as well with several shorter blocks of time scattered throughout your waking hours.
- Neuromonics is probably not for you if you cannot eliminate factors that make your tinnitus worse, whether physical or emotional, for example, if you work in a loud environment without proper ear protection.
- Finally, you need to have realistic expectations. Don't expect that your tinnitus will miraculously disappear. However, do expect that your tinnitus will become softer and less intrusive so it will not bother you much or at all.

## The Neuromonics Tinnitus Treatment Program

Neuromonics tinnitus treatment typically consists of a 6 to 12 month program of support, monitoring, counseling and education combined with daily wearing of the Neuromonics proprietary sound generator/sound processor called the *Oasis*.

There are 5 stages in the Neuromonics tinnitus treatment program:

- Comprehensive assessment of your hearing and tinnitus
- Configuring the sound processor
- Phase I (preconditioning stage)
- Phase II (active treatment stage)
- Maintenance stage [2]

## Comprehensive Assessment

During the assessment stage, your audiologist does a complete audiological evaluation of your hearing ability. You may have a high frequency hearing loss of which you're not even aware—but you brain is—and the result can be tinnitus. (More than 70% of the people with hearing loss also have tinnitus accompanying their hearing losses.)

Your audiologist will then "test" your tinnitus to determine its frequency and perceived loudness. During this initial assessment, you will also fill out the Tinnitus Reaction Questionnaire (TRQ). Neuromonics uses the 26-item TRQ to subjectively measure how much tinnitus is affecting the quality of your life. You can see/take the TRQ on the Neuromonics website at http://neuromonics.com/trq2/.

For each of the 26 questions on the TRQ you rate them between 0 and 4 with 0 being "not at all", 1 "a little of the time" and up to 4, "almost all of the time".

You answer each question as to how your tinnitus has affected you only **over the past week**. Since you'll be taking this questionnaire at various points throughout the Neuromonics program, you can measure your progress—the more your score drops, the better your progress.

Incidentally, a lowered score does not necessarily reflect any change in the loudness of your tinnitus, but it does reflect a lessened impact of your tinnitus on the quality of your life.

Here are four of the statements on this questionnaire to give you a feel for the kinds of questions it asks.

- My tinnitus makes me feel tense.
- My tinnitus has led me to avoid quiet situations.
- My tinnitus has interfered with my ability to work.
- My tinnitus has interfered with my sleep.

Possible scores range from 0 to 104 with a score of 17 or greater being considered clinically significant.[3] Incidentally, when I took this questionnaire (just for fun), I was surprised to discover that my score was 0. I'm so thoroughly habituated to my tinnitus that I do not let it bother me although my ears are "ringing away" every waking moment, and "ring" louder whenever I write about, or help people with their tinnitus, which seems to happen almost daily.

During the initial meeting, your audiologist will develop a comprehensive profile of your hearing loss and tinnitus. This information is needed in order to program the Neuromonics sound generator to meet your specific needs.

Your audiologist also will explain about tinnitus and how your autonomic nervous system and limbic (emotional) system play a very important role in how intrusive you perceive your tinnitus.

In addition to the information on tinnitus you receive in your initial session, you will receive another 8 to 10 hours of information and counseling, either face to face, via email or by telephone, with the bulk of this coming in the first six months you are on the Neuromonics program. This helps keep you on track.

By the end of the initial session you will know whether the Neuromonics program is something you want to try or not.

## Configuring the Sound Processor

If you decide to proceed with the Neuromonics program, your audiologist will send your tinnitus/hearing loss profile to the Neuromonics headquarters. There, a technician will program your new Neuromonics *Oasis* sound generator/ sound processor to fit both your hearing loss and your tinnitus profile.

The *Oasis* sound generator/sound processor looks somewhat like an MP3 player that you listen to via special high-quality earphones. It contains several hours of highly modified Baroque and New Age music customized specifically to fit your profile. White noise is embedded in the music. Many people find white noise less "irritating" when it is embedded in music than listening to it alone like you do with the TRT program. The frequency range of these sounds lies between 100 Hz and 12,500 Hz.

It takes about two weeks from the time of your initial session until you will receive your customized Neuromonics sound processor.

## Phase I (Preconditioning Stage)

During the first phase of the Neuromonics tinnitus treatment program, which lasts between 2 and 6 months, you listen to the Neuromonics sound generator for a minimum of two hours a day, but in order to get optimal benefits you should listen to it for 4 hours each day. One study revealed that 75% of the people listening for 2 hours per day achieved at least a 40% reduction in their TRQ score, whereas 100% of the people that listened for more than 2 hours per day achieved this same result.[4] You can break up your listening sessions—you do not have to find a single four-hour block of time.

During the listening sessions, you want to be reasonably relaxed, not hard at physical work, or doing a task that requires your full mental concentration. You can typically listen while you go about your normal (unhurried) daily tasks. It is not something you have to stop and listen to—using up precious hours each day. For example, you could be eating your lunch or reading a book. You could also fit your listening times into relaxed travel times, or quiet work in order to meet your daily listening requirements.

The highly-customized "easy listening" Baroque and New Age music needs to be familiar to fit into the background of your conscious mind, rather than requiring active listening on your part. This music promotes relaxation in addition to its main purpose of auditory retraining.

The audio program (music) includes an acoustic neural stimulus (a fancy way of saying it contains white noise). This white noise is intermittent and varies in intensity. It is set a bit louder than your tinnitus. By setting the volume a bit louder than you hear your tinnitus, it masks your tinnitus and can bring you almost immediate relief while you are listening to it. For example, one man went to a clinic to be evaluated for the Neuromonics program. He explained, "While there I had the Neuromonics headset on while talking, and in a short time my tinnitus was almost inaudible. Note, this was a stock unit. It was not set up for my particular sound and pitch." You have complete control over the volume and set it to a comfortable level that brings you the most relief.

The purpose of listening to a pattern of processed music interspersed with white noise is designed to retrain the neural pathways in your auditory system to ignore tinnitus through a process called neural plasticity. In short, it interrupts your preoccupation with tinnitus and relaxes you. Getting your mind off your tinnitus is critical to your success since it is your emotional response to your tinnitus that typically makes your tinnitus so intrusive in the first place.

## Phase II (Active Treatment Stage)

When you have gotten your tinnitus under control as indicated by a reducing TRQ score, you enter Phase II. During Phase II the white noise is eliminated from the music so your brain is intermittently exposed to your tinnitus and is trained to filter it out.

The way this happens is that without the white noise in the background, your tinnitus is now louder than the soft notes of the music you are listening to. Thus in the short intervals between the louder notes your tinnitus briefly "appears". Since you are listening to the music, not your tinnitus, you learn to ignore your tinnitus in these tiny gaps in the music in a process called acoustical desensitization.

Note: If for some reason your tinnitus flares up, you can always go back to Phase I to bring it under control, then switch over to Phase II again. Some people need to do this, some don't. Don't let it discourage you if you have to do this. The goal is to get your tinnitus under control, not to see how quickly you can move through the program.

During Phase II, you set the music level low enough so it won't disturb you. If you have normal hearing, you can still hear environmental sounds and conversations through this "background" music. If you have a significant hearing loss, this is not likely to happen.

As you progress through Phase II and you retrain your brain, you will find that your tinnitus becomes less and less intrusive, even when you are not wearing the Neuromonics sound generator.

### Maintenance Stage

Once you are desensitized to the disturbing quality of you tinnitus such that your tinnitus no longer bothers you, you have entered the maintenance phase. By this time you are typically 6 to 12 months into the Neuromonics program. At this point you can reduce your listening sessions to suit your needs.

Incidentally, when most people reach this stage, they do not even need to use the sound generator any more. If you do need to use the sound generator, you will find that just brief listening sessions each day are all you typically need, unless you are having a "bad" tinnitus day.

In addition to the *Oasis* sound generator, Neuromonics has come out with several other units including the *Haven*, *Sanctuary* and *Refuge*.

## Be Cautious of Those That Downplay Directive Counseling

Although the Neuromonics sound generator part of the program is basically the same wherever you go, it seems that a number of places providing Neuromonics are downplaying the importance of the directive counseling. They appear to be relying on the Neuromonics sound generator to carry the whole load. This is leaving out a critical part of the program.

The reason directive counseling is so important is that tinnitus is not just a "physical" thing in your auditory circuits that can be manipulated by sound generators or sound maskers, but the volume and intrusiveness of the tinnitus you experience is closely tied to your limbic (emotional) and autonomic nervous systems. Thus you need to learn how to control your mind and emotions in order to successfully habituate to your tinnitus. (In fact, for many people directive counseling may be all they need to bring their tinnitus under control—it's that important.)

Therefore, if you are thinking about taking the Neuromonics program, be sure your audiologist places a high value on the importance of the directive counseling part of the program. Otherwise, you may largely be wasting your money.

Another thing of which you need to be aware is that if you begin using the Neuromonics sound generator and your tinnitus gets worse, stop using it and talk to your audiologist. There may be some other factors that are contributing to your increasing tinnitus and need to be addressed. You don't want to continue to do anything that makes your tinnitus worse.

## What Kind of Results Should I Expect?

The goal of Neuromonics (and indeed, many of the other tinnitus treatments in this book) is not necessarily to cure tinnitus, but rather, to reduce the amount of time you are aware of your tinnitus and reduce the degree to which it impacts your quality of life.

Therefore, the correct expectation of the Neuromonics tinnitus treatment program is not that your tinnitus disappears completely (although it does for some people), but that the volume and intrusiveness of your tinnitus drops such that you typically are no longer bothered by your tinnitus. As a result, you may go for hours without even noticing your tinnitus. This is success!

Does Neuromonics work? Consider the case of Tim. His tinnitus started and rapidly escalated until he could no longer tolerate the level of sound generated when his family got together. It disrupted his sleep. He could think of nothing else.

After taking the Neuromonics treatment he explained, "If I consciously listen for my tinnitus, it's there, or in stressful situations it's there. But during most of the day I'm not even aware of it, and I can sleep now without any medication. I would say there is a 60% improvement."[5] Again, this is success!

About 90% of the people taking the Neuromonics treatment have at least a 40% reduction in their TRQ score. Success is defined as at least a 40% reduction in tinnitus disturbance as measured by the TRQ, an average improvement of 67% and a 2-month time frame for the benefits to be felt.[6]

In one study, 95% of the people at 6 months had a reduction in their tinnitus disturbance of at least 40%, while 79% reported that their tinnitus was no longer disturbing them (in other words it was not clinically significant, meaning their TRQ score was 16 or less).[7]

Neuromonics doesn't work for everyone—but it does help a high percentage of the people who **stick** with this treatment. A lot depends on the individual.

For example, one man reported, "I went for a hearing evaluation. They offered several alternatives to deal with my tinnitus. I am convinced that Neuromonics is the way to go for me. The program is $4500.00 [at that time]—costly—but if I get the relief, it is money well spent."

Neuromonics has a good success rate (so do other tinnitus treatment programs such as TRT). However, it seems to have a higher acceptability rate, and that means that people stick with the program—which ultimately leads to success.

To find a Neuromonics tinnitus treatment clinic near you, type your zip code into the appropriate box at http://neuromonics.com/clinic-locations/.[8]

---

**Chapter 23 Endnotes**

1 Shafer, 2009. Personal communication.
2 Diiulio, 2007. p. 1.
3 Sinopoli, 2007. p. 1.
4 Sinopoli, 2007. p. 1.
5 Smith, 2007. p. 1.
6 Diiulio, 2007. p. 1.
7 Sinopoli, 2007. p. 1.
8 Neuromonics, 2009. p. 1.

## Chapter 24

# BeyondTinnitus Therapy

Two doctors, Dr. Hamid Djalilian (otologist) and Dr. John McGuire (otolaryngologist) have recently (2011) developed a new approach to tinnitus treatment—called "BeyondTinnitus". This treatment protocol is based on the latest understanding of how our brains generate tinnitus (see Chapter 3).

Here's a quick recap of the essential points. Before chronic tinnitus begins, three things have to happen.

- First, there needs to be an increase in the spontaneous firing rate in the area in the brain corresponding with the damaged region (region of hearing loss) of the cochlea. This hyperactivity happens fairly quickly. The damaged area of the cochlea is called the "lesion projection zone".
- Second, the sound frequencies that border the damaged area in the cochlea become associated with the hyperactivity that is occurring in the lesion projection zone. These frequencies at the edge of the damaged area are appropriately called the "lesion edge frequencies".
- Third, neural plasticity must kick in and create new connections between the auditory and limbic systems.[1]

When these three events occur, you end up with annoying tinnitus.

Since the lack of sound signals in the damaged area of the cochlea results in tinnitus, it logically follows that the most effective sound frequencies used in treating the resulting tinnitus are the sound frequencies that are closest in frequency to your tinnitus. Research has borne this out.

However, listening to a sound similar to your tinnitus will itself be very annoying because it will sound just like your tinnitus.[2] If your tinnitus is already annoying you (and you wouldn't be seeking help if it didn't), then listening to another sound similar to your tinnitus will be just as annoying.

Fortunately, Drs. Djalilian and McGuire have come up with a novel way to not only help reduce your tinnitus using sound therapy, but one that is also pleasing to listen to.[3]

The goal of sound therapy is creating a real external sound that will induce your brain to stop its excessive spontaneous neuronal hyperactivity in the damaged area of the cochlea (lesion projection zone). This will provide tinnitus relief.

The most effective way to mask tinnitus is not to use a broadband white-noise approach, but rather, to focus all the acoustic energy on the lesion edge frequencies. The more closely the masking sound corresponds with the lesion edge frequencies, the more effectively it will suppress your tinnitus.[4]

The BeyondTinnitus therapy program includes a new customized masking strategy called "Harmonic Sound Therapy". This strategy delivers focused acoustic energy at the lesion edge frequencies, yet at the same time allows significant portions of the hearing spectrum to remain unmasked.[5]

Here's how it works. A special part of your brain, the "pitch cortex", processes pitch. It is organized like a helix. Each coil of the pitch cortex represents one octave. The essence of Harmonic Sound Therapy is to use the lesion edge frequency and its several sub-octave tones (tones that are at octave intervals lower than the lesion edge frequency) to decrease hyperactivity in the lesion projection zone via the pitch cortex.[6]

Using the sub-harmonic tones in addition to the tinnitus frequency tone avoids the noxious quality that would result if the BeyondTinnitus protocol only stimulated tones at the tinnitus frequency. The BeyondTinnitus protocol uses those sub-harmonic notes that most effectively lead to tinnitus masking—producing masking sounds that are both comfortable to listen to, and at the same time give you the most tinnitus relief.[7] The result is not just a single tone, but rather, "a band of structured noise that surrounds your tinnitus frequency and its sub-harmonics".[8]

This protocol takes into account the tinnitus frequency, the right ear-left ear balance, and the difference in hearing from low to high tones. It uses these factors to create a customized Harmonic Masking File for each user. Since each person's tinnitus is different, the harmonic sound file will also be different for each person. "The result is a file that sounds much like water running in the background. Those who use these customized masking sounds feel as if the file 'brings their head into balance', almost as if they are not listening to anything at all."[9]

The BeyondTinnitus treatment program consists of three parts.

First, the **preliminaries**: These include determining the loudness and frequency of your tinnitus, as well as determining which ear hears tinnitus louder. This is all done via software on the Internet. Based on this, you will receive a special customized Harmonic Masking File.

Second, the **induction stage**: During this stage you listen to the Harmonic Masking File (sound therapy file) for a minimum of 8 hours a day for two weeks (or even longer if you feel it necessary). You should soon notice a reduction in your tinnitus annoyance.

Third, the **maintenance stage**: During this stage you listen to the Harmonic Masking File for a minimum of 2 hours per day, and, in addition, any other time when your tinnitus is bothering you. Incidentally, as your tinnitus changes, so will your Harmonic Masking File, but you can easily update it over the Internet.

During this stage you can, and should, merge the kind of music you love with your Harmonic Masking File to produce Music Therapy files. (You can actually mix your favorite MP3 music with your customized Harmonic Masking File to create Music Therapy files on your computer.) Doing this allows you to listen to your favorite music and at the same time, let the sound therapy do its work in the background.[10] This will further help you transform your negative emotional states associated with tinnitus into the positive emotional states associated with music.

You can expect to remain in the maintenance stage for three to six months. However, as the months roll by, you will likely find that you don't need to listen to these files as much as you did at the start, and eventually you may not need to listen to them at all.[11]

One of the cool things about this program is that you do it all over the Internet—no doctors' appointments are necessary, so you can use this tinnitus treatment program no matter where you live in the world.

This program originally was designed for people that have tinnitus but do not have significant hearing loss. That is why the harmonic masking files and the music therapy files are meant to be listened to with special headphones

(AirDrives: see http://www.airdrives.com) that do not block your ears, so allow outside sounds in.

However, if you have a severe hearing loss and wear hearing aids, you can still use this program. All you need to do is couple your hearing aids via their t-coils to your MP3 player or iPod by plugging a neckloop into the earphone jack. Then you set your hearing aids to the combined microphone/t-coil setting so you can hear both the therapy files and yet still hear other sounds around you.

You will likely do very well on this program if you have constant tinnitus that can be frequency-matched; you have normal hearing, or mild to severe hearing loss; and you are not unduly anxious about your tinnitus.

If you are unduly anxious or depressed, in addition to the BeyondTinnitus program itself, you will probably need additional directive counseling regarding your attitudes towards your tinnitus in order to gain much benefit from this program.

Preliminary results indicate that 88% of the people completing this program will have reduced tinnitus impact, while it will not significantly affect the tinnitus of 12% of the people taking it. Of the people that are helped, about 75% of them will have at least a 25% reduction in their tinnitus while the remaining 25% will have a much more substantial reduction.

Dr. Djalilian emphasizes that this is not a miracle cure for tinnitus, but for many people this program will help reduce their tinnitus. If you are like most people, you will have to "work" at it. Remember, tinnitus has both a physical and a psychological component. This program addresses the physical component, but at the same time, you will have to address the psychological component so your tinnitus won't continue to bother you. The information contained in this book will go a long ways in helping you mentally/emotionally adjust to your tinnitus.

The BeyondTinnitus system is similar to Neuromonics. However, its big advantage over Neuromonics is that you can use your own MP3 music rather than listen to the same 4 tracks that Neuromonics has on their device.

Here's some more good news—this program is designed to be affordable. It doesn't cost an arm and a leg like some of the other tinnitus treatments do. For example, the BeyondTinnitus program only costs about one tenth as much as the Neuromonics program since it is delivered via the web. The standard six-month personalized sound therapy program will only set you back $399.99 (USD). You can learn more about the BeyondTinnitus treatment at http://www.beyondtinnitus.com.

### Chapter 24 Endnotes

1 BeyondTinnitus, 2011b. pp. 1-2.
2 BeyondTinnitus, 2011a. p. 1.
3 BeyondTinnitus, 2011a. p. 1.
4 BeyondTinnitus, 2011b. pp. 2-3.
5 BeyondTinnitus, 2011b. p. 3.
6 BeyondTinnitus, 2011b. pp. 3-4.
7 BeyondTinnitus, 2011b. p. 4.
8 BeyondTinnitus, 2011b. pp. 4-5.
9 BeyondTinnitus, 2011b. p. 5.
10 BeyondTinnitus, 2011a. p. 1.
11 BeyondTinnitus, 2011c. pp. 1-2.

Chapter 25

# Natural Remedies for Tinnitus

There are a number of different kinds of natural remedies for tinnitus including homeopathic remedies, vitamins, minerals, antioxidants and herbals. All have some merit, depending on the exact kind of tinnitus you have.

## Homeopathic Remedies

Homeopathy is not very common in North America, but it is a respected profession in much of Europe and elsewhere in the world. Note that homeopathy is not a new or passing fad. It has been around for almost 200 years. Basically, homeopathic remedies are very dilute preparations extracted from herbs. Because they are so dilute, there are no negative side effects.

Homeopathic preparations are not wonder drugs that promise results immediately. Rather, homeopathy is a slow process than needs time to work. As a result, people who persist with homeopathic treatments for two or three months or longer experience far greater success than those who simply stop after six weeks or so. In some cases, it can take three to six months for the benefits of a homeopathic remedy to become evident.

As a general rule, it takes about one month to provide complete relief from tinnitus for every year that you've suffered from the condition. Thus if you have had your tinnitus for ten years, you could expect it will take ten months of homeopathic treatment to eliminate your tinnitus, although you will likely see substantial improvements in your tinnitus within the first two months.

Even so, there is no guarantee homeopathic remedies will do the trick for you. Some people don't respond to these remedies, just like some people don't respond to one or more of the other treatments listed in this book. Thus, try homeopathy if you like. If it works for you—great. If not, go on to something else.

With homeopathy, sometimes at the beginning of a treatment the symptoms seem to get worse. Strange as it may seem, in some cases, you need to have this initial worsening of the symptoms before you get better. Unfortunately, at this point a number of people abandon the treatment as worthless—when, in fact, it is really working.

Most western doctors pooh-pooh homeopathy, but if you want to try it, the worst it will do is flatten your wallet a bit. However, a number of people swear by homeopathic remedies because their tinnitus has gone away completely after treatment, or was greatly reduced in volume. I don't argue with success!

There are three major homeopathic preparations designed specifically to help people with tinnitus about which I know at this time.

**T-Gone Tinnitus Remedies**: The people at T-Gone have studied tinnitus for a number of years and have done something unique. They have broken tinnitus down into several different categories—which makes a lot of sense to me. Then they have carefully formulated specific tinnitus remedies for each type of tinnitus. Thus if you correctly identify your tinnitus type (and they will help you), you have a better chance of reducing your tinnitus.

According to John Currie at T-Gone, something like 78% of people with tinnitus should experience complete relief from their tinnitus if they continue with their treatment to completion. The rest of the people should find their tinnitus reduced in volume and often in duration.

John cautions, "Most homeopathic remedies gain effect only to a certain point and after that, begin to cause a worsening of the condition—so you need to stop at this optimal point".

If you are interested in trying out T-Gone's homeopathic remedies for your tinnitus, go to John Currie's T-gone website at http://t-gone.org/. You can also download and read Ellen Currie's free 250 page book *Living Tinnitus Free* (http://t-gone.org/blog/tinnitus-book/) that gives their slant on understanding and treating tinnitus.

**RingStop**: RingStop has been on the market since 2002 and is specifically formulated for people with tinnitus. Bob Martin, DC, the man behind RingStop says, "I put in all the homeopathic remedies that have ever been shown to help different causes. Then I put in the supportive nutrients that will help auditory function as a base."[1] Thus, RingStop takes a shotgun approach to treating the various kinds of tinnitus in contrast to T-Gone's specific tinnitus remedy approach.

As with all homeopathic remedies, RingStop takes time to "work". Some people experience tinnitus reduction within 2 weeks, but most people don't notice any change until 3 to 6 weeks after they start RingStop. The recommendation is that you should take it continuously for 3 months before deciding how helpful it will be to you. Once your tinnitus starts reducing, it should continue to do so for several more months.

RingStop contains herbal extracts in addition to homeopathic ingredients. Herbal extracts such as Ginkgo act as blood thinners, so if you are already on a blood-thinner, check with your doctor before taking RingStop.

For more information on RingStop go to http://www.ringstop.net/.

**Clear Tinnitus**: This product is much the same as RingStop—half homeopathic remedies and half herbal extracts. You can learn more at http://www.clearproductsinc.com/clear-tinnitus-60-count/.

Note: Don't expect miracles from these homeopathic remedies, but if they work for you, be thankful. I took Clear Tinnitus faithfully for a 6 months or more to test it out—but in the end there was no difference to my tinnitus.

## Vitamin and Mineral Supplements

You can try vitamins and mineral supplements. Many people have tried using certain combinations of vitamins and minerals and claim it helps reduce their tinnitus. If your health is poor, taking vitamin and mineral supplements will have a beneficial effect on your whole body including your ears and may reduce your tinnitus in the process.

Generally vitamin and mineral supplements take time before they show positive results. Therefore, try them for several months before you conclude that they do not work for you.

Noise damage results in a lot of tinnitus. The good news is that an animal study at the University of Michigan showed that "a combination of high doses of vitamins A, C and E and magnesium, taken one hour before noise exposure and continued as a once-daily treatment for five days, was very effective at preventing permanent noise-induced hearing loss."[2]

Researchers noted that pre-treatment [with vitamins A, C and E and magnesium] had several positive effects:

- reduced the free radicals that form during and after noise exposure,
- reduced noise-induced constriction of blood flow to the inner ear,
- reduced neural excitotoxicity, or the damage to auditory neurons that can occur due to over-stimulation.

In addition, the post-noise nutrient doses apparently "scavenged" free radicals that continue to form long after this noise exposure ends.[3]

## Vitamins

**Vitamin A:** Vitamin A is found in high concentrations in the cochlea. In fact, the hair cells in your inner ears depend on Vitamin A in order to function properly. Several studies have reported substantial benefits to people suffering from tinnitus after taking Vitamin A supplements.[4] For example, in one study at Zurich University in 1952, people were given the equivalent of 300,000 IU of Vitamin A twice a week for 6 weeks. The result was that tinnitus was significantly improved in 39% of the cases, and completely cured in 27%. In another study at the University of Milan in 1951, 50,000 IU of vitamin A was injected 2 or 3 times a week. The results were similar to the above study—30% had a considerable lessening of their tinnitus, while in 25% their tinnitus completely disappeared.[5]

Warning: Vitamin A is toxic when taken in high quantities for long periods. Higher doses for short periods to knock down your tinnitus are apparently ok.

**Vitamin $B_3$ (Niacin):** Niacin (vitamin $B_3$) is a member of the vitamin B complex. It acts as a vasodilator and so allows more blood to reach your ears. Thus, it gives you a temporary flush. Some people take lecithin in combination with niacin. The idea is that lecithin, a fat emulsifier, helps break down the build-up of fats in your capillaries. At the same time the niacin helps dilate your capillaries to let the lecithin in and do its work. If your tinnitus is related to poor blood flow, this vitamin may help you.

**Vitamin $B_{12}$:** In one study, 47% of the people with tinnitus had a vitamin $B_{12}$ deficiency. All the people low on vitamin $B_{12}$ received injections of 1,000 micrograms weekly for about 4 months. At the end of that time, all of them reported some improvement in their tinnitus, including a decrease in loudness.[6]

## Minerals

**Magnesium:** The mineral magnesium plays an important part in hearing and ear health. Scientists have found that a magnesium deficiency increases susceptibility to noise damage, chronic tinnitus[7] and to sound sensitivity.[8]

Being exposed to loud sounds depletes your ears of magnesium, thus leaving your ears unprotected. Since tinnitus is often triggered by loud sounds, supplementing your magnesium intake could be beneficial.[9] Low magnesium levels can cause the tiny arteries in your inner ears to constrict, thus depriving them of an adequate supply of oxygen. When combined with noise exposure, this can deplete the delicate hearing cells of their energy stores thus leading to damage or death.[10]

There is evidence that high doses of magnesium taken soon after a sudden hearing loss can sometimes help restore hearing (and thus also help prevent tinnitus).[11]

Probably the best form of magnesium to take is magnesium threonate, followed by magnesium glycinate and magnesium citrate. You want to stay away from magnesium stearate.[12]

**Zinc:** The cochlea normally has a very high concentration of zinc. In fact, "the highest concentration of zinc in our bodies is in the inner ear".[13] If your body is low on zinc, it can affect your inner ears since your cochlea needs adequate zinc in order to function properly.

Even a slight to moderate zinc deficiency can cause tinnitus.[14] One otolaryngologist estimates that about 25% of the people he sees with severe tinnitus are deficient in zinc.[15]

In one study, 82% of the people who took zinc supplements (50 mg of zinc daily) found the severity of their tinnitus decreased by an average of 45%,[16] whereas the placebo group had no significant reduction in their tinnitus. Incidentally, at the beginning of this study 31% of the people had lower than normal zinc levels. In another study people with tinnitus and no hearing loss had significantly lower zinc levels than did the controls who did not have tinnitus.[17]

If you are going to take zinc supplements, make sure you take it in a form that is bioavailable and thus easy for your body to absorb. Look for zinc picolinate as its absorption rate is around 90%, in contrast to zinc oxide with an absorption rate of only 35% or so.[18]

If you take zinc supplements, note this well: taking too high a dosage of zinc is harmful and can lead to anemia and other nasty problems. Therefore, do not take more than 50 mg of zinc daily (30 mg is usually recommended), because zinc competes with copper and manganese for absorption. If you take higher doses of zinc, you can become deficient in these two important minerals.[19]

## Antioxidants: Natural Remedies for Noise Exposure

Exposing your ears to loud noise can result in tinnitus and hearing loss.

As mentioned previously, one of the major factors causing tinnitus and hearing loss from loud noise is excessive free radical activity. Free radicals form in your inner ears when you expose your ears to loud sounds. In part, this is because cell mitochondria in your inner ears churn out damaging free radicals in response to loud sounds. (In the medical literature, you may see this referred to as "oxidative stress".) These free radicals then zap the cells in your inner ears.

"Think of these free radicals as tiny enemy bullets. If they fatally damage a cell, it goes into a process called apoptosis in which the cell systematically shuts itself down and dies. If those cells are the hair cells in your inner ears, then you lose hearing when those hair cells die. This often brings on tinnitus as a result. Thus, it is important to zap the free radicals before they do their dastardly deeds."[20]

### Glutathione

The best way to zap free radicals is with powerful antioxidants. Glutathione is considered the most powerful natural antioxidant there is. Thus, it helps protect your ears from the effects of loud noise by protecting against free radical damage.

Your body makes this antioxidant naturally from compounds such as N-acetyl-cysteine and D-methionine which in turn are made from three amino acids–cysteine, glycine and glutamic acid.

If your body cannot make enough glutathione in time to zap all the free radicals created due to noise exposure, your inner ears can use a bit of extra help. Although glutathione is readily available as a supplement, taking glutathione supplements isn't very effective. This is because the digestive juices in your stomach break down the glutathione before your gut can absorb enough to help your ears.

All is not lost, however. You can take the basic building blocks of glutathione and let your body synthesize the glutathione it needs from these ingredients. The two most important of these ingredients are N-acetyl-cysteine and D-methionine.

## N-Acetylcysteine (NAC)

N-acetyl-cysteine (NAC) is a major glutathione precursor that is readily available in most health food stores or on-line.

According to Barbara Jenkins, Au.D., "The U.S. Navy has been researching the use of antioxidants to protect service members exposed to noise". N-acetyl-cysteine (NAC) was found to be very effective. The Navy found that NAC protected the cochlea after exposure to impulse noise, such as coming from gunfire, whose peak levels reached as high as 165 dB.[21]

If you take NAC immediately after being exposed to loud noise, your body can quickly make more glutathione and thus prevent a lot of damage that could otherwise result in long-lasting tinnitus. (If you don't have NAC handy, take Vitamins C and E. Both are also antioxidants—but not as good as NAC.)

**Note**: You don't want to overdose on N-acetyl-cysteine, as it can actually work "backwards" and cause more ear damage. I've seen figures that if you take more than 2,800 mg of N-acetyl-cysteine a day it can reverse its activity and become a pro-oxidant rather than the beneficial antioxidant. Your ears need some N-acetyl-cysteine, but too much can be dangerous.[22] Probably a conservative safe upper level would be around 1,800 mg a day.

## Acetyl-L-Carnitine (ALCAR)

Research papers have shown that NAC, together with acetyl-L-carnitine (ALCAR), reduces the amount of damage to the inner ear hair cells in animals after exposure to loud sounds, and that their protective benefit persists even one to four hours after exposure.[23] Even if you have accidentally exposed your ears to loud noise, "if you act quickly enough, the oxidative stress caused by noise damage can be reduced even after the fact".[24]

Therefore, you should consider taking acetyl-L-carnitine as well as NAC if you have exposed your ears to loud sounds. You can get NAC and ALCAR at health food stores and on-line.

## Herbal Remedies

There are a number of herbals that may help with your tinnitus. However, not all herbals are helpful. Some are just the opposite. Therefore, be aware that if you have tinnitus, you should **not** take herbs that mimic aspirin (which makes tinnitus worse) like willow bark (Salix spp.), meadowsweet (Filipendula ulmaria) and wintergreen (Gaultheria procumbens). Also, you might want to avoid taking Cinchona (Cinchona spp.) because it contains quinine, which is ototoxic and could negatively affect not only your tinnitus, but also your hearing and balance.[25]

Below are four helpful herbals for tinnitus.

**Black cohosh:** Black cohosh (Cimicifuga racemosa) taken as a tincture works for some people with tinnitus. Black cohosh and ginkgo taken together makes a good combination to fight tinnitus according to herbalist, Deb Soule.[26]

**Gingko biloba:** Ginkgo has had a lot of bad press by people out to prove that herbals don't work. I think it is time to set the record straight.

Ginkgo biloba extract is a powerful herbal extract that can do three things.

First, one primary reason Ginkgo biloba extract may be helpful for tinnitus is because it is a glutamate antagonist. Bilobalide, one component in Ginkgo extract, is a potent antagonist to glutamate release. Glutamate is a neurotransmitter used by the cochlea to transmit signals across the synapses leading to the brain. It is produced by the hair cells in the inner ear when converting sound vibrations into electrical signals. When the hair cells are damaged, they produce **excess** glutamate, which flood the neuroreceptors in the auditory nerve and brain. Excess glutamate overexcites the receptors and causes them to fire continuously until they become depleted and eventually die. This process is called glutamate neurotoxicity, and causes a kind of tinnitus called cochlear-synaptic tinnitus.

Now here's where Ginkgo comes in. Since Ginkgo is a powerful glutamate antagonist, it keeps excessive glutamate from being released. As a result you don't get run-away glutamate excitability leading to tinnitus and cell death.

Second, Ginkgo is a powerful antioxidant and enhances cellular metabolism.[27]. The Ginkgo flavonoids are powerful antioxidants and help prevent free radical damage to the auditory pathways. In addition, the terpenoids in Ginkgo can help reduce tinnitus by decreasing free-radical damage to the cochlea.[28]

Third, Ginkgo is a vasodilator. Taking Ginkgo increases blood circulation to the ears. It does this by dilating the blood vessels so they can carry more blood. It also inhibits platelet-aggravating factor, which causes the blood platelets to clump together and slow circulation. [29] Numerous studies have shown that Ginkgo increases blood flow in the brain and the extremities, and thus sometimes helps alleviate tinnitus.[30]

According to Dr. James Duke, hundreds of European studies have confirmed the use of standardized ginkgo extract for a variety of conditions including poor circulation, tinnitus and vertigo.[31]

There have been studies that show that Ginkgo does not work for tinnitus, but you need to check into these studies to see what level of Ginkgo extract was used. For example, one study of 978 people concluded that Ginkgo didn't work. However, the people in this study were only given 150 mg of Ginkgo extract a day, which is less than one third of the 480 mg per day needed to be clinically effective according to the German "Commission E", one of the foremost authorities in the world on herbal therapies,[32] including the use of Ginkgo.[33] Thus, if you are going to use Ginkgo, make sure you are taking an effective dose if you want effective results.

To be effective, Ginkgo extract should be standardized to contain a minimum of 24% flavone glycosides, 6% terpene lactones[34] and 2.6% bilobalide.[35] (The German Commission E tests showed the extract was characterized by 22 – 27% flavone glycosides, 5 – 7% terpene lactones and 2.6 – 3.2% bilobalide[36] so any Ginkgo extract that is in this ballpark should be effective.)

Furthermore, an effective dose for "vertigo and tinnitus of vascular or involutional [degenerative] origin" according to the German "Commission E" is "120 – 160 mg dry extract in 2 or 3 doses"[37]. Thus, the effective dose **begins** at a minimum of 240 and rises to 480 mg per day. Therefore, if you have tinnitus and want to see if Ginkgo can help you, it makes sense to go for the 480 mg dose per day.

"In my experience", says Jennifer Brett, ND, "Ginkgo improves tinnitus in about half the people who try it". "Even if you've had tinnitus for more than 3 years, Ginkgo can be effective, although it seems to be more helpful in people who haven't had tinnitus that long."[38]

Let me emphasize this again. Ginkgo does not work with every person who has tinnitus, but it does help some. Some study results show tinnitus improvement in 26% to 82% of the people taking an effective dose so you might want to give it a try.[39]

However, here's a word of caution. Don't go overboard on Ginkgo. As mentioned above, Ginkgo is a blood thinner, which can be good, but too much of a good thing can be bad. If you let your blood get too thin, you can bleed to death internally without realizing the damage you are doing to your body. The first sign that your blood is getting too thin may be frequent nosebleeds.

Furthermore, if you are an older adult and take an anti-coagulant (or a blood-thinner), or if you have any bleeding disorder, do **not** take Ginkgo without working together with your doctor to adjust your medications so you don't thin your blood too much.[40]

Therefore, based on the above, you should not take Ginkgo in the long term. Dr. Steven Nagler says, "There is general agreement that if Ginkgo has not been effective within three months, it will not become effective thereafter. Thus, Ginkgo should be discontinued after three months if ineffective."[41]

If you are interested, probably one of the best sources of "good" Ginkgo extract is Arches Tinnitus Formula. It contains effective levels of Ginkgo biloba extract, zinc and garlic. You can learn more about it at http://www.tinnitusformula.com.

**St. John's Wort**: If depression is causing or exacerbating your tinntus, as an alternative to prescription drugs, you might want to consider the natural herbal remedy, St. John's Wort. St. John's Wort is not ototoxic and has far fewer side effects than prescription drugs. Over 40 studies (so far) have reported it to be just as effective for mild to moderate depression as the drugs doctors typically prescribe.

You can get St. John's Wort at almost any drug store or health food store. Just be sure that the dose is standardized to between 0.3% - 0.7% hypericin, the active ingredient. St. John's Wort can take two weeks (and sometimes up to a month) to become effective.

Just be careful when mixing herbals and drugs. St. John's Wort interferes with some medications (including some anti-depressants and contraceptives), so work closely with your doctor if you are taking any other medications and want to take St. John's Wort.

**Hydergine**: This extract of a fungus (ergot derivative) grows on rye. It requires a prescription in the USA, but is sold as a non-prescription supplement in Europe. At a dosage of 10 - 15 mg. per day it alleviates tinnitus in some people.[42] In one small study of 20 people, after 30 to 90 days on just 4.5 mg/day, tinnitus improved by 57%.[43]

**Chapter 25 Endnotes**

1 Shepherd, 2002. p. 33.
2 Reuter, 2007.
3 Reuter, 2007.
4 Martin, 2001. p. 6.
5 Using Vitamin A to Treat Tinnitus, 1999.
6 Maleskey, 1999. p. 641.
7 Craggs-Hinton, 2007. p. 96.
8 Mayes, 2010. p. 172.
9 Treatment Possibilities, 1997. pp. 15-17.
10 Martin, 2001. p. 7.
11 Bauman, 2009a. pp. 2-3.
12 Mercola, 2015. p. 2.
13 Mayes, 2010. p. 177.
14 Keate, 2010b. p. 46.
15 Martin, 2001. p. 6.
16 Keate, 2010b. p. 46.
17 Sanders, 2004. pp. 5-6.
18 Keate, 2010b. p. 46.
19 Keate, 2010b. p. 46.
20 Bauman, 2009b. p. 1.
21 Jenkins, 2014. p. 28.
22 Bauman, 2009a. p. 2.
23 Jenkins, 2014. p. 28.
24 Jenkins, 2014. p. 29.
25 Duke, 1997. p. 423.
26 Duke, 1997. p. 422.
27 Martin, 2001. p. 5.
28 Tunkel, 2014. p. S27.
29 Keate, 2010b. p. 44.
30 Bilger, 1998.
31 Duke, 1997. p. 422.
32 German "FDA" Approves Ginkgo for Tinnitus. 1994. p. 1.
33 Keate, 2010b. p. 46.
34 PDR for Herbal Medicines, 2000. p. 344.
35 Keate, 2010b. p. 46.
36 German "FDA" Approves Ginkgo for Tinnitus. 1994. p. 1.
37 German "FDA" Approves Ginkgo for Tinnitus. 1994. p. 1.
38 Maleskey, 1999. p. 640.
39 Keate, 2010b. p. 46.
40 Tunkel, 2014. p. S27.
41 Nagler, 2003. p. 2.
42 Life Extension, 2011. p. 3.
43 Jimenez-Cervantes, 1990. p. 1.

Chapter 26

# Medical Treatments for Tinnitus

Medical doctors and researchers have various treatments they may use to try and control your tinnitus. Some of the below treatments are still experimental, but show promise.

## Vagus Nerve Stimulation

Vagus nerve stimulation (VNS) is a new experimental therapy for tinnitus that seems to work for some people that have not been helped by other tinnitus treatments.

VNS itself is not new. It is currently being used to treat roughly 50,000 people with epilepsy or depression.[1] What is new is using it to treat cases of intractable tinnitus.

Unlike many tinnitus treatments that work on reducing the symptoms of tinnitus, VNS works to fix the underlying cause of tinnitus.

Researchers believe that many types of tinnitus are caused by negative neural changes in the brain in response to ear trauma such as loud noise. "When sensory cells in the inner ear are damaged, such as from loud noise, the resulting hearing loss changes some of the signals sent from the ear to the brain. For reasons that are not fully understood, some people will develop tinnitus as a result."[2]

"Researchers Dr. Michael Kilgard and Dr. Navzer Engineer from The University of Texas at Dallas and University-affiliated biotechnology firm

MicroTransponder report that stimulation of the vagus nerve paired with sounds eliminates tinnitus."[3]

> "We believe the part of the brain that processes sounds—the auditory cortex—delegates too many neurons to some frequencies, and things begin to go awry," said Michael Kilgard, Ph.D., associate professor of behavior and brain sciences at UT-Dallas. "Because there are too many neurons processing the same frequencies, they are firing much stronger than they should be."
>
> In addition, the neurons fire in sync with one another and they also fire more frequently when it is quiet. According to Dr. Kilgard, it's these changing brain patterns that produce tinnitus.[4]

Thus, the solution was to repeatedly pair tones with brief pulses applied to the vagus nerve in the neck. This stimulation ultimately eliminated tinnitus by causing controlled, positive changes in the auditory cortex in the brain. The researchers were, in essence, retraining the brain to ignore the nerve signals that simulate ringing.[5]

In short, vagus nerve stimulation is similar to pressing a reset button in the brain. This helps retrain the part of the brain that interprets sound so that errant neurons revert back to their original state, and thus the tinnitus disappears.[6]

"This minimally invasive method of generating neural plasticity allows us to precisely manipulate brain circuits, which cannot be achieved with drugs," said Dr. Navzer Engineer. "Pairing sounds with VNS provides that precision by rewiring damaged circuits and reversing the abnormal activity that generates the phantom sound."[7]

Past research has shown that the severity of chronic pain and tinnitus is tied to the degree of plasticity in the brain's cortex. A previous study showed that repeatedly pairing sensory stimuli with electrical stimulation of a brain structure called the "nucleus basalis" generates powerful and long-lasting changes in cortical organization. Since the vagus nerve is easier to access for clinical use, and is known to trigger the release of molecules in the brain that promote neural changes, follow-up studies were performed on the vagus nerve.[8]

"How can the vagus nerve in the neck cause changes in the brain?" The vagus nerve is unlike any other nerve in the body. It directly connects to the brain and sends important signals to tell the brain what to learn. For example, when someone is exposed to a stressful event, a hormone called epinephrine is released into the bloodstream, which activates the vagus nerve. The vagus nerve then sends a signal to the brain to release the neurotransmitter norepinephrine in a region of the brain called the amygdala (part of the limbic system), which strengthens memory storage for the emotional feelings during that specific time. This is why people often vividly remember traumatic events in great detail. The vagus nerve is sending a signal, telling the brain what to learn and when to learn it."[9]

Researchers used this natural response system,

> ...by directly stimulating the vagus nerve while playing a sound, which tells the brain to 'pay attention' to that sound. This simultaneous pairing of a specific tone with vagus nerve stimulation strengthens auditory neurons representing that tone. Consistently pairing vagus nerve stimulation with all other tones except the tinnitus tone, reduces the expanded representation of the tinnitus tone. Over time, the brain learns to ignore the tinnitus tone. Pairing several of these tones (except the tinnitus tone) helped subdue the abnormal hyperactivity and restored the auditory cortex activity back to normal in a rat model of tinnitus. These changes persisted for several weeks after stopping the treatment.[10]

The researchers found that the VNS treatment paired with tones had not only reorganized the neurons in the rats' brains to respond to their original frequencies, but it also made their brain responses sharper, decreased excitability, and decreased synchronization of auditory cortex neurons.[11]

VNS worked well for lab rats in eliminating their tinnitus, so researchers decided to try as small study on humans. "Ten tinnitus patients who showed no benefit from previous audiological, drug, or neural stimulation treatments received a stimulation electrode directly on the vagus nerve."[12]

Unlike in the animal study, not all these 10 people benefited from the vagus nerve stimulation therapy. Interestingly enough, those people who did not show significant changes were on medications that might have prevented the beneficial effect of the VNS therapy.

> It is well-known that drugs can interfere with the acetylcholine and norepinephrine metabolism and release that are important to the promotion of plasticity changes and, therefore, could block the effect of vagus nerve stimulation.[13]

The good news was that even though the participants had not benefitted from other tinnitus treatments, VNS therapy was able to reduce tinnitus in 60% to 80% of the drug-free participants who had chronic, severe tinnitus.[14]

In another case, vagus nerve stimulation was used on a 59-year-old man who had suffered from bilateral tinnitus for 14 years that arose after a cervical fusion operation. Pharmacotherapy (drugs), transcranial magnetic stimulation, ıl direct current stimulation, neurofeedback, and bilateral auditory ulation via implanted electrodes had not improved his tinnitus. ter implanting the vagal nerve stimulator, this person received daily vagus nerve stimulation tone pairings for 4 weeks. At the end of therapy, he experienced a significant reduction in his tinnitus symptoms that lasted for 2 months after treatment.[15]

According to Dr. Kilgard, the key to vagus nerve stimulation therapy for tinnitus,

> ...is that, unlike previous treatments, we're not masking the tinnitus, we're not hiding the tinnitus. We are retuning the brain from a state where it generates tinnitus to a state that does not generate tinnitus. We are eliminating the source of the tinnitus![16]

Today's therapies for tinnitus have limited success and frequently must be modified over time because they become ineffective. "The VNS treatment would be an improvement over current therapies involving medications or counseling because it offers a possible permanent end to the condition and doesn't appear to cause any significant side effects," Kilgard said.[17]

Ongoing clinical trials will ultimately reveal whether VNS is a valid tinnitus treatment with results that prove to be permanent or at least long term, and therefore will be used in the future.

## Transcutaneous Electrical Nerve Stimulation (TENS)

Transcutaneous Electrical Nerve Stimulation (TENS) can provide relief from tinnitus for some people. TENS has been used for pain relief, and since there are many similarities between chronic tinnitus and chronic pain, numbers of people with tinnitus find a corresponding relief from their tinnitus.

TENS treatment is simple, non-invasive and painless. Each treatment basically consists of touching a probe to the skin on and around your ears, face or neck for a few minutes.

In a small study of 45 people treated with TENS, 62% had subjective improvement in their tinnitus. In this study, the people most helped by TENS were people with low-frequency tinnitus and those with mild hearing losses.[18]

In another study of 64 people with annoying tinnitus, after treatment with transcutaneous electrical stimulation, 47% reported some degree of improvement in their tinnitus.[19]

In a larger study, 500 people with annoying tinnitus underwent transcutaneous electrical stimulation. Here is how this treatment was done.

> Each patient was asked to judge his or her tinnitus on a subjective scale of 1-10, 1 being barely noticeable and 10 being intolerable. Patients were asked to do this before and after each treatment session. The instrument used to deliver the electrical stimulation was a Neuroprobe 500. This unit is used mainly in pain control and is available in many physical therapy clinics. The electrical stimulation is delivered by a hand-held probe with a small gold ball electrode. The patient is seated in a comfortable chair with the therapist at the patient's side, and the electrical stimulation then is delivered to the external ear, using 20 points around the external ear and tragus. In the protocol used, each point was stimulated for 30 seconds two times in each treatment. The waveform was an alternating current with an intensity of 0.5 to 1.0 mA. The number of visits for each patient was between 6 and 10.[20]

In this above study, 53% of the people had a reduction in their tinnitus of at least two points. Even better, 7% of the study participants had complete suppression of their tinnitus.

Approximately three months after the end of this study, 72% of the participants reported a sustained benefit from the electrical stimulation in decreasing their tinnitus.

Before this study, participants rated their tinnitus an average of eight, with a range between three and ten. After treatment, this average dropped to four, with a range of 0 - 10. Thus, the average participant in this study found their tinnitus dropped an average of four on the ten-point rating system.[21]

A 40% reduction in tinnitus is nothing to sneeze at. However, TENS is not for everyone. In this study 13 people found their tinnitus got worse, not better. Fortunately, upon stopping treatment, 11 of the 13 people found their tinnitus soon reverted to its old level, but unfortunately, two people were left with permanent, louder tinnitus.[22]

Why does electrical stimulation work? Here are some theories.

> One possible reason is a direct effect on the cochlea. A second reason might be improved cochlear blood flow, as this has been shown to take place in the different parts of the body with electrical stimulation, and a third possible reason could be related to the gate theory of pain. The gate theory of pain says that there are cutaneous fibers that might control central modifiers, and stimulation of the peripheral sensory nerves can modify the perception of pain. In the same manner then,

> electrical stimulation of the peripheral sensory nerves may have some control over a central gate that might modify the perception of pain.[23]

Not only can transcutaneous electrical nerve stimulation work for people with the common sensorineural kind of tinnitus, it can also work for people with somatosensory tinnitus.

In another study of 240 people with somatosensory tinnitus (tinnitus modulated by neck movements or by pressure on the head or face), researchers stimulated the upper cervical nerve (C2). Less than 1 in 5 (17.9%) had any improvement in their tinnitus. However, those that had reductions in the tinnitus had very significant improvement—an average of 43%—and 6 lucky people found their tinnitus completely disappeared.[24]

Unfortunately, TENS treatments don't last forever, so you may have to repeat them from time to time. In the above studies, most people that had reduced tinnitus found that their tinnitus reduction lasted to the final follow-up at one month or three months, depending on the study.[25]

## Repetitive Transcranial Magnetic Stimulation

Repetitive Transcranial Magnetic Stimulation (rTMS) is another relatively new treatment for tinnitus. Researchers developed it around 1993 or so.

Transcranial Magnetic Stimulation works on the principle that a varying magnetic field will induce an electrical current in nearby "structures". In this case, the nearby "structure" is the auditory cortex of your brain located just above and behind your ears.

When the magnetic pulses are delivered repetitively and rhythmically, this process is called repetitive Transcranial Magnetic Stimulation.[26]

A doctor typically places an electromagnet (basically a coil of wire encased in plastic) on your scalp over one temporal lobe near the auditory cortex and delivers magnetic pulses of about one Tesla[27] at the rate of one per second for about 30 minutes. This is done once each day for three to ten consecutive days. The treatment alters the biochemistry and firing patters of neurons in the cortex—that is, the part of your brain nearest the surface.

The frequency of the stimulation determines whether it speeds up or slows down the cortical activity in your brain. Low frequency stimulation (less than or equal to 1 Hz) tends to inhibit (slow down) neuronal activity, while high frequency stimulation (greater than or equal to 3 Hz) tends to excite (speed up) neuronal activity. Numerous studies have revealed that chronic tinnitus is associated with **increased** activity in the primary auditory cortex. Therefore, in the case of tinnitus, you want to **slow down** this activity by using low frequency rTMS.[28]

In some people, low-frequency (1 Hz) rTMS reduces the "excitability" of the cerebral cortex, and can cause long-lasting inhibitory effects in tinnitus perception—up to six months or more.

In one study, after five days of rTMS treatments, there was a highly significant reduction in tinnitus perception, whereas people who received the sham treatment did not show any significant changes.

Not all reports are as glowing. "Despite some very promising initial claims of long-term efficacy, subsequent investigations observed short-term effects (less than two weeks) even when rTMS treatment was applied for ten days."[29]

To extend the positive effects on tinnitus reduction, subsequent maintenance rTMS treatments consisting of one session a day for three consecutive days produced longer-lasting benefits in some people—extending the length of time of tinnitus inhibition anywhere from a few weeks to six months.[30] In practical terms, rTMS won't be ready for the "big time" until researchers find a way to consistently extend its inhibitory effect on tinnitus from weeks to months or years.

Although rTMS shows promise, it still isn't the solution for everyone with tinnitus. It works for some people, but not for everyone. For example, in one study it had good effects in 25% of the people studied, partial effects in 28% of the people, and no effect in 47%.[31] If this holds true for all people with tinnitus, then rTMS will only help about half of tinnitus sufferers. In another study of 32 people with tinnitus for more than 1 year, that were treated with rTMS, 18 people (56%) "found their symptoms were alleviated for a least six months".[32] Thus, rTMS definitely shows promise. If you are one of the lucky ones, you will receive partial or complete reduction in your tinnitus.

So far, no one is talking about any negative side effects, if any, from "slowing down" your brain. However, I feel rTMS is bound to have some effect on the brain's proper functioning in other nearby areas to the auditory cortex, so I'd suggest caution in using rTMS until researchers know for sure there are no unwanted side effects.

Even though rTMS is used in other countries, the FDA has yet to approve rTMS for regular use here. At the present time (2016), rTMS is only used in clinical trials in the USA.

## Hyperbaric Oxygen Therapy

Hyperbaric oxygen therapy (HBOT) is another tool in your tinnitus toolbox that you may choose to try. Although it is widely used in various European countries, it is not at all common in the USA, even though there is significant medical evidence supporting its use for recent sudden sensorineural hearing loss and tinnitus.[33]

### What Is Hyperbaric Oxygen Therapy?

"Hyperbaric" is just a fancy word that is made up of two words—the word "hyper" meaning "high", and "bar" from the Greek "baros" meaning "weight". It is used to refer to the weight of air or air pressure. Thus increasing the air pressure above normal atmospheric pressure would result in hyperbaric pressure.

Hyperbaric oxygen therapy consists of sitting in a hyperbaric chamber—basically a steel tank that is designed to withstand pressure several times standard atmospheric pressure. The air pressure in the chamber is raised to approximately twice atmospheric pressure while you breathe pure oxygen. Each treatment typically lasts from one to two hours.

"Due to the increased pressure inside the chamber, far more oxygen is dissolved in the bloodstream than under normal conditions. HBOT enables the oxygen content of the blood to reach up to 7%, which is 20 times higher than normal. Those parts of the body which suffered damage due to poorly supplied oxygen are now exposed to significant quantities."[34] This increased blood oxygen allows parts of your body that were oxygen deficient to have an abundance of oxygen to facilitate their biological processes. This can help fix problems in the inner ear and brain. Interestingly enough, in 40% of cases, improvement in the patient's condition continues even after treatment has stopped.[35]

### How Does Hyperbaric Oxygen Therapy Work for Tinnitus?

Hyperbaric oxygen therapy is used to treat various chronic conditions including tinnitus and pain.

Apparently chronic tinnitus and chronic pain share something in common—basically they form endless loops in the brain that keep them going even after the stimulus that caused them in the first place no longer exists.

An example of a condition that causes chronic pain is fibromyalgia. In one recent study of women with fibromyalgia, about 70% of the women who took part experienced symptoms that had to do with the interpretation of pain in their brains.[36] This is the same kind of problem many people with tinnitus have in respect to the sounds their brains produce.

Now, here's a surprising finding. Hyperbaric oxygen therapy was found to induce neuroplasticity that leads to repair of chronically impaired brain functions. This is because HBOT pushes more oxygen into the patient's bloodstream, which delivers it to the brain.[37] Thus, hyperbaric oxygen therapy treats the underlying cause—the brain pathology responsible for the fibromyalgia and results in brain repair, including neuronal regeneration.

For example, in one study, women with fibromyalgia received 40 HBOT treatments—one 90-minute treatment for 5 days each week spread over 2 months. Each treatment consisted of breathing pure oxygen at two times normal atmospheric pressure.[38]

The result was that these women were able to drastically reduce or even eliminate their use of pain medications. The HBOT actually reversed their condition.[39]

Since chronic tinnitus is caused by negative changes in the brain, it seems that HBOT should be able to reverse these negative changes, and cause positive changes to reduce or eliminate tinnitus, just like it does with fibromyalgia.

Most research on hyperbaric oxygen therapy related to ears has centered around recent sudden hearing loss and tinnitus. "Recent" being defined as within two weeks of the sudden hearing loss or tinnitus starting.

In 50 studies, a total of 4,109 patients suffering from sudden hearing loss and tinnitus underwent HBO therapy following unsuccessful conventional therapy. The results revealed that if the HBO treatment started between two and six weeks after the tinnitus started, 4% no longer experienced tinnitus, 81.3% had a decrease in their tinnitus, 13.5% noticed their tinnitus remained the same and 1.2% found their tinnitus got worse.

If hyperbaric oxygen therapy began between six weeks and three months following the onset of tinnitus, 7% no longer experienced tinnitus, 44% had a decrease in their tinnitus, and another 44% noticed no change in their tinnitus while 5% found their tinnitus got worse.

If the HBO therapy began more than three months after the onset of tinnitus (and up to several years later), 33% reported a decrease in their tinnitus, 60 - 62% reported no change in their tinnitus, and 4 - 7% noticed their tinnitus got worse.[40]

Thus, it appears that the sooner HBO therapy is started, the better the overall results will be.

Despite the stipulation that the best treatment results are seen in early onset cases, many people in Germany and Europe with chronic tinnitus are treated with HBO. In fact, in Germany there are approximately 80 multi-person hyperbaric oxygen chambers and 80% of the treatments are for inner ear dysfunction.[41]

Note that in the above studies, conventional tinnitus treatments had already been tried with no success. This indicates that hyperbaric oxygen therapy really works for numbers of people. Thus, if you have a hyperbaric chamber near you, this is one treatment you might want to try.

However, you'll be more successful in getting your tinnitus under control if, at the same time, you also choose one of the complementary psychological tinnitus treatments mentioned in previous chapters.

## Low-Level Laser Treatment

Another relatively new development involves using laser light to treat tinnitus. Low-level laser treatment has been used on tens of thousands of people in Europe that were suffering from tinnitus. It works on the principle that light heals and provides new energy to the cells of the body. This therapy is designed to use laser light to increase the inner-cellular energy of the cells in your cochlea (inner ear) that may have been damaged by excess noise, etc. This is probably why the people that have the most success in using low-level laser therapy to help their tinnitus are people who have tinnitus as the result of noise damage.

The low-level laser light energy stimulates the nerve and hair cells imparting to them increased energy in the form of increased production of the cell fuel, adenosine triphosphate (ATP). This enables the damaged cells to use their own biochemical processes to heal.

In 30 years of research, there have been no known adverse side effects. But there is one side effect that has been noted—a good side effect. Some of the people taking low-level laser treatment not only have their tinnitus reduced or eliminated, but they also actually have some of their hearing restored in the process. According to one study, the increase in hearing ran 11 dB.[42] So if a tinnitus treatment has to have any side effects, t effect you definitely want to have!

The results in Europe are impressive. Low-level laser therapy been used in Germany, Italy, France, Switzerland, Hungary, Russia, and the Scandinavian countries since the late 1980s. More than 20,000 people with tinnitus have been treated. One study revealed that after treatment 26% had no more tinnitus! An additional 36% reported their tinnitus reduced by more than 50%. Another 19% reported some reduction in their tinnitus—up to 50%.[43] This gives a success rate of 81%. Unfortunately, this low-level laser treatment doesn't work for about the one in five that try it.

Low-level laser therapy utilizes a non-surgical laser that emits a red beam of light that is cool to the touch. It causes no pain and does no damage to the human body.

Treatment consists of aiming the laser beam at your cochlea (contained in the mastoid bone behind your ear). Each treatment lasts for about one hour—30 minutes per ear. This protocol continues once a day for ten consecutive days.

By the end of the treatment, tinnitus is reduced by an average of 30% to 60%. Furthermore, the tinnitus continues to decrease and normally reaches maximum results from one to three months later. If you need further treatment because of your tinnitus, you can be retreated after three months have elapsed, or you can continue treatment at home with a "Home Treatment" unit.

## Treating Tinnitus Caused from Taking Ototoxic Drugs

If your ears start to ring after you begin taking a new drug or an increased dose of an existing drug, you should immediately report this to your doctor. Together you should then decide what to do. You basically have four options.

**1. Stop taking the drug.**

You need to decide whether the side effects of that drug are worse than any benefit you get from taking a given drug or not. That makes it obvious which way to choose.

For example, one man began taking Amitriptyline and soon noticed he had severe tinnitus. His tinnitus was driving him "buggy" so he contacted me for help. I suggested the Amitriptyline might be causing his tinnitus. With his doctor's permission, he stopped taking the drug. Twelve days later, he joyfully reported that his tinnitus had gone away. That was his choice and he is glad he made it.

**2. Continue with the same drug.**

If you decide that the benefits of taking a given drug outweigh the side effects, then you may choose to keep taking the drug and put up with the side effects, especially if you feel the side effects such as tinnitus are not bothering you much.

For example, a lady takes Celecoxib for her arthritis. When she takes it, her tinnitus gets louder, but her arthritis pain improves. She chooses the increased tinnitus (which doesn't really bother her) over the arthritis pain (which she definitely doesn't like). That is her choice, and she is content to live with it.

**3. Switch to a different drug.**

If a drug you are taking is causing your tinnitus or making your existing tinnitus worse, ask your doctor to switch you to a different drug that won't affect your tinnitus. This is often an effective strategy. Sometimes you can switch to a different drug in the same class of drugs. However, sometimes you need to switch to a different class of drugs in order to avoid tinnitus.

**4. Reduce the dose.**

Many drugs have what I call a "magic threshold" in terms of dosage below which you don't have any noticeable ototoxic side effects. (I call it your "magic threshold" because you don't know what that dosage level is below which you don't have ototoxic side effects. Furthermore, this "magic threshold" varies from person to person.) When you increase the dose such that it crosses your "magic threshold" level—wham—suddenly side effects (such as tinnitus) appear.

For example, when her doctor doubled her dose of Irbesartan, one lady found her existing tinnitus became noticeably louder. When she complained to her doctor, he reduced her dose to the old level (obviously below her "magic threshold" for this drug) and her tinnitus dropped to its previous level.

Thus, taking a lower dose means that you have a **much** better chance of flying below the radar of your "magic threshold"—whatever level it is.

When it comes to drugs, the trick is to try to put the odds in your favor. The way to do this is to follow these three rules of thumb.

1. Choose the least ototoxic drug that will do the job.

2. Take the lowest effective dose.

3. Take the drug for the shortest time possible.

You also need to understand that side effects for a given drug may be temporary or permanent depending on the person. This means that one person could take a given drug and find he has temporary tinnitus, while another person could take the same drug and discover his tinnitus never goes away—even after he stops taking the drug. That's just the way it is. There is currently no way to know this in advance.

This can even happen to the **same** person. For example, one man began taking a certain drug and reported to me that his ears began ringing. I suggested it might be the drug, so he stopped taking it for a week or so. He did this and found his tinnitus went away. Based on this experience, he decided to put up with the tinnitus while taking the drug for the full duration his doctor had prescribed, knowing that when he finished the drug, he could give it another week or so and his tinnitus would be gone. Imagine his shock when he did this—and discovered to his horror that his tinnitus refused to go away. It was now permanent!

If you find you have permanent tinnitus as the result of taking a drug or drugs, apart from stopping taking the offending drug, if your tinnitus bothers you, you should seek treatment much as you would for neurophysiologic tinnitus from other causes.

## Treating Existing Tinnitus with Drugs

Everyone wants the magic pill that stops tinnitus cold. However, in spite of the desire of millions of tinnitus sufferers for a safe and effective drug to cure or reduce the distress caused by tinnitus, currently neither the Food and Drug Administration (FDA) in the USA nor the European Medicines Agency (EMEA) has approved a single drug targeting tinnitus relief.[44] "There are presently no validated medications for tinnitus—nothing that can permanently silence the perception of tinnitus."[45]

Thus, the "best practices" *Clinical Practice Guideline: Tinnitus* state,

> Avoid the routine use of medications for tinnitus, as medications have not been shown to alleviate tinnitus and may have adverse effects. At this time, there are no medications approved by the US Food and Drug Administration (FDA) for treatment of tinnitus. No medications have been shown to reliably eliminate or reduce tinnitus perception.[46]

Furthermore, this above-mentioned guideline specifically recommended **against** antidepressants, anticonvulsants (such as Gabapentin [*Neurontin*]), anxiolytics (which includes the Benzodiazepines), or intratympanic medications for the routine treatment of patients with persistent, bothersome tinnitus.[47] For example, the *Clinical Practice Guidelines: Tinnitus* state that none of the studies of "anticonvulsants for tinnitus have shown a clear benefit".[48]

Even so, researchers keep on trying to find the "magic pill". For example, the article *New Drug Promises Relief from Tinnitus* in part, reads, "Neurophysiologists at the University of Connecticut have discovered a new drug that may prevent tinnitus by selectively affecting potassium channels in the brain". They go on to say that tinnitus is caused by overly excitable cells that flood the brain with an overload of signals that can lead to phantom ringing in the ears (tinnitus).

One of the more effective drugs, Retigabine, helps open KCNQ potassium channels, which serve as the "brakes" that shut down the signaling of overly excited nerves. Retigabine, however, has terrible side effects. Thus, they decided to create a new drug. The new drug, SF0034, was chemically identical to Retigabine, but included an extra fluorine atom. The first thing they had to do was determine whether SF0034 works on KCNQ potassium channels the same way Retigabine does, and if so, if it would be better or worse.

There are five different kinds of KCNQ potassium channels in the body, but only two are important in tinnitus—KCNQ2 and KCNQ3. The problem with Retigabine is that it acts on other KCNQ potassium channels as well. When testing SF0034 in neurons, the researchers found that it was more selective than Retigabine. It appeared to only open KCNQ2 and KCNQ3 potassium channels, and to not affect others. The results are promising and they hope to start FDA trials with SF0034 to test its safety and efficacy in people in the near future.[49]

The chances that this new drug will be the magic pill are almost nil. For example, the KCNQ2 and KCNQ3 potassium channels no doubt affect other parts of the body besides just slowing the neurons down in the auditory circuits to reduce or eliminate tinnitus. Thus, other unrelated serious side effects are bound to show up—and so, yet another "magic pill" bites the dust.

Dr. Hazell cautions, "Our new understanding of tinnitus makes it unlikely that any one drug will permanently switch off tinnitus. Your brain treats tinnitus sounds like warning signals, so an instant cure would indicate a fault in your security system!" However, it is likely that some drugs will speed up the retraining therapy by acting on the chemicals used in passing messages between brain cells. Work in this area is already underway.

People who suffer extreme distress, depression or sleeplessness may need short term drugs to deal with this aspect of the problem.[50] Unfortunately, many people with severe tinnitus are just treated with strong anti-depressants and anti-anxiety drugs to try and help them cope, but this ultimately does nothing for their tinnitus. As tinnitus, researcher Fatima Husain, Ph.D. explains, "These psychoactive drugs are used to lessen the patient's emotional reaction to tinnitus, not to silence the tinnitus signal itself".[51]

If you are going to give drugs a try in spite of the above, note that the effective dose for treating tinnitus is often well below that usually used for treating non-tinnitus conditions. Therefore you need to work with your doctor to find the lowest dose that will work for you.[52]

Using such drugs is not without its own pitfalls. It is possible to become so overmedicated with sedatives and tranquilizers that you are too "zonked out" to enjoy life. In addition, you may not have enough strength and willpower left to cope with your tinnitus. Furthermore, such drugs may take away your own natural ability to sleep.

Thus, it is generally better to try to learn to manage your tinnitus without drugs. However, if severe tinnitus, stress and insomnia are having a major effect on your life, using sedatives and tranquilizers may be helpful in the **short** term.[53] (Note: When you hear the words "short term", think two weeks or less, not a period of several months or years.)

Never forget, **all** drugs have harmful side effects of which you should be aware. Also, some drugs actually make your tinnitus worse, in addition to creating addictions and personality changes. So, seriously question whether the consequences of a possible cure, including drug-dependency, are worth the benefits.

## Anesthetics

**Lidocaine** (*Xylocaine*): Although Lidocaine is one of the many drugs that can cause tinnitus, one study suggests that Lidocaine injections actually can help control tinnitus.

In 2000, Dr. John Shea of the Shea Ear Clinic in Memphis, Tennessee reported that injections of Lidocaine, both into the ear and intravenously, repeated on three consecutive days, had resulted in partial or complete tinnitus relief.

This treatment worked for people with tinnitus deriving from conditions involving disturbed hair cells such as Meniere's disease, positional vertigo and the side effects of taking *Aspirin*, as well as for those with hearing loss.

Treating tinnitus with Lidocaine seems to be quite effective. According to Shea, "almost all patients get immediate relief". What is even more impressive is that a month after the treatment, 70% of the patients still reported either complete or partial relief from their tinnitus.

In a later study, Shea showed that with Lidocaine perfusion of the inner ear plus intravenous Lidocaine, 70% of the "ears" in the study showed a decrease in their tinnitus. This figure rose to 77% after 3 months and to 83% by 12 months.

Lidocaine does have some side effects including temporary paralytic spontaneous nystagmus, so it is not risk-free. However, Shea concludes, "Lidocaine perfusion plus intravenous Lidocaine is a safe and effective treatment of intractable tinnitus".[54]

Shea adds, "Most patients with tinnitus are also depressed". Therefore, in order for the tinnitus treatment to be effective, patients need to be treated for **both** conditions.[55]

In spite of its apparent initial success, Lidocaine tinnitus therapy has not caught on due to a major drawback. In further testing, few people found long-lasting relief from their tinnitus. Thus, the treatment needed to be done frequently—and not many people are willing to be "stuck by a needle" repeatedly for short-term tinnitus relief.[56] Furthermore, in two studies participants reported side effects including severe vertigo, nausea and vomiting. Thus the *Clinical Practice Guideline: Tinnitus* report does not recommend Lidocaine injections for controlling tinnitus.[57]

## Anti-Insomnia Drugs

Benzodiazepines are both anti-insomnia and anti-anxiety agents. When used safely, benzodiazepines are effective for **short-term** management of **sleep**. Examples of benzodiazepines used for sleep management include Estazolam (*ProSom*), Flurazepam (*Dalmane*), Quazepam (*Doral*), Temazepam (*Restoril*) and Triazolam (*Halcion*).[58]

In the short-term these drugs promote sleep, but their disadvantage is that they may also cause daytime drowsiness.

**Gatifloxacin**
*Gengraf* **(Cyclosporine)**
*Genotropin* **(Somatropin)**
**Gentamicin**
*Geodon* **(Ziprasidone)**
*Gin Pain Pills* **(Sodium salicylate)**
**Glatiramer**
*Gleevec* **(Imatinib)**
Glibenclamide **(Glyburide)**
**Gliclazide**
**Glipizide**
**Glisoxepide**
*Glucoben* **(Glisoxepide)**
*Gluco-K* **(Potassium gluconate)**
*Glucotrol* **(Glipizide)**
*Glucotrol* **(Glipizide)**
**Glyburide**
**Grepafloxacin**
**Guanabenz**
**Guanfacine**
**Gusperimus**

**H**

*Habitrol* **(Nicotine)**
*Halcion* **(Triazolam)**
*HCTZ* **(Hydrochlorothiazide)**
*Helidac* **(Bismuth subsalicylate)**
*Hemabate* **(Carboprost)**
**Hepatitis B vaccine**
*Hexamine* **(Methenamine)**
*Hiprex* **(Methenamine)**
*Histase* **(Methapyrilene)**
*Hivid* **(Zalcitabine)**
**Homatropine**
*Horizant* **(Gabapentin)**
*Hp-PAC* **(Lansoprazole)**
*Humatin* **(Paromomycin-Aminosidine)**
*Humatrope* **(Somatropin)**
*Humira* **(Adalimumab)**
*Hycodan* **(Hydrocodone)**
*Hydeltrasol* **(Prednisolone)**
*Hydeltra-TBA* **(Prednisolone)**
**Hydrocodone**
*HydroDIURIL* **(Hydrochlorothiazide)**
*Hydromorph Contin* **(Hydromorphone)**
**Hydromorphone**
*Hydropres* **(Hydrochlorothiazide)**
Hydroxychloroquine
**Hydroxyzine**
*Hygroton* **(Chlorthalidone)**
*Hyperstat* **(Diazoxide)**
*Hytrin* **(Terazosin)**
*Hyzaar* **(Losartan)**

**I**

**Ibandronate**
*Ibandronic acid* **(Ibandronate)**
*IBU* **(Ibuprofen)**
**Ibuprofen**
*Idarac* **(Floctafenine)**
**Iloperidone**
*Ilosone* **(Erythromycin)**
*Ilotycin* **(Erythromycin)**
**Imatinib**
*Imdur* **(Isosorbide)**
**Imidapril**
**Imipenem—Cilastatin**
**Imipramine**
*Imitrex* **(Sumatriptan)**
*Imovax* **(Rabies vaccine)**
**Indapamide**
*Indera* **(Propranolol)**
*Inderal-LA* **(Propranolol)**
*Inderide* **(Propranolol)**

*Indocid* **(Indomethacin)**
*Indocin* **(Indomethacin)**
**Indomethacin**
**Indoprofen**
*Indotec* **(Indomethacin)**
*Infergen* **(Interferon alfacon-1)**
Influenza vaccine
*INH* **(Isoniazid)**
*Inhibace* **(Cilazapril)**
*Innopran XL* **(Propranolol)**
*Intal* **(Cromolyn sodium)**
**Interferon alfa-2a**
**Interferon alfa-2b**
**Interferon alfacon-1**
**Interferon alfa-n3**
**Interferon beta-1a**
**Interferon beta-1b**
*Intron A* **(Interferon alfa-2b)**
*Invirase* **(Saquinavir)**
**Iodixanol**
**Iohexol**
*Ionsys* **(Fentanyl)**
**Iotrolan**
**Ioversol**
**Ipratropium**
**Irbesartan**
*Isepacin* **(Isepamicin)**
**Isepamicin**
*Ismo* **(Isosorbide)**
**Isoniazid**
**Isoproterenol**
*Isoptin* **(Verapamil)**
*Isopto Homatropine* **(Homatropine)**
**Isosorbide**
*Isotamine* **(Isoniazid)**
**Isotretinoin**
**Isoxicam**
**Isradipine**
*Isuprel* **(Isoproterenol)**
Itraconazole

**K**

*Kaletra* **(Ritonavir)**
**Kanamycin**
*Kantrex* **(Kanamycin)**
*Kapidex* **(Dexlansoprazole)**
*Keflex* **(Cephalexin)**
*Kefurox* **(Cefuroxime)**
*Kenacomb* **(Neomycin)**
*Keral* **(Dexketoprofen)**
*Kerlone* **(Betaxolol)**
**Ketoconazole**
**Ketoprofen**
**Ketorolac**
*Klonopin* **(Clonazepam)**

**L**

**Labetalol**
**Lacosamide**
*Lactisal* **(Salicylic acid)**
*Lamictal* **(Lamotrigine)**
*Lamisil* **(Terbinafine)**
**Lamotrigine**
**Lansoprazole**
*Lariam* **(Mefloquine)**
*Lasix* **(Furosemide)**
*L-Deprenyl* **(Selegiline)**
*Lederfen* **(Fenbufen)**
*Legatrin* **(Quinine)**
**Leuprolide**
*Levaquin* **(Levofloxacin)**
*Levitra* **(Vardenafil)**
**Levobetaxolol**
**Levobupivacaine**

**Levofloxacin**

**Levonorgestrel—Ethinyl estradiol**

*Lexapro* **(Escitalopram)**

*Lexiscan* **(Regadenoson)**

*Lexxel* **(Enalapril)**

*Lialda* **(Mesalamine)**

*Librium* **(Chlordiazepoxide)**

**Lidocaine**

*Lidoderm* **(Lidocaine)**

*Lidone* **(Molindone)**

*Limbitrol* **(Amitriptyline)**

*Lincocin* **(Lincomycin)**

Lincomycin

*Lincorex* **(Lincomycin)**

*Linessa 28* **(Ethinyl estradiol)**

**Linezolid**

*Lioresal* **(Baclofen)**

*Lipidil* **(Fenofibrate)**

*Lipitor* **(Atorvastatin)**

**Liposomal daunorubicin**

**Liposomal doxorubicin**

**Lisinopril**

*Lithane* **(Lithium)**

**Lithium**

*Lithobid* **(Lithium)**

*Lodine* **(Etodolac)**

*Loestrin* **(Ethinyl estradiol)**

**Lomefloxacin**

*Lopinavir* **(Ritonavir)**

*Lopresor* **(Metoprolol)**

*Lopressor* **(Metoprolol)**

*Lopressor HCT* **(Metoprolol)**

**Loratadine**

**Lorazepam**

*Lorelco* **(Probucol)**

**Lornoxicam**

*[illegible]* **(Hydrocodone)**

**Losartan**

*Losec* **(Omeprazole)**

*Lotemax* **(Loteprednol)**

*Lotensin* **(Benazepril)**

*Lotensin HCT* **(Benazepril)**

**Loteprednol**

*Lotrel* **(Amlodipine)**

*Loxapac* **(Loxapine)**

**Loxapine**

*Loxitane* **(Loxapine)**

*Lozide* **(Indapamide)**

*Lozol* **(Indapamide)**

*Ludiomil* **(Maprotiline)**

*Lunesta* **(Eszopiclone)**

*Lupron* **(Leuprolide)**

*Lupron Depot* **(Leuprolide)**

*Luvox* **(Fluvoxamine)**

*Lyrica* **(Pregabalin)**

**M**

*Maalox Total Stomach Relief* **(Bismuth subsalicylate)**

*Macugen* **(Pegaptanib)**

**Magnesium salicylate**

*Magnevist* **(Gadopentetate)**

*Malarone* **(Atovaquone/Proguanil)**

*Malarone* **(Proguanil)**

*Mandelamine* **(Methenamine)**

*Manerix* **(Moclobemide)**

**Maprotiline**

*Marcaine* **(Bupivacaine)**

*Marinol* **(Dronabinol)**

*Marvelon* **(Ethinyl estradiol)**

*Marzine* **(Cyclizine)**

*Mavik* **(Trandolapril)**

*Maxalt* **(Rizatriptan)**

*Maxaquin* **(Lomefloxacin)**

*Maxicam* **(Isoxicam)**

**Mebendazole**
**Mechlorethamine**
**Meclizine**
**Meclofenamate**
*Meclomen* (**Meclofenamate**)
*Medrone* **(Medroxyprogesterone)**
**Medroxyprogesterone**
**Mefenamic acid**
**Mefloquine**
**Melitracen**
**Meloxicam**
**Memantine**
**Mephentermine**
**Mepivacaine**
*Mepron* **(Atovaquone/Proguanil)**
*Mepron* **(Proguanil)**
*Meridia* **(Sibutramine)**
*Mersyndol with Codeine* **(Doxylamine)**
*Mervan* **(Alclofenac)**
**Mesalamine**
*Metadate* **(Methylphenidate)**
**Methapyrilene**
**Methazolamide**
**Methdilazine**
**Methenamine (Hexamine)**
*Methergine* **(Methylergonovine)**
**Methotrexate**
**Methrazone (Feprazone)**
**Methyclothiazide**
**Methyl salicylate**
**Methylergonovine**
*Methylin* **(Methylphenidate)**
**Methylnaltrexone**
**Methylphenidate**
**Metolazone**
**Metoprolol**
*Metreton* **(Prednisone)**
*Metrogel-Vaginal* **(Metronidazole)**
**Metronidazole**
**Mexiletine**
*Mexitil* **(Mexiletine)**
*Mezavant* **(Mesalamine)**
*Miacalcin* **(Calcitonin)**
*Micardis* **(Telmisartan)**
*Micardis HCT* **(Telmisartan)**
*Micardis Plus* **(Telmisartan)**
**Micronomicin**
*Microzide* **(Hydrochlorothiazide)**
*Midamor* **(Amiloride)**
**Midazolam**
*Midol Extra Strength* **(Pyrilamine)**
*Migranal* **(Dihydroergotamine)**
**Milnacipran**
*Milophene* **(Clomiphene)**
*Mimims Homatropine* **(Homatropine)**
*Minestrin* **(Ethinyl estradiol)**
*Minipress* **(Prazosin)**
*Minizide* **(Prazosin)**
*Minocin* **(Minocycline)**
**Minocycline**
*Mintezol* **(Thiabendazole)**
*Mirapex* **(Pramipexole)**
*Mircette* **(Ethinyl estradiol)**
**Mirtazapine**
**Misonidazole**
**Misoprostol**
*Moban* **(Molindone)**
*Mobic* **(Meloxicam)**
*Mobicox* **(Meloxicam)**
*Mobiflex* **(Tenoxicam)**
**Moclobemide**
*Moduret* **(Amiloride)**
*Moduretic* **(Amiloride)**
**Moexipril**

**Molindone**

*Momentum Backache Relief* **(Magnesium salicylate)**

**Mometasone**

*Monitan* **(Acebutolol)**

*Monocor* **(Bisoprolol)**

*Mono-Gesic* **(Salsalate)**

*Monoket* **(Isosorbide)**

*Monopril* **(Fosinopril)**

*Monopril HCT* **(Fosinopril)**

**Montelukast**

**Moricizine**

*Motrin* **(Ibuprofen)**

**Moxifloxacin**

*MSD Enteric coated ASA* **(Acetylsalicylic acid)**

*MultiHance* **(Gadobenate)**

**Muromonab-CD3**

*Mustargen* **(Mechlorethamine)**

*Mycifradin* **(Neomycin)**

**Mycophenolate**

*Mykrox* **(Metolazone)**

*Mylan-Nifedipine Extended Release* **(Nifedipine)**

*Myobloc* **(Botulinum Toxin Type B)**

*Myocet* **(Doxorubicin)**

*Myoflex* **(Triethanolamine)**

**N**

**Nabilone**

**Nabumetone**

**Nadolol**

*Nafidimide* **(Amonafide)**

*Nalfon* **(Fenoprofen)**

**Naltrexone**

*Namenda* **(Memantine)**

*Naprelan* **(Naproxen)**

*Naprosyn* **(Naproxen)**

**Naproxen**

**Naratriptan**

*Nardil* **(Phenelzine)**

*Naropin* **(Ropivacaine)**

*Nasonex* **(Mometasone)**

*Nebcin* **(Tobramycin)**

**Nebivolol**

*Necon 1/35* **(Ethinyl estradiol)**

**Nefazodone**

**Neomycin**

*Neoral* **(Cyclosporine)**

*Neosporin* **(Neomycin)**

*Neptazane* **(Methazolamide)**

*Nesacaine* **(Chloroprocaine)**

**Netilmicin**

*Netromycin* **(Netilmicin)**

*Neupro* **(Rotigotine)**

*Neurontin* **(Gabapentin)**

*Nexavar* **(Sorafenib)**

*Nexium* **(Esomeprazole)**

**Niacin**

*Niaspan* **(Niacin)**

**Nicardipine**

*Nicoderm* **(Nicotine)**

*Nicorette* **(Nicotine)**

**Nicotine**

*Nicotrol* **(Nicotine)**

*NidaGel* **(Metronidazole)**

**Nifedipine**

**Nilotinib**

**Nilotinib**

**Nilvadipine**

**Nimodipine**

*Nimotop* **(Nimodipine)**

*Nipent* **(Pentostatin)**

**Nisoldipine**

**Nitrendipine**

*Nitrepin* **(Nitrendipine)**
*Nitrogen mustard* **(Melchlorethamine)**
*Nivadil* **(Nilvadipine)**
*Nizoral* **(Ketoconazole)**
*Norco* **(Hydrocodone)**
*Norditropin* **(Somatropin)**
**Norelgestromin**
*Norethindrone—Ethinyl estradiol* **(Ethinyl estradiol)**
*Norflex* **(Orphenadrine)**
**Norfloxacin**
*Norgesic* **(Acetylsalicylic acid)**
**Norgestimate—Ethinyl estradiol**
*Normodyne* **(Labetalol)**
*Normodyne* **(Labetalol)**
*Noroxin* **(Norfloxacin)**
*Norpramin* **(Desipramine)**
**Nortriptyline**
*Norvasc* **(Amlodipine)**
*Norvir* **(Ritonavir)**
*Novo-Amiodarone* **(Amiodarone)**
*Novo-AZT* **(Zidovudine)**
*Novo-Butazone* **(Phenylbutazone)**
*Novocain* **(Procaine)**
*Novo-Clopate* **(Clorazepate)**
*Novo-Cycloprine* **(Cyclobenzaprine)**
*Novo-Difenac* **(Diclofenac)**
*Novo-Diltazem* **(Diltiazem)**
*Novo-Divalproex* **(Divalproex)**
*Novo-Famotidine* **(Famotidine)**
*Novo-Fluoxetine* **(Fluoxetine)**
*Novo-Fluvoxamine* **(Fluvoxamine)**
*Novo-Gabapentin* **(Gabapentin)**
*Novo-Minocycline* **(Minocycline)**
*Novo-Moclobemide* **(Moclobemide)**
*Novo-Norfloxacin* **(Norfloxacin)**
*Novo-Selegiline* **(Selegiline)**
*Novo-Veramil* **(Verapamil)**
*Nplate* **(Romiplostim)**
*Nuprin* **(Ibuprofen)**
*NuvaRing* **(Ethinyl estradiol)**
*Nytol* **(Diphenhydramine)**

**O**

*Occlusal* **(Salicylic acid)**
**Octreotide**
**Ofloxacin**
Oil of Wintergreen **(Methyl Salicylate)**
**Olanzapine**
*Oleptro* **(Trazodone)**
Olmesartan
*Olmetec* **(Olmesartan)**
*Olmetec Plus* **(Olmesartan)**
**Olsalazine**
**Omeprazole**
*Omnipaque* **(Iohexol)**
*Omniscan* **(Gadodiamide)**
*Onabotulinum* **(Botulinum Toxin)**
*OptiMARK* **(Gadoversetamide)**
*Optimine* **(Azatadine)**
*Optiray* **(Ioversol)**
*Orafen* **(Ketoprofen)**
*Oraflex* **(Benoxaprofen)**
*Orapred* **(Prednisolone)**
*Orencia* **(Abatacept)**
*Oretic* **(Hydrochlorothiazide)**
*Orinase* **(Tolbutamide)**
*Ornade Spansule* **(Phenylpropanolamine)**
**Orphenadrine**
*Ortho* **(Ethinyl estradiol)**
*Ortho 7/7/7* **(Ethinyl estradiol)**
*Ortho-Cept* **(Ethinyl estradiol)**
*Orthoclone OKT3* **(Muromonab-CD3)**
*Orudis* **(Ketoprofen)**
*Oruvail* **(Ketoprofen)**

*Osmovist* **(Iotrolan)**
*Ostoforte* **(Ergocalciferal)**
**Oxaprozin**
**Oxazepam**
**Oxcarbazepine**
**Oxprenolol**
*Oxy IR* **(Oxycodone)**
**Oxybutynin**
**Oxycodone**
*OxyContin* **(Oxycodone)**
**Oxymetazoline**

**P**
*Pabalate* **(Sodium salicylate)**
*Pacerone* **(Amiodarone)**
**Paclitaxel**
*Pacyl* **(Isoxicam)**
**Palonosetron**
*Pamelor* **(Nortriptyline)**
*Panectyl* **(Trimeprazine)**
*Panimycin* **(Dibekacin)**
*Pan-Streptomycin* **(Streptomycin)**
*Panto* **(Pantoprazole)**
*Panto IV* **(Pantoprazole)**
*Pantoloc* **(Pantoprazole)**
**Pantoprazole**
*Parafon Forte* **(Acetaminophen)**
*Paraplatin* **(Carboplatin)**
**Parecoxib**
*Pariet* **(Rabeprazole)**
*Parnate* **(Tranylcypromine)**
**Paromomycin—Aminosidine**
**Paroxetine**
*Paxil* **(Paroxetine)**
*Paxil CR* **(Paroxetine)**
*PBZ* **(Tripelennamine)**
*PCE* **(Erythromycin)**
*Pediapred* **(Prednisolone)**
*Pediazole* **(Erythromycin)**
*Pediotic* **(Neomycin)**
**Pegaptanib**
*Pegasys* **(Peginterferon alfa-2a)**
*Pegasys RBV* **(Peginterferon alfa-2a)**
*Pegetron* **(Peginterferon alfa-2b)**
**Peginterferon alfa-2a**
**Peginterferon alfa-2b**
*PEG-Intron* **(Peginterferon alfa-2b)**
*Penetrex* **(Enoxacin)**
**Penicillamine**
**Penicillin/Penicillin G**
*Pennsaid* **(Diclofenac)**
*Pentacarinat* **(Pentamidine)**
Pentamidine
*Pentamycetin* **(Chloramphenicol)**
*Pentasa* **(Mesalamine)**
**Pentazocine**
**Pentosan**
**Pentostatin**
*Pepcid* **(Famotidine)**
*Pepcid AC* **(Famotidine)**
*Pepto-Bismol Original* **(Bismuth subsalicylate)**
*Percocet* **(Oxycodone)**
*Percodan* **(Oxycodone)**
**Perflutren**
**Pergolide**
*Periactin* **(Cyproheptadine)**
**Perindopril**
*Permax* **(Pergolide)**
*Persantine* **(Dipyridamole)**
*Pertofrane* **(Desipramine)**
**Phenelzine**
*Phenergan* **(Promethazine)**
**Pheniramine**
**Phenylbutazone**

**Phenylpropanolamine**
*Phrenilin* **(Butalbital)**
*Phrenilin Forte* **(Butalbital)**
*Phrenilin with Caffeine and Codeine* **(Butalbital)**
**Pilocarpine**
**Pindolol**
**Piperacillin—Tazobactam**
*Pipracil* **(Piperacillin—Tazobactam)**
**Piroxicam**
**Pirprofen**
*Plaquenil* **(Hydroxychloroquine)**
*Platinol* **(Cisplatin)**
*Plendil* **(Felodipine)**
*Pletal* **(Cilostazol)**
*PMS-Lithium Carbonate* **(Lithium)**
*Polocaine* **(Mepivacaine)**
**Polymyxin B**
*Ponstan* **(Mefenamic acid)**
*Ponstel* **(Mefenamic acid)**
*Pontocaine* **(Tetracaine)**
**Posaconazole**
*Posanol* **(Posaconazole)**
**Potassium gluconate**
**Pramipexole**
*Pravachol* **(Pravastatin)**
**Pravastatin**
**Prazosin**
**Prednisolone**
**Pregabalin**
*Prelone* **(Prednisolone)**
*Premarin* **(Estradiol)**
*Premique* **(Medroxyprogesterone)**
*Premplus* **(Medroxyprogesterone)**
*Prempro* **(Medroxyprogesterone)**
*Preservex* **(Aceclofenac)**
*Prevacid* **(Lansoprazole)**
*PREVPAC* **(Lansoprazole)**
*Prialt* **(Ziconotide)**
**Prilocaine**
*Prilosec* **(Omeprazole)**
*Primaxin* **(Imipenem—Cilastatin)**
*Prinivil* **(Lisinopril)**
*Prinzide* **(Lisinopril)**
*Pristiq* **(Desvenlafaxine)**
*ProAir HFA* **(Albuterol)**
**Probucol**
**Procainamide**
**Procaine**
*Procan* **(Procainamide)**
*Procanbid* **(Procainamide)**
*Procardia* **(Nifedipine)**
*Proclim* **(Medroxyprogesterone)**
*Pro-Diaban* **(Glisoxepide)**
**Progesterone**
**Proglumetacin**
*Prograf* **(Tacrolimus)**
**Proguanil**
*ProHance* **(Gadoteridol)**
*Proloprim* **(Trimethoprim)**
**Promethazine**
*Prometrium* **(Progesterone)**
*Pronestyl* **(Procainamide)**
**Propafenone**
**Propofol**
**Propoxyphene**
**Propranolol**
**Proquazone**
*Prosed* **(Methenamine)**
*ProSom* **(Estazolam)**
*Protaxon Forte* **(Proglumetacin)**
*Prothiaden* **(Dothiepin)**
*Protonix* **(Pantoprazole)**
*Protopic* **(Tacrolimus)**
*Protostat* **(Metronidazole)**

**Protriptyline**
*Proventil* **(Albuterol)**
*Provera* **(Medroxyprogesterone)**
*Prozac* **(Fluoxetine)**
**Prozepam**
**Pseudoephedrine**
*Pyribenzamine* **(Tripelennamine)**
**Pyrilamine**

**Q**

**Quazepam**
*Questran* **(Cholestyramine)**
**Quetiapine**
*Quinaglute* **(Quinidine)**
*Quinamed* **(Amonafide)**
**Quinapril**
*Quinate* **(Quinidine)**
*Quinidex* **(Quinidine)**
**Quinidine**
**Quinine**
*Q-Vel* **(Quinine)**

**R**

*RabAvert* **(Rabies vaccine)**
**Rabeprazole**
**Rabies vaccine**
*Ralivia* **(Tramadol)**
**Ramipril**
*Ranexa* **(Ranolazine)**
**Ranitidine**
**Ranolazine**
*Rantudil Retard* **(Acemetacin)**
*Rapamune* **(Sirolimus)**
*ratio-Fentanyl* **(Fentanyl)**
*ratio-Glyburide* **(Glyburide)**
*Raxar* **(Grepafloxacin)**
*Reactine* **(Cetirizine)**
*Rebetol* **(Ribavirin)**
*Rebetron* **(Interferon alfa-2b)**
*Rebif* **(Interferon beta-1a)**
*Reclast* **(Zoledronic acid)**
*Recombivax HB* **(Hepatitis B vaccine)**
*Redux* **(Dexfenfluramine)**
**Regadenoson**
*Relafen* **(Nabumetone)**
*Relistor* **(Methylnaltrexone)**
*Relpax* **(Eletriptan)**
*Remeron* **(Mirtazapine)**
*Remeron RD* **(Mirtazapine)**
*Remeron SolTab* **(Mirtazapine)**
*Reminyl* **(Galantamine)**
*Renedil* **(Felodipine)**
*Rengasil* **(Pirprofen)**
*Replagal* **(Agalsidase alfa)**
*ReQuip* **(Ropinirole)**
*Rescriptor* **(Delavirdine)**
*Restasis* **(Cyclosporine)**
*Restoril* **(Temazepam)**
*Retrovir* **(Zidovudine)**
*Revatio* **(Sildenafil)**
*ReVia* **(Naltrexone)**
*Rexolate* **(Sodium thiosalicylate)**
*Rheumatrex* **(Methotrexate)**
*Rheumox* **(Azapropazone)**
*Rhodacine* **(Indomethacin)**
*Rhodis* **(Ketoprofen)**
*RhotralSectral* **(Acebutolol)**
*Rhotrimine* **(Trimipramine)**
*Rhovail* **(Ketoprofen)**
**Ribavirin**
*Ridaura* **(Auranofin)**
*Rifadin* **(Rifampin)**
*Rifamate* **(Rifampin)**
**Rifampin**

*Rifater* **(Rifampin)**
**Rifaximin**
*Rimactane* **(Rifampin)**
*Rimadyl* **(Carprofen)**
**Rimantadine**
**Risedronate**
*Risperdal* **(Risperidone)**
**Risperidone**
*Ritalin* **(Methylphenidate)**
**Ritonavir**
*Rituxan* **(Rituximab)**
**Rituximab**
**Rivastigmine**
*Rivotril* **(Clonazepam)**
**Rizatriptan**
*Robaxisa* **(Acetylsalicylic acid)**
*Rocephin* **(Ceftriaxone)**
*Rofact* **(Rifampin)**
**Rofecoxib**
*Roferon-A* **(Interferon alfa-2a)**
*Romazicon* **(Flumazenil)**
**Romiplostim**
**Ropinirole**
**Ropivacaine**
**Rotigotine**
*Roubac* **(Trimethoprim)**
*Rowasa* **(Mesalamine)**
*Roxicet* **(Oxycodone)**
**Roxithromycin**
*Royflex* **(Triethanolamine)**
*Rulid* **(Roxithromycin)**
*Rulide* **(Roxithromycin)**
*Rynatan* **(Azatadine)**
*Rythmol* **(Propafenone)**
*Ryzolt* **(Tramadol)**

**S**
*Sabril* **(Vigabatrin)**
*Sagamicin* **(Micronomicin)**
*Saizen* **(Somatropin)**
*Salac* **(Salicylic acid)**
*Salacid* **(Salicylic acid)**
*Salagen* **(Pilocarpine)**
*Salazopyrin* **(Sulfasalazine)**
*Salbutamol* **(Albuterol)**
*Salflex* **(Salsalate)**
**Salicylic acid**
*Salofalk* **(Mesalamine)**
**Salsalate**
*Sandimmune* **(Cyclosporine)**
*Sandostatin* **(Octreotide)**
*Sandostatin LAR* **(Octreotide)**
*SangCya* **(Cyclosporine)**
**Saquinavir**
*Sarafem* **(Fluoxetine)**
*Sativex* **(Dronabinol)**
*Savella* **(Milnacipran)**
*Scandonest* **(Mepivacaine)**
*Seasonale* **(Ethinyl estradiol)**
*Sedapap* **(Butalbital)**
*Select* **(Ethinyl estradiol)**
*Select 1/35* **(Ethinyl estradiol)**
**Selegiline**
*Sensorcaine* **(Bupivacaine)**
*Septocaine* **(Articaine)**
*Septra* **(Trimethoprim)**
*Septrin* **(Trimethoprim)**
*Serax* **(Oxazepam)**
*Serophene* **(Clomiphene)**
*Seropram* **(Citalopram)**
*Seroquel* **(Quetiapine)**
*Serostim* **(Somatropin)**
**Sertraline**

*Serzone* **(Nefazodone)**
**Sibutramine**
**Sildenafil**
*Simply Sleep* **(Diphenhydramine)**
**Simvastatin**
*Sinequan* **(Doxepin)**
*Singulair* **(Montelukast)**
**Sirolimus**
**Sitaxsentan**
*Skelid* **(Tiludronate)**
*Slow-Trasicor* **(Oxprenolol)**
*Sobril* **(Oxazepam)**
*Sodium cromoglycate* **(Cromolyn Sodium)**
**Sodium oxybate**
**Sodium salicylate**
**Sodium thiosalicylate**
*Soliris* **(Eculizumab)**
*Solodyn* **(Minocycline)**
*Solupred* **(Prednisolone)**
**Somatropin**
*Sonata* **(Zaleplon)**
**Sorafenib**
*Soriatane* **(Acitretin)**
*Sotacor* **(Sotalol)**
**Sotalol**
*Spanidin* **(Gusperimus)**
**Sparfloxacin**
*Spiroben* **(Chl[illegible])**
*Sporanox* **(Itraconazole)**
*Sprycel* **(Dasatinib)**
*St. Joseph Aspirin* **(Acetylsalicylic acid)**
*Stadol* **(Butorphanol)**
*Stadol NS* **(Butorphanol)**
*Starnoc* **(Zaleplon)**
*Stilnoct* **(Zolpidem)**
*Stilnox* **(Zolpidem)**
**Streptomycin**
*Stugeron* **(Cinnarizine)**
*Suboxone* **(Buprenorphine)**
*Sudafed* **(Pseudoephedrine)**
*Sudafed Sinus Advance* **(Ibuprofen)**
*Sular* **(Nisoldipine)**
**Sulfadiazine**
**Sulfadoxine—Pyrimethamine**
**Sulfamethizole**
**Sulfamethoxazole**
**Sulfasalazine**
**Sulfisoxazole**
**Sulindac**
**Sumatriptan**
*Supeudol* **(Oxycodone)**
*Supracaine* **(Tetracaine)**
*Suprefact* **(Buserelin)**
*Suprefact Depot* **(Buserelin)**
*Surgam* **(Tiaprofenic acid)**
*Surlid* **(Roxithromycin)**
*Surmontil* **(Trimipramine)**
*Sustiva* **(Efavirenz)**
*Sylatron* **(Peginterferon alfa-2b)**
*Symbyax* **(Olanzapine)**
*Synacthen Depot* **(Cosyntropin)**
*Synphasic* **(Ethinyl estradiol)**
*Systral C* **(Chlorphenoxamine)**

**T**

*[illegible]* **(Dihydralazine)**
**Tacrine**
**Tacrolimus**
**Tadalafil**
*Tagamet* **(Cimetidine)**
*Talacen* **(Pentazocine)**
*Talwin* **(Pentazocine)**
*Talwin Compound* **(Pentazocine)**
*Talwin Nx* **(Pentazocine)**

*Tambocor* **(Flecainide)**
**Tamsulosin**
*Tanatril* **(Imidapril)**
*Targocid* **(Teicoplanin)**
*Tarka* **(Trandolapril)**
*Taro-Carbamazepine* **(Carbamazepine)**
*Tasigna* **(Nilotinib)**
*Tasigna* **(Nilotinib)**
*Tasmar* **(Tolcapone)**
*Tavist* **(Clemastine)**
*Tavor* **(Lorazepam)**
*Taxol* **(Paclitaxel)**
*Tazocin* **(Piperacillin—Tazobactam)**
*Tecta* **(Pantoprazole)**
*Tegretol* **(Carbamazepine)**
**Teicoplanin**
*Tekamlo* **(Amlodipine)**
**Telmisartan**
*Temaril* **(Trimeprazine)**
**Temazepam**
*Temgesic* **(Buprenorphine)**
*Temodal* **(Temozolomide)**
*Temodar* **(Temozolomide)**
**Temozolomide**
*Tenex* **(Guanfacine)**
*Tenfortan* **(Amezinium)**
*Tenolin* **(Atenolol)**
*Tenoretic* **(Atenolol)**
*Tenormin* **(Atenolol)**
**Tenoxicam**
*Tequin* **(Gatifloxacin)**
**Terazosin**
**Terbinafine**
**Terbutaline**
**Tetracaine**
**Tetracycline**
*Teveten* **(Eprosartan)**
*Teveten HCT* **(Eprosartan)**
**Thalidomide**
*Thalitone* **(Chlorthalidone)**
*Thalomid* **(Thalidomide)**
*Thelin* **(Sitaxsentan)**
*Theo-24* **(Theophylline)**
*Theochron* **(Theophylline)**
*Theo-Dur* **(Theophylline)**
*Theolair* **(Theophylline)**
**Theophylline**
**Thiabendazole**
**Thiethylperazine**
*Thiocyl* **(Sodium thiosalicylate)**
*Thiosulfil Forte* **(Sulfamethizole)**
**Thonzylamine**
**Thymoxamine**
**Tiagabine**
**Tiaprofenic acid**
*Tiazac* **(Diltiazem)**
*Tiazac XC* **(Diltiazem)**
*Ticlid* **(Ticlopidine)**
**Ticlopidine**
**Tiludronate**
*Timolide* **(Timolol)**
**Timolol**
*Timoptic* **(Timolol)**
*Timoptic-XE* **(Timolol)**
*Timpilo* **(Timolol)**
**Tirapazamine**
**Tizanidine**
*TOBI* **(Tobramycin)**
*Tobradex* **(Tobramycin)**
**Tobramycin**
**Tocainide**
*Tofranil* **(Imipramine)**
**Tolbutamide**
**Tolcapone**

*Tolectin* **(Tolmetin)**
**Tolmetin**
*Tonamil* **(Thonzylamine)**
*Tonocard* **(Tocainide)**
*Topamax* **(Topiramate)**
**Topiramate**
*Topril* **(Ramipril)**
*Toprol-XL* **(Metoprolol)**
*Toradol* **(Ketorolac)**
**Torasemide (Torsemide)**
*Torecan* **(Thiethylperazine)**
**Torsemide**
**Tositumomab**
*Tracleer* **(Bosentan)**
*Tramacet* **(Tramadol)**
**Tramadol**
*Trandate* **(Labetalol)**
*Trandate* **(Labetalol)**
**Trandolapril**
*Tranxene* **(Clorazepate)**
**Tranylcypromine**
*Trasicor* **(Oxprenolol)**
*Travatan* **(Travoprost)**
**Travoprost**
**Trazodone**
**Tretinoin**
*Treximet* **(Sumatriptan)**
*Triacomb* **(Neomycin)**
*Triavil* **(Amitriptyline)**
**Triazolam**
*Tricor* **(Fenofibrate)**
*Tri-Cyclen* **(Ethinyl estradiol)**
*Tridural* **(Tramadol)**
**Triethanolamine**
*Trileptal* **(Oxcarbazepine)**
*Trilisate* **(Choline magnesium trisalicylate)**
**Trimazosin**
**Trimeprazine**
**Trimethoprim**
**Trimipramine**
*Trinalin* **(Azatadine)**
**Tripelennamine**
*Triptil* **(Protriptyline)**
*Triquilar 28* **(Ethinyl estradiol)**
*Trisenox* **(Arsenic trioxide)**
*Trolamine* **(Triethanolamine)**
**Trovafloxacin**
*Trovan* **(Trovafloxacin)**
*Trudexa* **(Adalimumab)**
*Tusal* **(Sodium thiosalicylate)**
*Tussend* **(Hydrocodone)**
*Twinrix* **(Hepatitis B vaccine)**
*Tylenol* **(Acetaminophen)**

**U**

*Uloric* **(Febuxostat)**
*Ultracaine* **(Articaine)**
*Ultracet* **(Tramadol)**
*Ultradol* **(Etodolac)**
*Ultram* **(Tramadol)**
*Uniphyl* **(Theophylline)**
*Uniretic* **(Moexipril)**
*Unitron PEG* **(Peginterferon alfa-2b)**
*Univasc* **(Moexipril)**
*Uracel* **(Sodium salicylate)**
*Urasal* **(Methenamine)**
*Urex* **(Methenamine)**
*Urised* **(Methenamine)**
*Urobiotic* **(Sulfamethizole)**
*Uromax* **(Oxybutynin)**

**V**

*Valcyte* **(Valganciclovir)**
**Valdecoxib**

**Valganciclovir**
*Valium* **(Diazepam)**
**Valproate**
**Valproic acid**
**Valsartan**
*Vancenase* **(Beclomethasone)**
*Vanceril* **(Beclomethasone)**
*Vancocin* **(Vancomycin)**
**Vancomycin**
*Vanquish Extra Strength Pain Reliever* **(Acetylsalicylic acid)**
*Vantin* **(Cefpodoxime)**
**Vardenafil**
**Varenicline**
*Vascor* **(Bepridil)**
*Vaseretic* **(Enalapril)**
*Vasotec* **(Enalapril)**
*Vaxigrip* **(Influenza vaccine)**
*Vectren* **(Isoxicam)**
*Vectrin* **(Minocycline)**
*Veetids* **(Penicillin/Penicillin G)**
*Velban* **(Vinblastine)**
*Velbe* **(Vinblastine)**
*Venapulse* **(Atenolol)**
**Venlafaxine**
*Ventolin* **(Albuterol)**
*Veramyst* **(Fluticasone)**
**Verapamil**
*Verelan* **(Verapamil)**
*Versed* **(Midazolam)**
*Verukan* **(Salicylic acid)**
*Vesanoid* **(Tretinoin)**
*Vfend* **(Voriconazole)**
*Viagra* **(Sildenafil)**
*Vibra-Tabs* **(Doxycycline)**
*Vicodin* **(Hydrocodone)**
*Vicoprofen* **(Ibuprofen)**
*Videx* **(Didanosine)**
**Vigabatrin**
*Vigamox* **(Moxifloxacin)**
*Viibryd* **(Vilazodone)**
**Vilazodone**
*Vimpat* **(Lacosamide)**
**Vinblastine**
*Vioxx* **(Rofecoxib)**
*Virazole* **(Ribavirin)**
*Visipaque* **(Iodixanol)**
*Viskazide* **(Pindolol)**
*Visken* **(Pindolol)**
*Vistaril* **(Hydroxyzine)**
*Vistide* **(Cidofovir)**
*Vitamin D2* **(Ergocalciferal)**
*Vivactil* **(Protriptyline)**
*Vivelle-dot* **(Estradiol)**
*Volmax* **(Albuterol)**
*Voltaren* **(Diclofenac)**
*Voltaren Rapide* **(Diclofenac)**
*Voltaren SR* **(Diclofenac)**
**Voriconazole**
*Vytorin* **(Simvastatin)**

**W**

*Wellbutrin* **(Bupropion)**
*Wellbutrin SR* **(Bupropion)**
*Wellbutrin XL* **(Bupropion)**
*Wyamine* **(Mephentermine)**
*Wytensin* **(Guanabenz)**

**X**

*Xalacom* **(Timolol)**
*Xanax* **(Alprazolam)**
*Xanax TS* **(Alprazolam)**
*Xatral* **(Alfuzosin)**
*Xefo* **(Lornoxicam)**
*Xeomin* **(Botulinum Toxin Type A)**

*Xifaxan* **(Rifaximin)**
*Xylocaine* **(Lidocaine)**
*Xylocard* **(Lidocaine)**
*Xyrem* **(Sodium oxybate)**

**Y**
*Yasmin 28* **(Ethinyl estradiol)**
*Yaz* **(Ethinyl estradiol)**

**Z**
*Zagam* **(Sparfloxacin)**
**Zalcitabine**
**Zaleplon**
*Zanaflex* **(Tizanidine)**
*Zantac* **(Ranitidine)**
*Zaroxolyn* **(Metolazone)**
*Zebeta* **(Bisoprolol)**
*Zegerid* **(Omeprazole)**
*Zeldox* **(Ziprasidone)**
*Zelmid* **(Zimeldine)**
*Zepelin* **(Feprazone)**
*Zestoretic* **(Lisinopril)**
*Zestril* **(Lisinopril)**
*Zetia* **(Ezetimibe)**
*Ziac* **(Bisoprolol)**
**Ziconotide**
**Zidovudine**
**Zimeldine**
*Zinacef* **(Cefuroxime)**
**Ziprasidone**
*Zithromax* **(Azithromycin)**
*Zocor* **(Simvastatin)**
**Zoledronic acid**
**Zolmitriptan**
*Zoloft* **(Sertraline)**
**Zolpidem**
*Zomaril* **(Iloperidone)**
*Zomax* **(Zomepirac)**
**Zomepirac**
*Zomig* **(Zolmitriptan)**
*Zonegran* **(Zonisamide)**
**Zonisamide**
*Zosyn* **(Piperacillin—Tazobactam)**
**Zuclopenthixol**
*Zyban* **(Bupropion)**
*Zydone* **(Hydrocodone)**
*Zyloprim* **(Allopurinol)**
*Zymar* **(Gatifloxacin)**
*Zyprexa* **(Olanzapine)**
*Zyrtec* **(Cetirizine)**
*Zytram XL* **(Tramadol)**
*Zyvox* **(Linezolid)**
*Zyvoxam* **(Linezolid)**

## Herbals

*Herbal Common Name* **(Botanical Name)**
or **Botanical Name** (only)

*American wormseed* **(Chenopodium ambrosioides)**
*Ayahuasca* **(Banisteriopsis caapi)**
**Banisteriopsis caapi**
**Cannabis sativa**
**Chenopodium ambrosioides**
**Chrysanthemum cinerariifolium**
*Cinchona* **(Cinchona pubescens)**
Cinchona pubescens
*Hemp* **(Cannabis sativa)**
**Lactuca virosa**
*Lactucarium* **(Lactuca virosa)**
*Marijuana* **(Cannabis sativa)**
*Prickly lettuce* **(Lactuca virosa)**
*Pyrethrum* **(Chrysanthemum cinerariifolium)**

*Quinine* **(Cinchona pubescens)**
*Wormseed oil* **(Chenopodium ambrosioides)**
*Yage* **(Banisteriopsis caapi)**

## Chemicals

*Chemical Name* **(Common Name)**
or **Common Name** (only)

*1,1,2,2-Tetrachloroethane* **(Tetrachloroethane)**
*2-Hexanone* **(Hexanone)**
*3-Cresol* **(Cresol mixture)**
*4-Bromoaniline* **(Bromoaniline)**
*4-Cresol* **(Cresol mixture)**
*4-Hydroxyloluene* **(Cresol mixture)**
*4-Methylphenol* **(Cresol mixture)**
*6-Amino nicotinamide* **(Amino nicotinamide)**
*6-AN* **(Amino nicotinamide)**

### A

*Acetylene tetrachloride* **(Tetrachloroethane)**
*Acetylene trichloride* **(Trichloroethylene)**
*Agrocide* **(Lindane)**
*Alcanfor* **(Camphor)**
*Alcohol* **(Ethanol)**
*Algofrene* **(Dichlorodifluoromethane)**
*Algylen* **(Trichloroethylene)**
*Alpha-difluromethylornithine* **(Difluromethylornithine)**
*Alpha-hydroquinone* **(Hydroquinone)**
**Amino nicotinamide**
*Aminobenzene* **(Aniline)**
*AminoSweet* **(Aspartame)**
*Anhydrol* **(Ethanol)**
**Aniline**
**Arsenic**
*Arsenic chloride* **(Arsenic)**
*Arsenic trioxide* **(Arsenic)**
**Aspartame**

### B

*Benzenamine* **(Aniline)**
**Benzene**
*Benzene hexachloride* **(Lindane)**
*Benzenol* **(Phenol)**
*Benzinol* **(Trichloroethylene)**
*Benzohydroquinone* **(Hydroquinone)**
*Benzol* **(Benzene)**
*Benzolene* **(Benzene)**
*Beta-quinol* **(Hydroquinone)**
*Blue oil* **(Aniline)**
*Bonoform* **(Tetrachloroethane)**
**Bromoaniline**
*Butoflin* **(Deltamethrin)**
*Butoss* **(Deltamethrin)**
*Butyl methyl ketone* **(Hexanone)**

### C

**Camphor**
*Carbinol* **(Methyl alcohol)**
*Carbolic acid* **(Phenol)**
*Carbon dichloride* **(Tetrachloroethylene)**
**Carbon monoxide**
*Cellon* **(Tetrachloroethane)**
*Chlorilen* **(Trichloroethylene)**
*Chloromethane* **(Methyl chloride)**
*Cislin* **(Deltamethrin)**
*CO* **(Carbon monoxide)**
*Columbian spirit* **(Methyl alcohol)**
*Crackdown* **(Deltamethrin)**
**Cresol mixture**
*Cyanol* **(Aniline)**
**Cyclohexane**

**D**

*D-Camphor* **(Camphor)**
*Decis* **(Deltamethrin)**
**Deltamethrin**
*DFMO* **(Difluromethylornithine)**
**Dichlorodifluoromethane**
*Dichloromethane* **(Methylene chloride)**
**Difluromethylornithine**
*Dihydroxybenzene* **(Hydroquinone)**
*Dipropyl* **(Hexane)**
*Dukeron* **(Trichloroethylene)**

**E**

*Equal* **(Aspartame)**
*Eskimon 12* **(Dichlorodifluoromethane)**
**Ethanol**
*Ethenylbenzene* **(Styrene)**
*Ethyl alcohol* **(Ethanol)**
*Ethyl hydrate* **(Ethanol)**
*Ethylene tetrachloride* **(Tetrachloroethylene)**
*Ethylene trichloride* **(Trichloroethylene)**

**F**

*Fluorocarbon* **(Dichlorodifluoromethane)**
*Freon* **(Dichlorodifluoromethane)**
*Frigen 12* **(Dichlorodifluoromethane)**

**G**

*Germalgene* **(Trichloroethylene)**
*Grain alcohol* **(Ethanol)**

**H**

*Hexahydrobenzene* **(Cyclohexane)**
*Hexamethylene* **(Cyclohexane)**
*Hexanaphthene* **(Cyclohexane)**
**Hexane**
**Hexanone**
*Hexit* **(Lindane)**
*Hexyl hydride* **(Hexane)**
**Hydroquinone**
*Hydroxybenzene* **(Phenol)**

**K**

*K-Otek* **(Deltamethrin)**
*K-Othrin* **(Deltamethrin)**
*Kwell* **(Lindane)**
*Kyanol* **(Aniline)**

**L**

*L-Asparty-L-phenylalanine methyl ester* **(Aspartame)**
*L-Camphor* **(Camphor)**
**Lead**
**Lindane**

**M**

*M-,P-Cresol mixture* **(Cresol mixture)**
**Mercury**
*Methacide* **(Toluene)**
*Methane dichloride* **(Methylene chloride)**
**Methyl chloride**
*Methyl hydroxide* **(Methyl alcohol)**
*Methyl N-butyl keytone* **(Hexanone)**
*Methylbenzene* **(Toluene)**
*Methylbenzol* **(Toluene)**
**Methylene chloride**
*Mineral naphtha* **(Benzene)**
*Molasses alcohol* **(Ethanol)**
*Monochloromethane* **(Methyl chloride)**

**N**

*Narcogen* **(Trichloroethylene)**
*Narkotil* **(Methylene chloride)**
*N-Hexane* **(Hexane)**
*NutraSweet* **(Aspartame)**

**O**

*Octafluoropropane* **(Perfluoropropane)**
*Oxybenzene* **(Phenol)**

**P**

*P-Benzenediol* **(Hydroquinone)**
*P-Bromoaniline* **(Bromoaniline)**
*P-Bromophenylamine* **(Bromoaniline)**
*P-Cresylic acid* **(Cresol mixture)**
*Perchlor* **(Tetrachloroethylene)**
*Perchloroethylene* **(Tetrachloroethylene)**
*Perclene* **(Tetrachloroethylene)**
**Perfluoropropane**
*Perklone* **(Tetrachloroethylene)**
*Petzinol* **(Trichloroethylene)**
**Phenol**
*Phenyl hydroxide* **(Phenol)**
*Phenylethylene* **(Styrene)**
*Phenylic acid* **(Phenol)**
*Phenylmethane* **(Toluene)**
*Potato alcohol* **(Ethanol)**
*P-Oxytoluene* **(Cresol mixture)**
*Pyrobenzol* **(Benzene)**

**Q**

*Quinol* **(Hydroquinone)**

**S**

*Skellysolve B* **(Hexane)**
*Solaesthin* **(Methylene chloride)**
*Spirits of wine* **(Ethanol)**
**Styrene**
*Styrol* **(Styrene)**

**T**

*Tecquinol* **(Hydroquinone)**
*Tetracap* **(Tetrachloroethylene)**
**Tetrachloroethane**
**Tetrachloroethylene**
*Tetroguer* **(Tetrachloroethylene)**
*Threthylene* **(Trichloroethylene)**
**Toluene**
*Toluol* **(Toluene)**
*Trichloran* **(Trichloroethylene)**
**Trichloroethylene**
*Trilene* (**Trichloroethylene**)

**V**

*Vestrol* (**Trichloroethylene**)

**W**

*Westron* (**Tetrachloroethane**)
*Wood alcohol* **(Methyl alcohol)**
*Wood naphtha* (**Methyl alcohol**)

# Literature Cited

> **Obsolete URLs**
>
> **Note**: Many of the URLs from which information was cited no longer exist. Obsolete URLs (as of February 2016) are shown in square brackets. The information obtained from now obsolete links may still exist on the Internet at another URL if you want to try and track down that particular information.

AdvancedWellness. 2012. The Whiplash Syndrome: Ringing in the Ears. http://www.advanced-wellness.net/blog/the-whiplash-syndrome-ringing-in-the-ears.

All About Tinnitus. 2001. Acoustic Neuroma Archive. [http://www.anarchive.org/tinnitus.htm].

American Sleep Association. 2007. Exploding Head Syndrome. [http://www.sleepassociation.org/index.php?p=explodingheadsyndrome].

American Tinnitus Association. 2002. Frequently Asked Questions. [http://www.ata.org/about_tinnitus/consumer/faq.html].

Atkinson, Cheryl & Doug. 2008. Salicylate Intolerance Information. http://magicref.tripod.com/health/salicylate.htm.

Auditory Disorders. 1997. Conner's Corner. [http://www.ccnet.com/~njones/auditory.html#table].

Bartels, H. et al. 2007. Tinnitus and Neural Plasticity of the Brain. Otology and Neurotology 2007 Feb. 28 (2): 178-184. [http://dissertations.ub.rug.nl/FILES/faculties/medicine/2008/h.bartels/01_c1.pdf].

Basic Information about Auditory Integration Training. 1997. Society for Auditory Integration Training. [http://www.elaine.teleport.com/~sait/basic.html].

Bauman, Neil. 2002a. Large Vestibular Aqueduct Syndrome (LVAS). http://hearinglosshelp.com/blog/large-vestibular-aqueduct-syndrome.

Bauman, Neil. 2009a. Loud Music and Hearing Loss. http://hearinglosshelp.com/blog/loud-music-and-hearing-loss.

Bauman, Neil. 2009b. Vitamins A, C & E Combined with Magnesium Help Prevent Noise-Induced Hearing Loss. http://hearinglosshelp.com/blog/vitamins-a-c-e-combined-with-magnesium-help-prevent-noise-induced-hearing-loss.

Bauman, Neil. 2010a. Ototoxic Drugs Exposed. 3rd Edition. Integrity First Publications. 49 Piston Court. Stewartstown, PA. 17363. http://hearinglosshelp.com/shop/ototoxic-drugs-exposed.

Bauman, Neil. 2010b. Reduce Your Tinnitus by Listening to Your Favorite (Notched) Music. May 29, 2010. http://hearinglosshelp.com/blog/reduce-your-tinnitus-by-listening-to-your-favorite-notched-music.

Bauman, Neil. 2011a. The Agony of Meniere's Disease—Please Make My World Stop Spinning. 3rd Edition Integrity First Publications. 49 Piston Court. Stewartstown, PA. 17363. http://hearinglosshelp.com/shop/the-agony-of-menieres-disease.

Bauman, Neil. 2011b. Phantom Voices, Ethereal Music & Other Spooky Sounds. 2nd Edition. Integrity First Publications. 49 Piston Court. Stewartstown, PA. 17363. http://hearinglosshelp.com/shop/phantom-voices-ethereal-music-and-other-spooky-sounds.

Bauman, Neil. 2013. Do I Have Tonic Tensor Tympani Syndrome (TTTS)? http://hearinglosshelp.com/blog/do-i-have-tonic-tensor-tympani-syndrome-ttts.

Bauman, Neil. 2015. Atlas Adjustments Alleviate Meniere's Disease. http://hearinglosshelp.com/blog/atlas-adjustments-alleviate-menieres-disease.

Beck, Douglas, et. al. Issues in Tinnitus: 2014-2015. October, 2014. HearingReview.Com.

Beck, Douglas. 2015. Clinical Aspects of Tinnitus: An Interview with David Baguley, Ph.D. Dec. 23, 2015. The Hearing Review. http://www.hearingreview.com/2015/12/clinical-aspects-tinnitus-interview-david-baguley-phd.

Bedrich Smetana. 2004. Bedrich Smetana. http://members.tripod.com/~Nash_K/bio.html.

BeyondTinnitus. 2011a. Acoustic Neural Stimulation for Tinnitus. http://www.beyondtinnitus.com/acoustic-neural-stimulation-tinnitus.

BeyondTinnitus. 2011b. Tinnitus Cause. [http://www.beyondtinnitus.com/tinnitus-cause].

BeyondTinnitus. 2011c. BeyondTinnitus Treatment Protocol. [http://www.beyondtinnitus.com/tinnitus-treatment-protocol].

Bilger, Burkhard. May 1998. Natural Remedies That Really Work. In: *Health*. Published in Reader's Digest.

Blair Upper Cervical—Dr. William G. Blair. 2002. http://www.upcspine.com/tech3.htm.

Buchanan, Greg. 2002. Introduction to Upper Cervical Techniques. http://www.upcspine.com/approach1.htm.

Burcon, Michael, 2014. Cervical Specific Protocol & Results for 300 Meniere's Patients. Presented at the New Zealand College of Chiropractic, Upper Cervical Conference. http://www.burconchiropractic.com/g5-bin/client.cgi?G5button=626&subcategoryID=2525.

Busto, Usoa. 1988. Protracted Tinnitus After Discontinuation of Long-Term Therapeutic Use of Benzodiazepines. New England Journal of Medicine. 315:854-859. http://www.benzo.org.uk/busto.htm.

California Tinnitus Assessment Center. 1997. CTAC News & Notes—Volume 1. San Diego, CA. 92120. [http://www.earinfo.com/ctac/news297.html].

Centore, Linda. 2010. A Guide to Pharmacologic Management of Target Symptoms of Severe Tinnitus. The Hearing Journal. New York, NY. November, 2010, Vol. 63. No. 11.

Coexisting with Tinnitus by Masking. 1997. Tinnitus FAQ. [http://www.cccd.edu/faq/tinnitus/coexist.html].

Cognitive Behavioral Treatment of Tinnitus. ~2011. eNetMD. http://www.enetmd.com/content/cognitive-behavioral-treatment-tinnitus.

Cognitive Therapy for Tinnitus. 2002. RNID Factsheets. Royal National Institute for the Deaf. [http://www.rnid.org.uk/html/factsheets/tin_cognitive.htm].

Cohn, Neville. 2004. Triumph over Adversity. Zartsreview. Jan. 2004. [http://members.ozemail.com.au/~ozartsreview/Features/disabled.html].

Coleman, Thomas. 2009. Tinnitus Miracle. http://www.tinnitusmiracle.com.

Compendium of Pharmaceuticals and Specialties. 2000. 35th Edition. Canadian Pharmacists Association. 1785 Alta Vista Drive. Ottawa, Ontario. Canada K1G 3Y6.

Connor, Frederick. 2003. Tinnitus: A Preliminary Investigation of the Experience and Its Psychological Effects. Liverpool John Moores University. http://www.angelfire.com/pro/tinnitusstudy/Preliminary_Investigation.pdf.

Craggs-Hinton, Christine. 2007. Coping with Tinnitus. Sheldon Press. London SW1P 4ST.

Cullen, Theresa, Au.D. 2014. Questions and Answers. Tinnitus Today. Vol. 39, Number 3, Winter 2014.

Currie, John. 2005. Homeopathic Remedies for Tinnitus Relief. T-Gone Remedies, Inc. http://t-gone.org.

De Ridder, Dirk, et al. 2005. Transcranial Magnetic Stimulation for Tinnitus: Influence of Tinnitus Duration on Stimulation Parameter Choice and Maximal Tinnitus Suppression. Otology & Neurotology. 26(4): 616-619.

De Ridder, Dirk, et. al. 2015. Placebo-Controlled Vagus Nerve Stimulation Paired with Tones in a Patient with Refractory Tinnitus: A Case Report. Otol Neurotol. 2015 Apr;36(4):575-80. PubMed. http://www.ncbi.nlm.nih.gov/pubmed/25689839.

Diiulio, Renee. October, 2007. It's All in Your Head. Hearing Products Report. [http://www.hearingreview.com/issues/articles/hpr_2007-10_03.asp].

Discovering and Understanding Tinnitus. 1997. Tinnitus FAQ. [http://www.cccd.edu/faq/tinnitus/discover.html].

Disorders of the Inner Ear. 2000. Chapter 8. Hearing and Balance; the Inner Ear. Department of Neurophysiology. University of Wisconsin-Madison. http://www.neurophys.wisc.edu/~ychen/textbook/chap-8.html.

Dobie, Robert, et al. "Tinnitus, Depression, and Aging" Geriatric Otorhinolaryngology.

Dornhoffer, John and Mark Mennemier. 2010. Using Repetitive Transcranial Magnetic Stimulation for the Treatment of Tinnitus. The Hearing Journal. Nov. 2010. Vol. 63, No. 11.

Drugs and Tinnitus. 2001. Factsheets. Royal National Institute for the Deaf. [http://www.rnid.org.uk/html/Factsheets/tin_drugs.htm].

Duke, James. 1997. The Green Pharmacy. Rodale Press. Emmaus, Pennsylvania.

Exploding Head Syndrome. 2011. Wikipedia. http://en.wikipedia.org/wiki/Exploding_head_syndrome.

FAQ. 2002. Upper Cervical Chiropractic. http://www.upper-cervical.com/html/faq.htm.

Folmer, Robert, et. al. 2015. Repetitive Transcranial Magnetic Stimulation Treatment for Chronic Tinnitus: A Randomized Clinical Trial. JAMA Otolaryngology - Head & Neck Surgery, 2015 DOI: 10.1001/.jamaoto.2015.1219. https://www.sciencedaily.com/releases/2015/07/150716124118.htm.

Forstag, Ben. 2014. Head Noise: Tinnitus and the Human Brain. Tinnitus Today. Summer, 2014.

Fractal Tones via Amplification for Tinnitus Relief. 2010. American Academy of Audiology. http://www.audiology.org/news/Pages/20101202.aspx.

Functional Magnetic Resonance Imaging. Nov. 2000. Online Newsletter. Royal National Institute for the Deaf. [http://www.rnid.org.uk/html/information/tinnitus/newsletter/nov2000_fmri.htm].

Gans, Jennifer. 2010. Mindfulness-Based Tinnitus Therapy Is an Approach with Ancient Roots. The Hearing Journal. November, 2010. Vol. 63. No. 11.

Gans, Jennifer. 2014. Mindfulness: Changing the Brain to Change Our Perception of Tinnitus. Tinnitus Today. Spring, 2014.

Gans, Jennifer. 2015. Mindfulness Based Tinnitus Stress Reduction: Unraveling the Gordian Knot of Tinnitus. HearingReview.com. July, 2015.

German “FDA” Approves Ginkgo for Tinnitus. 1994. Excerpted from the Complete Commission E Monographs: Therapeutic Guide to Herbal Medicine. Ginkgo Biloba Leaf Extract. http://www.tinnitusformula.com/library/german-fda-approves-ginkgo-for-tinnitus/#.VZkVokYenLU.

Gibrin, P. C., et. al. Prevalence of Tinnitus Complaints and Probable Association with Hearing Loss, Diabetes Mellitus and Hypertension in Elderly. CoDAS (December, 2013). Reported in: Tinnitus Today. Spring 2014.

Goldstein, Barbara, Abraham Shulman, et al. 2001. Long-term Inhibition of Tinnitus by UltraQuiet™ Therapy—Preliminary Report. International Tinnitus Journal, Volume 7, Number 2. [http://www.tinnitus.vcu.edu/Pages/Tinnitus.pdf].

Greenspan, Kenneth. 1998. Treating Tinnitus & Hyperacusis: An Integrated Approach. Hearing Health. Ingleside, Texas. Vol. 14. No. 1. Jan/Feb 1998.

Greuel, Dr. Hans. 1997. Biomental Therapy. Teleklinik, Kaiser Wilhelm Ring 37. D-40545. Dusseldorf, Germany. http://www.teleklinik.com.

Guimaraes, A. C., et. al.. 2014. Study of the Relationship Between the Degree of Tinnitus Annoyance and the Presence of Hyperacusis. Brazilian Journal of Otorhinolaryngology (Jan-Feb 2014). As reported in Tinnitus Today. Summer, 2014.

Hain, Timothy. 2001. Ototoxic Medications. [http://www.tchain.com/otoneurology/disorders/bilat/ototoxicns.html].

Haybach, Patty J. 1998. Ototoxicity for Nurses. [http://www.geocities.com/otolithic/ototox.htm].

Haybach, Patty J. 1999. Balance and Hearing: At Risk from Drugs. Course #170. [http://nurse.cyberchalk.com/nurse/COURSES/NURSEWEEK/NW170/menu.html].

Hazell, Jonathan W. P. Tinnitus. CHIP Background Information for Speechreading Instructors. Extracted from various issues of the British publication, *Catchword*.

Hazell, Jonathan. 1997a. Tinnitus Retraining Therapy. Information for All. Royal National Institute for the Deaf. London, UK. [http://www.ucl.ac.uk/~rmjg101/tin2.htm].

Hazell, Jonathan. 1997b. Questions about Tinnitus. Royal National Institute for the Deaf. London, UK. [http://www.ucl.ac.uk/~rmjg101/rnidqa.htm].

Hazell, Jonathan. 1997c. Retraining Therapy for Tinnitus and Hyperacusis. Royal National Institute for the Deaf. London, UK. [http://www.ucl.ac.uk/~rmjg101/tinnitus1.html].

HearingReview.Com. October, 2014. "Caffeine Linked with Lower Levels of Tinnitus in Younger and Middle-Aged Women".

HearingReview.Com. September, 2015. "New Drug Promises Relief from Tinnitus, Epilepsy ".

Henry, James, A., et. al. 2010a. How to Manage Your Tinnitus: A Step-by-Step Workbook. Third Edition. http://www.ncrar.research.va.gov/Education/Documents/TinnitusDocuments/HowToManageYourTinnitus.pdf.

Henry, James, A., et. al. 2010b. Progressive Tinnitus Management: Clinical Handbook for Audiologists. Dept. of Veterans Affairs. Employee Education System. http://www.ncrar.research.va.gov/Education/Documents/TinnitusDocuments/ClinicalHandbookAndSupplements.asp.

Herzfeld, Melanie, et. al. 2014. Clinical Trial on the Effectiveness of Widex Zen Therapy for Tinnitus. HearingReview.Com. November, 2014.

Hickish, Gordon. How GP's Can Help Tinnitus Sufferers. CHIP Background Information for Speechreading Instructors. Extracted from various issues of the British publication, *Catchword*.

Hobbs, Jay. 2014. What Is the Therapy to Remove Trigger Points of Tinnitus?. Tinnitus Synergy. http://tinnitussynergy.com/wp-content/uploads/2014/10/WhatistheTherapytoRemoveTriggerPointsofTinnitus.pdf.

Hogan, Kevin. 1998. Tinnitus: Turning the Volume Down. Proven Strategies for Turning the Noise Down in Your Head. Network 3000 Publishing Co. Eagan, MN 55123.

How Is Tinnitus Diagnosed? October, 2004. [http://yourmedicalsource.com/library/tinnitus/TIN_diagnosis.html].

Information About Tinnitus. 1988. American Tinnitus Association. Portland, Oregon.

Info-Tinnitus, Causes and Factors in the Hearing System. 1990. Tinnitus Association of Ottawa. Dorval, Quebec.

Info-Tinnitus, Relaxation. 1990. Tinnitus Association of Ottawa. Dorval, Quebec.

Info-Tinnitus, Solutions. 1990. Tinnitus Association of Ottawa. Dorval, Quebec.

Info-Tinnitus, the Holistic Approach. 1990. Tinnitus Association of Ottawa. Dorval, Quebec.

Jastreboff, Pawel J. 1997a. Overview. Tinnitus & Hyperacusis Center. University of Maryland at Baltimore. http://www.tinnitus-pjj.com.

Jastreboff, Pawel J. 1997b. Theoretical Basis of the Approach and Main Practical Guidelines. Tinnitus & Hyperacusis Center. University of Maryland at Baltimore. [http://www.tinnitus-pjj.com/overview.html].

Jastreboff, Pawel J. 1997c. A New Look at Tinnitus. Hearing Health Magazine. Feature Article # 2. [http://www.hearinghealthmag.com/feature2.htm].

Jenkins, Barbara. 2014. Reduce Your Risk. Hearing Health Magazine. Summer, 2014.

Jimenez-Cervantes, Nicolas. 1990. Hydergine in Pathology of the Inner Ear. An Otorrinolaringol Ibero AM. 1990 17(1):85-98. http://www.ncbi.nlm.nih.gov/pubmed/2334027.

Johnson, Marsha. 1999. Pulsatile Tinnitus Brief. Oregon Tinnitus and Hyperacusis Treatment Center. [http://www.tinnitus-audiology.com/articles/pulse.htm].

Johnson, Sharon. 2007. New Treatment for Tinnitus Brings Relief of Symptoms. The New York Times. [http://www.tinnitusphase-out.com/news.html].

Jun, H. J. and M. K. Park. 2013. Cognitive Behavioral Therapy for Tinnitus: Evidence and Efficacy. Korean Journal of Audiology (December, 2013). Reported in: Tinnitus Today. Summer, 2014.

Kaltenbach, James. 2011. The Brain Playing Tricks—An Update on the Origins of Tinnitus. Hearing Health. A publication of the Deafness Research Foundation. Winter 2011.

Kaute, Bernd, 1998. The Influence of Atlas Therapy on Tinnitus. International Tinnitus Journal, Vol. 4, No. 2, 165-167 (1998). http://www.tinnitusjournal.com/imagebank/pdf/v4n2a18.pdf.

Keate, Barry. 2010a. Diet and Tinnitus: What to Eat...and What Not to Eat. http://www.tinnitusformula.com/library/diet-and-tinnitus/#.VsNHheYel30.

Keate, Barry. 2010b. Arches Tinnitus Formula: What It Contains and Some Findings on Its Effectiveness. The Hearing Journal. November, 2010. Vol. 63. No. 11.

Keate, Barry. 2013. Hyperbaric Oxygen Therapy for Tinnitus. http://www.tinnitusformula.com/library/hyperbaric-oxygen-therapy-for-tinnitus/#.Vo5jM1Iemb0.

Keate, Barry. 2016. How Insulin Resistance and Diabetes Cause Tinnitus. http://www.tinnitusformula.com/library/how-insulin-resistance-and-diabetes-cause-tinnitus.

Klemons, Ira. 2010. Successful Treatment of Tinnitus in Patients with TMJ Dysfunction. http://www.tinnitusformula.com/library/tinnitus-and-tmj-dysfunction/#.VsNIE-Yel30.

Koren, Tedd. 2004. Tinnitus. World Chiropractic Today. http://worldchiropractictoday.com/Tinnitus.htm.

Kurian, Jills K. 2014. International Conference Explores Hyperacusis. In: Tinnitus Today. Spring, 2014.

Lacerte Marketing. 1997. Sound Therapy for the Walkman—At the Lacerte Mall. [http://www.lacerte.com/steele/search/081197.htm].

Lamm, K., et. al. 1998. Effect of Hyperbaric Oxygen Therapy in Comparison to Conventional or Placebo Therapy or No Treatment in Idiopathic Sudden Hearing Loss, Acoustic Trauma, Noise-Induced Hearing Loss and Tinnitus. A Literature Survey. Adv. Otorhinolaryngol 1998, 54:86-99. http://www.ncbi.nlm.nih.gov/pubmed/9547879.

Lean, Sandra. 2004. Sandra Lean Offers These Notes on Bewich Fallcaster's 92 Variations on the Tinnitus Theme. [http://btinternet.com/~paul.melia/tin.html].

Leaver, Amber, et al. 2011a. Dysregulation of Limbic and Auditory Networks in Tinnitus. Neuron 69, 33-43. Elsevier Inc. January 13, 2011.

Leaver, Amber. 2011b. Tinnitus: Current Neuroscience Research and Theories. Presentation made at the Hearing Loss Association of America National Convention at Crystal City, VA. June 18, 2011.

Lee, S.K., et. al. 2014. Effectiveness of Transcutaneous Electrical Stimulation for Chronic Tinnitus. Acta Otolaryngol. 2014 Feb;134(2):159-67. http://www.ncbi.nlm.nih.gov/pubmed/24215217.

Levine, Robert, MD. 1999. Somatic Modulation Appears to be a Fundamental Attribute of Tinnitus. Massachusetts Eye and Ear Infirmary. Boston, MA.

Levine, Robert, MD. 2000. Diagnostic Issues in Tinnitus: a Neuro-Otological Perspective. Eaton-Peabody Laboratory. Massachusetts Eye and Ear Infirmary, Boston, MA. [http://epl.harvard.edu/~ral/Baguley.Seminar.pdf].

Levine, Robert, MD., et al. 2003. All that Rings is Not from the Ear: Somatic Tinnitus in Non-Clinical Subjects and the Profoundly Deaf. Massachusetts Eye and Ear Infirmary. Boston, MA.

Levine, Robert, MD. 2004. p. 108. Somatic Tinnitus. Chapter 9. Tinnitus: Theory & Management. BC Decker.

Lidocaine Helps Relieve Ringing in the Ears. May 19, 2000. Reuters Health.

Life Extension. 2011. Tinnitus. Life Extension Foundation. http://www.lef.org/protocols/prtcl-105.shtml.

Lockwood, A. H., et al. 1999. Positron Emission Tomographic (PET) Studies of Gaze-Evoked Tinnitus. Abstract #472. Date 2/16/99, Session O, Podium, 4:30p. [http://www.aro.org/archives/1999/472.html].

Lockwood, Alan H. 2001a. Eye Movements Linked to Tinnitus; Ringing in Ears. American Academy of Neurology. [http://www.newswise.com/articles/2001/2/NEURLOGY.VAR.html].

Lockwood, A. H., et al. 2001b. The Functional Anatomy of Gaze-Evoked Tinnitus and Sustained Lateral Gaze. Neurology 56. February (2 of 2) 2001. [http://www.smbs.buffalo.edu/neu/GET_paper.pdf].

Luo, H., et. al. Blast-Induced Tinnitus and Spontaneous Firing Changes in the Rat Dorsal Cochlear Nucleus. Journal of Neuroscience Research (June, 2014). Reported in: Tinnitus Today. Summer, 2014.

Maleskey, Gale. 1999. Nature's Medicines. Prevention Health Books. Rodale Inc.

Martin, Robert, DC. 2001. Ringing in the Ears. [www.earinc.com/RingStop-Guide.doc].

Mayes, J. L. 2010. Tinnitus Treatment Toolbox—A Guide for People with Ear Noise. Trafford Publishing. [http://www.trafford.com].

McCall, Rosemary. 1991. Hearing Loss?—A Guide to Self-help. Robert Hale Limited. London.

McCarthy, Michael. 1997. Auditory Integration Training. Autism/A.D.D. Resources Inc. Vashon Island, Washington. 98070. [http://www.vashonisland.com/brainresources/ait.htm].

McCombe, A., et. al. 1999. Guidelines for the grading of tinnitus severity: the results of a working group commissioned by the British Association of Otolaryngologists, Head and Neck, Surgeons, 1999. Clin. Otolaryngol. 26, 388-393.

McKenna, Laurence, 2007. Changing Reactions to Tinnitus. [http://www.hearingreview.com/issues/articles/2007-08_01.asp?]

Mercola, Joseph. 2015. Magnesium—A Key Nutrient for Health and Disease Prevention. http://articles.mercola.com/sites/articles/archive/2015/12/28/magnesium-atp.aspx.

MicroTransponder. 2015. How Stimulating a Nerve in the Neck Treats Tinnitus. http://www.microtransponder.com/technology/how-it-works.

Mindfulness-Based Cognitive Therapy. 2011. Wikipedia. http://en.wikipedia.org/wiki/Mindfulness-based_cognitive_therapy.

Moller, Aage R., et al. Textbook of Tinnitus. 2011. Springer. New York.

Multicenter Study Finds S–Tones Beat Broadband Noise in Tinnitus Relief. HearingReview.Com. October, 2014.

Nagler, Stephen, MD. 2003. Ginkgo—A Word of Caution. Dr. Nagler's Tinnitus Site. [http://www.tinn.com/ginkgo.html].

Nerves in Head and Neck Linked to Tinnitus. 2008. The Hearing Review. Vol. 15, No. 2, February, 2008. [http://www.hearingreview.com/issues/articles/2008-02_08.asp].

Neuromonics. 2009. http://www.neuromonics.com.

Newman, C. W., et. al. 1996. Development of the Tinnitus Handicap Inventory. Arch Otolaryngol Head Neck Surg. 122, 143-148.

Noise, Its Effects on Hearing and Tinnitus. 1988. American Tinnitus Association. Portland, Oregon.

O'Dell, Alexandra. 2015. Sound Therapy and Addressing the Gap in Tinnitus Care. Tinnitus Today. Spring, 2015.

Okamoto, Hidehiko et al. Listening to Tailor-Made Notched Music Reduces Tinnitus Loudness and Tinnitus-Related Auditory Cortex Activity. Proc Natl. Acad. Sci. USA. 2010 January 19; 107(3): 1207–1210. http://www.ncbi.nlm.nih.gov/pmc/articles/PMC2824261.

Olsson, Robert. 1997a. Your Doctor Said "Live with It." CTAC Says Different. California Tinnitus Assessment Center. San Diego, CA. 92120. [http://www.earinfo.com/ctac/index1.html#anchor2213775].

Olsson, Robert. 1997b. California Tinnitus Assessment Center's Frequently Asked Questions. California Tinnitus Assessment Center. San Diego, CA. 92120. [http://www.earinfo.com/ctac/faqs.html].

Pape, J. et. al. 2014. Playing and Listening to Tailor-Made Notched Music: Cortical Plasticity Induced by Unimodal and Multimodal Training in Tinnitus Patients. Reported in: Tinnitus Today. Summer, 2014.

PDR for Herbal Medicines. 2nd Edition. 2000. Medical Economics Company, Inc. Montvale, NJ 07645-1742.

Phua, Peter, MD. 2015. What Are the Most Common Tinnitus Frequencies? http://www.audionotch.com/blog/tinnitus-research-2/what-are-the-most-common-tinnitus-frequencies.

Piskosz, Michael, et. al. June, 2015. Flexible and Personalized Sound Therapy. HearingReview.Com.

Powers, Leanne, et. al. June, 2015. Acoustic Therapy for the Treatment of Tinnitus: A Primer. HearingReview.Com.

Press, Linda & Jack Vernon. 1997. Tinnitus in the Elderly. Hearing Health. Volume 13, Number 6.

Prochazka, Miroslav & Renata Tejnska. 1999. Non-Invasive Laser in Therapy of Tinnitus. [http://www.jarov.cz/prednasky/tinit_en.htm].

Pulsatile Tinnitus. 2001. Royal National Institute for the Deaf. [http://www.rnid.org.uk/html/factsheets/tin_pulsatile.htm].

Pulsatile Tinnitus. 2003. British Tinnitus Association/Royal National Institute for the Deaf.

## Appendix

# Listing of Prescription Medications, Over-the-Counter Drugs, Herbals and Chemicals Associated with Tinnitus

The following list contains all the drugs, herbals and chemicals that have been associated with tinnitus and were known to the author at the time of compilation.

Although this list is one of the most complete listings of drugs associated with tinnitus, no list of this kind can ever be totally complete. New drugs are coming to the market all the time. Furthermore, some existing drugs not listed here will be found to cause tinnitus in the future. Therefore, use this list as a guide and discussion tool with your doctor, and as a springboard to further research on any drugs you may be taking or are considering taking.

At least 597 drugs, herbals and chemicals are currently associated with tinnitus. However, just because a drug is listed here does not mean that you will automatically get tinnitus or exacerbate your existing tinnitus if you take it.

Some drugs result in tinnitus occurring in a high percentage of those taking it. With other drugs, tinnitus only seems to occur rarely. Sometimes the resulting tinnitus is permanent. Other times the tinnitus goes away in a few days to a few weeks. Sometimes the tinnitus is mild. Other times it can be so loud that it is debilitating.

Whether or not you experience tinnitus after taking one of the listed drugs or herbals, or after being exposed to one of the listed chemicals, depends on many factors such as your own body chemistry, your sensitivity to drugs, your emotional makeup, the dose you take, the length of time you take the drug, etc. Therefore, use this listing as a preliminary tool in your quest to discover whether one of the drugs listed here is causing your tinnitus or making your existing tinnitus worse.

For more detailed information on the probability (risk) of getting tinnitus from taking any drug, as well as a guide to the likely severity and permanence of any resulting tinnitus for any drug, herbal or chemical listed here, see the latest edition of the author's comprehensive book, *Ototoxic Drugs Exposed*, listed in the back of this book. In addition to listing tinnitus side effects, *Ototoxic Drugs Exposed* lists information about the other ototoxic (ear-damaging) side effects of these drugs such as hearing loss, hyperacusis, ear infections, ear pain and a number of balance problems.

If you experience tinnitus (or any other side effects), you should **not** discontinue taking any prescribed medication without contacting your prescribing physician.

Drug brand names are *italicized*. Generic drug names are in **bold**. Please note that not every brand name is included as some drugs have numerous brand names.

## Medications & Drugs

*Drug Brand Name* **(Generic Drug Name)**
or **Generic Drug Name** (only)

*222* **(Acetylsalicylic acid)**
*282* **(Acetylsalicylic acid)**
*282 MEP* **(Acetylsalicylic acid)**
*292* **(Acetylsalicylic acid)**
*5-ASA* **(Mesalamine)**
*692* **(Acetylsalicylic acid)**

**A**

**Abatacept**
*Abelcet* **(Amphotericin B)**
*Abilify* **(Aripiprazole)**
**Acamprosate**
*AccuNeb* **(Albuterol)**
*Accupril* **(Quinapril)**
*Accuretic* **(Quinapril)**
*Accutane* **(Isotretinoin)**
**Acebutolol**
**Aceclofenac**
**Acemetacin**
*Aceon* **(Perindopril)**
**Acetaminophen**
**Acetazolamide**
**Acetylsalicylic acid**
*Achromycin* **(Tetracycline)**
*Aciphex* **(Rabeprazole)**
**Acitretin**
*Aclasta* **(Zoledronic acid)**
*Acthar* **(Corticotropin)**
*Actifed* **(Pseudoephedrine)**
*Actiq* **(Fentanyl)**
*Actonel* **(Risedronate)**
*Adalat* **(Nifedipine)**
**Adalimumab**
*Adapin* **(Doxepin)**
*Adcirca* **(Tadalafil)**
*Adipex-P* **(Phentermine)**
*Adriamycin* **(Doxorubicin)**
*Advagraf* **(Tacrolimus)**
*Advair Diskus* **(Fluticasone)**
*Advil* **(Ibuprofen)**
*Advil Cold & Sinus* **(Ibuprofen)**
*Aerosporin* **(Polymyxin B)**
*Afloxan* **(Proglumetacin)**
*Afrin* **(Oxymetazoline)**
**Agalsidase alfa**
**Agalsidase beta**
*Aggrenox* **(Acetylsalicylic acid)**
*Agrylin* **(Anagrelide)**
*Airomir* **(Albuterol)**
Alatrofloxacin **(Trovafloxacin)**
*Albert Tiafen* **(Tiaprofenic acid)**
**Albuterol**
**Alclofenac**
*Aldoril* **(Hydrochlorothiazide)**
*Aleve* **(Naproxen)**
*Alferon N* **(Interferon alfa-n3)**
**Alfuzosin**
*Alka-Seltzer* **(Acetylsalicylic acid)**
*Allegra* **(Fexofenadine)**
*Allegra-D* **(Fexofenadine)**
*Aller-Chlor* **(Chlorpheniramine)**
**Allopurinol**
*Almogran* **(Almotriptan)**
**Almotriptan**

*Aloxi* **(Palonosetron)**
**Alprazolam**
*Altace* **(Ramipril)**
*Alumadrine* **(Phenylpropanolamine)**
*Ambien* **(Zolpidem)**
*Ambien CR* **(Zolpidem)**
*AmBisome* **(Amphotericin B)**
*Amen* **(Medroxyprogesterone)**
*Amerge* **(Naratriptan)**
**Amezinium**
*Amicar* **(Aminocaproic acid)**
**Amikacin**
*Amikin* **(Amikacin)**
**Amiloride**
**Aminocaproic acid**
**Aminopyrine**
**Aminosidine—Paromomycin**
**Amiodarone**
**Amitriptyline**
**Amlodipine**
*Amoebriz* **(Mebendazole)**
**Amonafide**
**Amoxapine**
**Amoxicillin**
*Amphotec* **(Amphotericin B)**
**Amphotericin B**
*Ampyrone* **(Aminopyrine)**
*Amrix* **(Cyclobenzaprine)**
**Amtolmetin**
*Amturnide* **(Amlodipine)**
Anacin **(Acetylsalicylic acid)**
*Anafranil* **(Clomipramine)**
**Anagrelide**
*Anaprox* **(Naproxen)**
*Andante* **(Bunazosin)**
*Anexate* **(Flumazenil)**
*Angeliq* **(Estradiol)**
*Ansaid* **(Flurbiprofen)**
*Antivert* **(Meclizine)**
*Antizol* **(Fomepizole)**
*Anzemet* **(Dolasetron)**
*Aplenzin* **(Bupropion)**
*Apo-Acebutolol* **(Acebutolol)**
*Apo-Amiloride* **(Amiloride)**
*Apo-Beclomethasone* **(Beclomethasone)**
*Apo-Butorphanol* **(Butorphanol)**
*Apo-Carvedilol* **(Carvedilol)**
*Apo-Cetirizine* **(Cetirizine)**
*Apo-Clorazepate* **(Clorazepate)**
*Apo-Diltiaz* **(Diltiazem)**
*Apo-Divalproex* **(Divalproex)**
*Apo-Doxepin* **(Doxepin)**
*Apo-Etodolac* **(Etodolac)**
*Apo-Fenofibrate* **(Fenofibrate)**
*Apo-Feno-Micro* **(Fenofibrate)**
*Apo-Floctafenine* **(Floctafenine)**
*Apo-Fluvoxamine* **(Fluvoxamine)**
*Apo-Gabapentin* **(Gabapentin)**
*Apo-Hydro* **(Hydrochlorothiazide)**
*Apo-Indapamide* **(Indapamide)**
*Apo-Keto* **(Ketoprofen)**
*Apo-Ketorolac* **(Ketorolac)**
*Apo-Lisinopril* **(Lisinopril)**
*Apo-Loratadine* **(Loratadine)**
*Apo-Mefenamic* **(Mefenamic acid)**
*Apo-Methazolamide* **(Methazolamide)**
*Apo-Midazolam* **(Midazolam)**
*Apo-Misoprostol* **(Misoprostol)**
*Apo-Moclobemide* **(Moclobemide)**
*Apo-Nabumetone* **(Nabumetone)**
*Apo-Norflox* **(Norfloxacin)**
*Apo-Nortriptyline* **(Nortriptyline)**
*Apo-Oxaprozin* **(Oxaprozin)**
*Apo-Phenylbutazone* **(Phenylbutazone)**

*Apo-Prazo* **(Prazosin)**
*Apo-Selegiline* **(Selegiline)**
*Apo-Sotalol* **(Sotalol)**
*Apo-Temazepam* **(Temazepam)**
*Apo-Tenoxicam* **(Tenoxicam)**
*Apo-Timol* **(Timolol)**
*Apo-Trimethoprim* **(Trimethoprim)**
*Apo-Valproic* **(Valproic acid)**
**Aprepitant**
*Apresazide* **(Hydrochlorothiazide)**
*Apri 28* **(Ethinyl estradiol)**
*Apriso* **(Mesalamine)**
*Aralen* **(Chloroquine)**
*Arcoxia* **(Etoricoxib)**
*Arestin* **(Minocycline)**
*Aricept* **(Donepezil)**
**Aripiprazole**
**Arsenic trioxide**
**Artemether/Lumefantrine**
*Arthrotec* **(Diclofenac)**
**Articaine**
*Artromed* **(Amtolmetin)**
*ASA* **(Acetylsalicylic acid)**
*Asacol* **(Mesalamine)**
*Asasantine* **(Acetylsalicylic acid)**
*Ascriptin* **(Acetylsalicylic acid)**
*Asendin* **(Amoxapine)**
*Asmanex* **(Mometasone)**
*Asmavent* **(Albuterol)**
*Aspirin* **(Acetylsalicylic acid)**
Aspirin *Backache* **(Acetylsalicylic acid)**
*Astelin* **(Amoxicillin)**
*Astepro* **(Amoxicillin)**
**Astromicin**
*Atacand* **(Candesartan)**
*Atacand HCT* **(Candesartan)**
*Atacand Plus* **(Candesartan)**
*Atarax* **(Hydroxyzine)**
**Atenolol**
*Ativan* **(Lorazepam)**
**Atorvastatin**
**Atovaquone/Proguanil**
*Atretol* **(Carbamazepine)**
*Atripla* **(Efavirenz)**
*Atrohist* **(Pyrilamine)**
*Atrohist Plus* **(Phenylpropanolamine)**
*Atrovent* **(Ipratropium)**
*Augmentin* **(Amoxicillin)**
**Auranofin**
*Avalide* **(Irbesartan)**
*Avamys* **(Fluticasone)**
*Avapro* **(Irbesartan)**
*Avelox* **(Moxifloxacin)**
*Aventyl* **(Nortriptyline)**
*Avlosulfon* **(Dapsone)**
*Avonex* **(Interferon beta-1a)**
*Axert* **(Almotriptan)**
*Axocet* **(Butalbital)**
*Azactam* **(Aztreonam)**
**Azapropazone**
**Azatadine**
**Azelastine**
**Azithromycin**
*AZT* **(Zidovudine)**
**Aztreonam**
*Azulfidine* **(Sulfasalazine)**

**B**

*Backache Caplets* **(Magnesium salicylate)**
**Baclofen**
*Bactrim* **(Trimethoprim)**
*Bayer Aspirin* **(Acetylsalicylic acid)**
*BC Powder* **(Acetylsalicylic acid)**
**Beclomethasone**

*Beconase* **(Beclomethasone)**
*Benadryl* **(Diphenhydramine)**
**Benazepril**
*Bendectin* **(Doxylamine)**
**Bendroflumethiazide**
*BenGay* **(Methyl salicylate)**
*Benicar* **(Olmesartan)**
*Benoral* **(Benorilate)**
**Benorilate**
*Benorylate* **(Benorilate)**
**Benoxaprofen**
**Bepridil**
*Betaloc* **(Metoprolol)**
*Betapace* **(Sotalol)**
*Betaseron* **(Interferon beta-1b)**
**Betaxolol**
*Betaxon* **(Levobetaxolol)**
*Betimol* **(Timolol)**
*Betoptic* **(Betaxolol)**
*Bextra* **(Valdecoxib)**
*Bexxar* **(Tositumomab)**
*Biarison* **(Proquazone)**
*Biaxin* **(Clarithromycin)**
*Bicillin* **(Penicillin/Penicillin G)**
*Biphentin* **(Methylphenidate)**
*Biquin* **(Quinidine)**
**Bismuth subsalicylate**
**Bisoprolol**
*Blenoxane* **(Bleomycin)**
**Bleomycin**
*Blocadren* **(Timolol)**
*Bonamine* **(Meclizine)**
*Bondormin* **(Brotizolam)**
*Bonine* **(Meclizine)**
*Boniva* **(Ibandronate)**
**Bosentan**
*Botox* **(Botulinum Toxin Type A)**
*Botox Cosmetic* **(Botulinum Toxin Type A)**
**Botulinum Toxin**
**Botulinum Toxin Type A**
**Botulinum Toxin Type B**
*Brethaire* **(Terbutaline)**
*Brevicon* **(Ethinyl estradiol)**
*Brexido* **(Piroxicam)**
*Bricanyl* **(Terbutaline)**
**Bromodiphenhydramine**
**Brotizolam**
*Bufferin* **(Acetylsalicylic acid)**
**Bumetanide**
*Bumex* **(Bumetanide)**
**Bunazosin**
**Bupivacaine**
*Buprenex* **(Buprenorphine)**
**Buprenorphine**
**Bupropion**
*Burinex* **(Bumetanide)**
**Buserelin**
*BuSpar* **(Buspirone)**
**Buspirone**
**Butalbital**
**Butorphanol**
*Butrans* **(Buprenorphine)**
*Bystolic* **(Nebivolol)**

**C**

*Cadithro* **(Roxithromycin)**
*Caduet* **(Amlodipine)**
*Caelyx* **(Doxorubicin)**
*Caffedrine* **(Caffeine)**
**Caffeine**
*Calan* **(Verapamil)**
**Calcitonin**
*Campral* **(Acamprosate)**
**Candesartan**

*Capastat* **(Capreomycin)**
*Capoten* **(Captopril)**
*Capozide* **(Captopril)**
*Capozide 25* **(Captopril)**
**Capreomycin**
**Carbamazepine**
*Carbatrol* **(Carbamazepine)**
*Carbex* **(Selegiline)**
*Carbocaine* **(Mepivacaine)**
*Carbolith* **(Lithium)**
**Carboplatin**
**Carboprost**
*Cardene* **(Nicardipine)**
*Cardif* **(Nitrendipine)**
*Cardioquin* **(Quinidine)**
*Cardizem* **(Diltiazem)**
*Cardovar BD* **(Trimazosin)**
*Cardura* **(Doxazosin)**
*Cardura-2* **(Doxazosin)**
**Carprofen**
**Carteolol**
*Cartia XT* **(Diltiazem)**
*Cartrol* **(Carteolol)**
**Carvedilol**
*Cataflam* **(Diclofenac)**
*Catapres* **(Clonidine)**
*CDDP* **(Cisplatin)**
**Cefpodoxime**
**Cefprozil**
*Ceftin* **(Cefuroxime)**
**Cefuroxime**
*Cefzil* **(Cefprozil)**
*Celebrex* **(Celecoxib)**
**Celecoxib**
*Celectol* **(Celiprolol)**
*Celexa* **(Citalopram)**
**Celiprolol**
*CellCept* **(Mycophenolate)**
*Cenestin* **(Estradiol)**
*Centrax* **(Prozepam)**
*Cepastat* **(Acetylsalicylic acid)**
**Cephalexin**
*Cerebyx* **(Fosphenytoin)**
*Cerumenex* **(Triethanolamine)**
*Cesamet* **(Nabilone)**
**Cetirizine**
**Cetuximab**
**Cevimeline**
*Champix* **(Varenicline)**
*Chantix* **(Varenicline)**
*Chibroxin* **(Norfloxacin)**
*Children's Tylenol* **(Acetaminophen)**
*Chirocaine* **(Levobupivacaine)**
**Chloramphenicol**
**Chlordiazepoxide**
*Chloromycetin* **(Chloramphenicol)**
**Chloroprocaine**
**Chloroquine**
**Chlorpheniramine**
**Chlorphenoxamine**
**Chlorthalidone**
*Chlor-Trimeton* **(Chlorpheniramine)**
*Chlor-Tripolon* **(Chlorpheniramine)**
*Chlor-Tripolon Decongestant* **(Chlorpheniramine)**
*Chlor-Tripolon N.D.* **(Loratadine)**
**Cholestyramine**
**Choline magnesium trisalicylate**
*Choloxin* **(Dextrothyroxine)**
*Chronovera* **(Verapamil)**
*Cialis* **(Tadalafil)**
*Cicatrin* **(Neomycin)**
*Cidecin* **(Daptomycin)**
**Cidofovir**
*Cidomycin* **(Gentamicin)**

**Cilazapril**
**Cilostazol**
**Cimetidine**
**Cinnarizine**
*Cinobac* **(Cinoxacin)**
**Cinoxacin**
*Cipralex* **(Escitalopram)**
*Cipramil* **(Citalopram)**
*Cipro* **(Ciprofloxacin)**
*Cipro XL* **(Ciprofloxacin)**
*Ciprodex* **(Ciprofloxacin)**
**Ciprofloxacin**
*Ciproxin* **(Ciprofloxacin)**
**Cisplatin**
**Citalopram**
*Citanest* **(Prilocaine)**
**Clarithromycin**
*Claritin* **(Loratadine)**
*Claritin Extra* **(Loratadine)**
*Claritin Liberator* **(Loratadine)**
*Claritin-D* **(Loratadine)**
*Clarus* **(Isotretinoin)**
**Clemastine**
*Cleocin* **(Clindamycin)**
*Climara* **(Estradiol)**
**Clindamycin**
*Clinoril* **(Sulindac)**
*Clomid* **(Clomiphene)**
**Clomiphene**
**Clomipramine**
**Clonazepam**
**Clonidine**
*Clopixol* **(Zuclopenthixol)**
**Clorazepate**
*Clorpres* **(Clonidine)**
*Co-Actifed* **(Pseudoephedrine)**
*Coartem* **(Artemether/Lumefantrine)**
*Coated Aspirin* **(Acetylsalicylic acid)**
**Codeine**
*Codeine Contin* **(Codeine)**
*Cognexv* **(Tacrine)**
*Colazal* **(Mesalamine)**
*Combigan* **(Timolol)**
*Combipres* **(Clonidine)**
*Combivent* **(Ipratropium)**
*Combivir* **(Zidovudine)**
*Compound W* **(Salicylic acid)**
*Concerta* **(Methylphenidate)**
*Copaxone* **(Glatiramer)**
*Coptin* **(Sulfadiazine)**
*Cordarone* **(Amiodarone)**
*Coreg* **(Carvedilol)**
*Corgard* **(Nadolol)**
*Coricidin D* **(Phenylpropanolamine)**
**Corticotropin**
*Cortisporin* **(Neomycin)**
*Cortrosyn* **(Cosyntropin)**
*Corzide* **(Bendroflumethiazide)**
*Cosopt* **(Timolol)**
**Cosyntropin**
*Covera-HS* **(Verapamil)**
*Coversyl* **(Perindopril)**
*Coversyl Plus* **(Perindopril)**
*Cozaar* **(Losartan)**
*Crestor* **(Rosuvastatin)**
**Cromolyn sodium**
*Cubicin* **(Daptomycin)**
*Cuprimine* **(Penicillamine)**
*Cyclen* **(Ethinyl estradiol)**
**Cyclizine**
**Cyclobenzaprine**
**Cyclosporine**
*Cycrin* **(Medroxyprogesterone)**
*Cymbalta* **(Duloxetine)**

**Cypropheptadine**
*Cytotec* **(Misoprostol)**
*Cytovene* **(Ganciclovir)**

**D**

*Dalacin* **(Clindamycin)**
*Dalgan* **(Dezocine)**
*Dalmane* **(Flurazepam)**
**Dapsone**
**Daptomycin**
*Daranide* **(Dichlorphenamide)**
*Darvon* **(Propoxyphene)**
*Darvon Compound-65* **(Acetylsalicylic acid)**
*Darvon-N* **(Propoxyphene)**
**Dasatinib**
**Daunorubicin**
*DaunoXome* **(Daunorubicin)**
*Daypro* **(Oxaprozin)**
*Deanxit* **(Melitracen)**
*Debrox* **(Acetylsalicylic acid)**
*Declomycin* **(Demeclocycline)**
*De-Congestine* **(Chlorpheniramine)**
**Deferoxamine**
*Definity* **(Perflutren)**
*Dehydral* **(Methenamine—Hexamine)**
**Delavirdine**
Delta-9-tetrahydrocannabinol **(Dronabinol)**
*Deltasone* **(Prednisone)**
*Demadex* **(Torsemide)**
**Demeclocycline**
Demethylchlortetracycline **(Demeclocycline)**
*Demulen* **(Ethinyl estradiol)**
*Dentantol* **(Bunazosin)**
*Depacon* **(Valproate)**
*Depakene* **(Valproic acid)**
*Depakote* **(Divalproex)**
*Depakote ER* **(Divalproex)**
*Depen* **(Penicillamine)**
*Depo-Medrol with Lidocaine* **(Lidocaine)**
*Depo-Provera* **(Medroxyprogesterone)**
*Deprenyl* **(Selegiline)**
*Deproic* **(Valproic acid)**
*Desferal* **(Deferoxamine)**
*Desferroxamine* **(Deferoxamine)**
**Desipramine**
**Desogestrel—Ethinyl estradiol**
**Desvenlafaxine**
*Desyrel* **(Trazodone)**
**Dexfenfluramine**
*Dexilant* **(Dexlansoprazole)**
**Dexketoprofen**
**Dexlansoprazole**
**Dextrothyroxine**
**Dezocine**
*DHE* **(Dihydroergotamine)**
*Diamicron* **(Gliclazide)**
*Diamicron MR* **(Gliclazide)**
*Diamox* **(Acetazolamide)**
*Diane-35* **(Ethinyl estradiol)**
*Diastat* **(Diazepam)**
*Diazemuls* **(Diazepam)**
**Diazepam**
**Diazoxide**
**Dibekacin**
**Dichlorphenamide**
*Diclectin* **(Doxylamine)**
**Diclofenac**
**Diclofensine**
**Didanosine**
**Diflunisal**
**Dihydroergotamine**
*Dilacor* **(Diltiazem)**

*Dilaudid* **(Hydromorphone)**
*Dilaudid-HP* **(Hydromorphone)**
**Dilevalol**
**Diltiazem**
**Dimenhydrinate**
*Diochloram* **(Chloramphenicol)**
*Diovan* **(Valsartan)**
*Diovan HCT* **(Valsartan)**
*Dipentum* **(Olsalazine)**
**Diphenhydramine**
*Diprivan* **(Propofol)**
*Diprosalic* **(Salicylic acid)**
**Dipyridamole**
*Dipyrone* **(Aminopyrine)**
**Dirithromycin**
*Disalcid* **(Salsalate)**
*Diuretin* **(Sodium salicylate)**
**Divalproex**
*Dixarit* **(Clonidine)**
*Dixeran* **(Melitracen)**
*Dizac* **(Diazepam)**
*Doan's Analgesic Caplets* **(Magnesium salicylate)**
*Dodd's Pills* **(Sodium salicylate)**
**Dolasetron**
*Dolobid* **(Diflunisal)**
**Donepezil**
*Doral* **(Quazepam)**
*Dosulepin* **(Dothiepin)**
*Dotarem* **(Gadoterate)**
**Dothiepin**
**Doxazosin**
**Doxepin**
*Doxil* **(Doxorubicin)**
**Doxorubicin**
**Doxycycline**
**Doxylamine**
*Dramamine* **(Dimenhydrinate)**
*Drisdol* **(Ergocalciferal)**
*Dristan Sinus* **(Ibuprofen)**
**Dronabinol**
**Drospirenone—Ethinyl estradiol**
**Duloxetine**
*DuoFilm* **(Salicylic acid)**
*DuoTrav* **(Travoprost)**
*Duraclon* **(Clonidine)**
*Duragesic* **(Fentanyl)**
*Duralith* **(Lithium)**
*Duranest* **(Etidocaine)**
*Dyclone* **(Dyclonine)**
**Dyclonine**
*Dynabac* **(Dirithromycin)**
*Dynacin* **(Minocycline)**
*DynaCirc* **(Isradipine)**
*Dynastat* **(Parecoxib)**

**E**

*E.E.S.* **(Erythromycin)**
*Easprin* **(Acetylsalicylic acid)**
*Ebixa* **(Memantine)**
*EC-Naprosyn* **(Naproxen)**
*Ecotrin Enteric-coated Aspirin* **(Acetylsalicylic acid)**
**Eculizumab**
*Edecrin* **(Ethacrynic acid)**
*Edluar* **(Zolpidem)**
**Efavirenz**
*Effexor* **(Venlafaxine)**
*Effexor XR* **(Venlafaxine)**
*ELA-Max* **(Lidocaine)**
*Elavil* **(Amitriptyline)**
*Elavil Plus* **(Amitriptyline)**
*Eldepryl* **(Selegiline)**
**Eletriptan**
*Eligard* **(Leuprolide)**
*Elmiron* **(Pentosan)**

*Elocon* **(Mometasone)**
*Emadine* **(Emedastine)**
**Emedastine**
*Emend* **(Aprepitant)**
*Emend IV* **(Aprepitant)**
*Emflex* **(Acemetacin)**
*Emla* **(Lidocaine)**
*Emsam* **(Selegiline)**
*E-Mycin* **(Erythromycin)**
**Enalapril**
*Enalaprilat* **(Enalapril)**
*Enbrel* **(Etanercept)**
*Enduron* **(Methyclothiazide)**
*Engerix-B* **(Hepatitis B vaccine)**
**Enoxacin**
*Entrophen* **(Acetylsalicylic acid)**
*Epiject* **(Divalproex)**
*Epival* **(Divalproex)**
**Eprosartan**
*Equetro* **(Carbamazepine)**
*Erbitux* **(Cetuximab)**
**Ergocalciferal**
*Ergometrine* **(Ergonovine)**
**Ergonovine**
*Ergotrate* **(Ergonovine)**
*Eryc* **(Erythromycin)**
*Ery-Ped* **(Erythromycin)**
*Ery-Tab* **(Erythromycin)**
*Erythrocin* **(Erythromycin)**
**Erythromycin**
**Escitalopram**
*Esgic-Plus* **(Butalbital)**
*Esidrix* **(Hydrochlorothiazide)**
*Esimil* **(Hydrochlorothiazide)**
*Eskalith* **(Lithium)**
**Esomeprazole**
**Estazolam**
*Estraderm* **(Estradiol)**
**Estradiol**
*Estring* **(Estradiol)**
**Eszopiclone**
**Etanercept**
**Ethacrynic acid**
**Ethinyl estradiol**
*Ethmozine* **(Moricizine)**
**Etidocaine**
**Etodolac**
*Etonogestrel—Ethinyl estradiol* **(Ethinyl estradiol)**
**Etoricoxib**
*Etrafon* **(Amitriptyline)**
*Eufans* **(Amtolmetin)**
*Euglucon* **(Glyburide)**
*Evoxac* **(Cevimeline)**
*Evra* **(Norelgestromin)**
*Exbenzol* **(Mebendazole)**
*Excedrin Back & Body* **(Acetylsalicylic acid)**
*Excedrin Extra Strength* **(Acetylsalicylic acid)**
*Excedrin Migraine* **(Acetylsalicylic acid)**
*Exelon* **(Rivastigmine)**
*Exforge* **(Amlodipine)**
*Exforge HCT* **(Amlodipine)**
*Extavia* **(Interferon beta-1b)**
Ezetimibe
*Ezetrol* **(Ezetimibe)**

**F**

*Fabrazyme* **(Agalsidase beta)**
**Famotidine**
*Fanapt* **(Iloperidone)**
*Fanapta* **(Iloperidone)**
*Fansidar* **(Sulfadoxine—Pyrimethamine)**
*Farlutal* **(Medroxyprogesterone)**

**Febuxostat**
*Feldene* **(Piroxicam)**
**Felodipine**
*Femtran* **(Estradiol)**
**Fenbufen**
**Fenofibrate**
**Fenoprofen**
**Fentanyl**
*Fentora* **(Fentanyl)**
**Feprazone**
**Fexofenadine**
*Fioricet* **(Butalbital)**
*Fioricet with Codeine* **(Butalbital)**
*Fiorinal* **(Butalbital)**
*Fiorinal with Codeine* **(Butalbital)**
*Fiorinal-C* **(Butalbital)**
*Flagyl* **(Metronidazole)**
**Flecainide**
*Flexeril* **(Cyclobenzaprine)**
**Floctafenine**
*Flomax* **(Tamsulosin)**
*Flonase* **(Fluticasone)**
*Florazole* **(Metronidazole)**
*Flovent* **(Fluticasone)**
*Floxicam* **(Isoxicam)**
*Floxin* **(Ofloxacin)**
*Fluarix* **(Influenza vaccine)**
*Flulaval* **(Influenza vaccine)**
*Flumadine* **(Rimantadine)**
**Flumazenil**
**Fluoxetine**
**Flurazepam**
**Flurbiprofen**
*FluShield* **(Influenza vaccine)**
**Fluticasone**
**Fluvoxamine**
*Fluzone* **(Influenza vaccine)**
**Fomepizole**
*Fortimicin* **(Astromicin)**
*Fortovase* **(Saquinavir)**
*Fosamax* **(Alendronate)**
*Fosaprepitant* **(Aprepitant)**
*Fosavance* **(Alendronate)**
**Foscarnet**
*Foscavir* **(Foscarnet)**
**Fosinopril**
*Fosint* **(Indoprofen)**
**Fosphenytoin**
*Fradiomycin* **(Neomycin)**
*Froben* **(Flurbiprofen)**
*Frova* **(Frovatriptan)**
**Frovatriptan**
*Frusemide* **(Furosemide)**
*Fungizone* **(Amphotericin B)**
Furosemide

**G**

**Gabapentin**
*Gabitril* **(Tiagabine)**
**Gadobenate**
**Gadodiamide**
**Gadopentetate**
**Gadoterate**
**Gadoteridol**
**Gadoversetamide**
**Galantamine**
**Gallium nitrate**
**Ganciclovir**
*Ganite* **(Gallium nitrate)**
*Gantanol* **(Sulfamethoxazole)**
*Gantrisin* **(Sulfisoxazole)**
*Garamycin* **(Gentamicin)**
*Garasone* **(Gentamicin)**
*Gastrocrom* **(Cromolyn sodium)**

Rabau, S., et. al. Changes over Time of Psychoacoustic Outcome Measurements Are Not a Substitute for Subjective Outcome Measurements in Acute Tinnitus. European Archives of Oto-Rhino-Laryngology (January 2014). Reported in: Tinnitus Today. Spring 2014.

Researchers Map Tinnitus in Human Brain During Surgery. HearingReview. Com. July, 2015.

Results from ATA's Membership Survey. Tinnitus Today. Spring, 2014.

Reuter, Anne. 2007. Nutrients Might Prevent Hearing Loss in War Zones, Concert Halls and Workplaces, New Animal Study Suggests. University of Michigan Health System. http://www.med.umich.edu/opm/newspage/2007/hearingloss.htm.

Rezen, Susan & Carl Hausman. 1985. Coping with Hearing Loss: a Guide for Adults and Their Families. Dembner Books, New York, N.Y.

Rizer, Franklin, MD. 2004. Inner Ear, Tinnitus. eMedicine. [http://emedicine.com/ent/topic235.htm].

Robb, Michael, M.D. 2015. A Silver Jubilee Tribute to Pawel J. Jastreboff, Ph.D., Sc.D., MBA. Tinnitus Today, Winter 2015.

Rocha, Carina. 2015. When Should a Patient with Tinnitus be Referred to a Physiotherapist? Audiology WorldNews. June 18, 2015. http://www.audiology-worldnews.com/focus-on/1362-when-should-a-patient-with-tinnitus-be-referred-to-a-physiotherapist.

Salicylate Sensitivity—Info2. 2011. http://salicylatesensitivity.com/info2.

Salicylate Sensitivity—Info3. 2011. http://salicylatesensitivity.com/info3.

Salicylate Sensitivity—Info4. 2011. http://salicylatesensitivity.com/info4.

Sanchez, Tanit Ganz, and Carina Bezerra Rocha. "Diagnosis and Management of Somatosensory Tinnitus: Review Article." *Clinics* 66.6 (2011): 1089–1094. *PMC*. Web. 24 Dec. 2015. http://www.ncbi.nlm.nih.gov/pmc/articles/PMC3129953.

Sanders, Barbara. 2004. A Year's Worth of Tinnitus Research. From Healthy Hearing, January 5, 2004.

Sauer, Elaine. 1992. Life with Tinnitus. Listen. Summer, 1992. Canadian Hard of Hearing Association.

Schleuning, Alexander. ~2003. Notes from *Otolaryngology Head and Neck Surgery*, Eighth Edition. [http://www.tinnitusearringing.com/pulsitile_tinnitus2.htm].

Shafer, James, Au. D. 2009. Personal Communication. A C Tinnitus—Hearing and Balance Center, Inc.. 1776 S. Queen St. York, PA. 17403. http://www.actinnitus.com.

Shatner, William. 1997. Sound of Silence. People. [http://www.pathfinder.com/people/970519/features/shatner.html].

Shea, John. ~2004. Lidocaine Perfusion—A Detailed Look. Shea Ear Clinic. Memphis, TN. [http://www.sheaclinic.com/services_9.asp].

Shellock, Frank. 2015. Acoustic Noise and MRI Procedures. http://www.mrisafety.com/SafetyInfov.asp?SafetyInfoID=252.

Shepherd, N. L. 2002. Hearing Products Report. Nov/Dec 2002.

Sinopoli, Teri et al. August, 2007. Tinnitus: Addressing Neurological, Audiological, and Psychological Aspects with Customized Therapy. The Hearing Review. [http://www.hearingreview.com/issues/articles/2007-08_03.asp].

Smith, Pohla. November, 2007. Music Therapy Shows Promise for Tinnitus Sufferers. http://www.post-gazette.com/pg/07332/837125-114.stm.

Some Theories of AIT. 1997. Society for Auditory Integration Training. Salem, Oregon 97302. [http:///www.sait.org/theories.html].

SoundCure. 2015. The Science. http://www.soundcure.com/for-patients/the-science.

Source of "Ringing of the Ears" Extends Beyond Hearing Systems. Feb. 27, 2001. Science News. [http://www.cosmiverse.com/science02270104.html].

Steenerson, Ronald, et. al. 1999. The Treatment of Annoying Tinnitus with Electrical Stimulation. The International Tinnitus Journal. Vol. 5. No. 1. http://www.tinnitusjournal.com/detalhe_artigo.asp?id=253.

Stanten, Michele. 1996. 150 Secrets to Erase the Signs of Aging. Rodale Press. Emmaus, PA.

Stracke, Henning, et al. 2010. Customized Notched Music Training Reduces Tinnitus Loudness. Communicative & Integrative Biology 3:3, 1-4;

May/June 2010. http://www.landesbioscience.com/journals/cib/StrackeCIB3-3.pdf.

Steele & Steele. 1997a. Hearing Loss and Sound Therapy. [http://www.intouchmag.com/soundtherapy1.html].

Steele & Steele. 1997b. Tinnitus, Vertigo and Sound Therapy. [http://www.intouchmag.com/soundtherapy5.html].

Study Explores Mindfulness-based Tinnitus Relief. 2015. Hearing Review. June, 2015.

Swain, Anne R, et. al. 1985. Salicylates in foods. http://www.slhd.nsw.gov.au/rpa/Allergy/research/salicylatesinfoods.pdf.

Sweetow, Robert. 1998. Tinnitus. University of California, San Francisco. [http://www.audiology.org/tinnitus.htm].

Sweetow, Robert, et. al. 2015a. Do Tinnitus Patients Continue to Use Amplification and Sound Therapy Post Habilitation? HearingReview.Com. March, 2015.

Sweetow, Robert, et. al. 2015b. A Controlled Study on the Effectiveness of Fractal Tones on Subjects with Minimal Need for Amplification. HearingReview.Com. September, 2015.

Tanase, Adam. 2015. Tinnitus (Ringing in the Ear). St. Louis Chiropractor. http://www.chiropracticstl.com/tinnitus-vertigo-relief.

Teachey, William S., et. al. 2012. Tinnitus of Myofascial Origin. International Tinnitus Journal. Vol. 17. No. 1. http://www.tinnitusjournal.com/imagebank/pdf/v17n1a13.pdf.

Thong, J. F., et. al. 2014. Habituation Following Tinnitus Retraining Therapy in Tinnitus Sufferers. Annals, Academy of Medicine, Singapore. Reported in: Tinnitus Today. Spring 2014.

Tinnitus 1-2-3. 2012. Chiropractic Treatment for Tinnitus—Can Spinal Adjustment Help with Ringing Ears? http://www.tinnitus123.com/chiropractic-treatment-for-tinnitus.

Tinnitus & Your Hearing. 1998. Health Touch Online. [http://www.healthouch.com/level1/leaflets/hhirr/hhirr016.htm].

Tinnitus and Hearing Loss. 2011. http://ehealthmd.com/library/tinnitus/TIN_loss.html.

Tinnitus Archive. 2004. Pocket Summary Data Set 1. Oregon Health & Science University. http://www.tinnitusArchive.org.

Tinnitus Association of Calgary. Calgary, AB.

Tinnitus Attributes; 1996. Pocket Summary Data Set 1. Oregon Hearing Research Center. Oregon Health & Science University. [http://gems.tinnitusarchive.org:81/www/pocketSummaryDataSet1.pdf].

Tinnitus Functional Index. 2015. Audiology.Org. http://www.audiology.org/news/tinnitus-functional-index.

Tinnitus: Is This What Happens When the Brain's Gatekeeper Breaks Down? 2011. [http://www.nidcd.nih.gov/news/releases/11/031611.htm].

Tinnitus Resources. 2002. Seattle Acoustic Neuroma Group. References & Resources on Acoustic Neuroma. [http://acousticneuromaseattle.org/refrestinnitus.html].

Tinnitus Synergy. 2014. What Is the Therapy to Remove Trigger Points of Tinnitus? http://tinnitussynergy.com/wp-content/uploads/2014/10/WhatistheTherapytoRemoveTriggerPointsofTinnitus.pdf.

Tinnitus Treatment Options. 2002. American Tinnitus Association. [http://www.ata.org/about_tinnitus/consumer/treatment.html].

Trauma of Sensory Loss.

Treatment Possibilities. 1997. Tinnitus FAQ. [http://www.cccd.edu/faq/tinnitus/treatment.html].

Tunkel, David. E., et. al. 2014. Clinical Practice Guideline: Tinnitus. Otolaryngology—Head and Neck Surgery. http://oto.sagepub.com/content/151/2_suppl/S1.full.pdf+html.

UB Study Finds That "Crossed Wires" in Brain Pathways Controlling Vision and Hearing Play a Role in Tinnitus. 2002. University at Buffalo. [http://www.buffalo.edu/research/6neurology.shtml].

University of Leicester. 2012. Key Cellular Mechanisms Behind the Onset of Tinnitus Identified. In: ScienceDaily. http://www.sciencedaily.com/releases/2012/05/120510100044.htm.

University of Texas at Dallas. 2011. Tinnitus Treatment: Rebooting the Brain Helps Stop the Ring of Tinnitus in Rats. ScienceDaily. January 13, 2011. http://www.sciencedaily.com/releases/2011/01/110112132130.htm.

Using Vitamin A to Treat Tinnitus. 1999. [http://www.alphatinnitusformulas.com/tinnitus_vitamin_a.asp].

Vanneste, Sven, et. al. 2010. Transcutaneous Electrical Nerve Stimulation (TENS) of Upper Cervical Nerve (C2) for the Treatment of Somatic Tinnitus. SpringerLink. Research Note. July 2010, Vol. 204. Issue 2, pp. 283-287. http://link.springer.com/article/10.1007%2Fs00221-010-2304-5#/page-1.

Vanneste, Sven. 2014. Tuning the Tinnitus Brain. Hearing Journal. September, 2014.

Vernick, David M. & Constance Grzelka. 1993. The Hearing Loss Handbook. Consumer Reports Books. Yonkers, N.Y.

Wade, Dr. Phillip S. 1995. Tinnitus Update–1995. Vibes. December, 1995. The Canadian Hearing Society. 271 Spadina Road. Toronto, Ontario M5R 2V3.

Walsh, Paul. 1997. Psychological Approach. Oto-calm Tinnitus Clinic. [http://www.otocalm.net.au/psy.htm].

Wenger, Jennifer. 2011. Rebooting the Brain Helps Stop the Ring of Tinnitus in Rats. NIDCD. January 12, 2011. http://www.nidcd.nih.gov/news/releases/11/Pages/011211.aspx.

"'We Cannot Do Anything About Your Tinnitus.' This is Simply Not True" January 28, 2016. Audiology WorldNews. http://www.audiology-worldnews.com/focus-on/1547-we-cannot-do-anything-about-your-tinnitus-this-is-simply-not-true?showall=&limitstart=.

Whittaker, Jason. 2013. How Can a Chiropractor Help with Tinnitus? http://entertogetwell.ca/tinnitus.

Wilden, Lutz & Dirk Ellerbrock. 1999. On the Effectiveness of Low-Level Laser Light (LLLL) in the Inner Ear. [http://www.dr-wilden.de/ehtmls/puben1.html].

Williams, Mike. 2015. Hyperbaric Hope for Fibromyalgia Sufferers. Rice University. http://news.rice.edu/2015/06/02/hyperbaric-hope-for-fibromyalgia-sufferers-2.

Zagolski, O., p. Strek. Tinnitus Pitch and Minimum Masking Levels in Different Etiologies. International Journal of Audiology (March 2014). As reported in: Tinnitus Today. Summer, 2014. All about Tinnitus. 2001. Acoustic Neuroma Archive. http://www.anarchive.org/tinnitus.htm.

# Good Books on Hearing Loss

**Integrity First Books** in the series:

***Everything You Wanted to Know About Your Hearing Loss But Were Afraid to Ask***
***(Because You Knew You Wouldn't Hear the Answers Anyway!)***
**by Neil G. Bauman, Ph.D.**

If you have enjoyed this book and would like to learn more about hearing loss and how you can successfully live with it, you may be interested in some helpful books by Dr. Neil. Each book is packed with the things you need to know in order to thrive in spite of your various hearing loss issues. The direct link to the following books is at http://hearinglosshelp.com/shop/category/books/.

***Ototoxic Drugs Exposed—The Shocking Truth About Prescription Drugs, Medications, Chemicals and Herbals That Can (and Do) Damage Our Ears*** ($52.45; eBook $39.95)

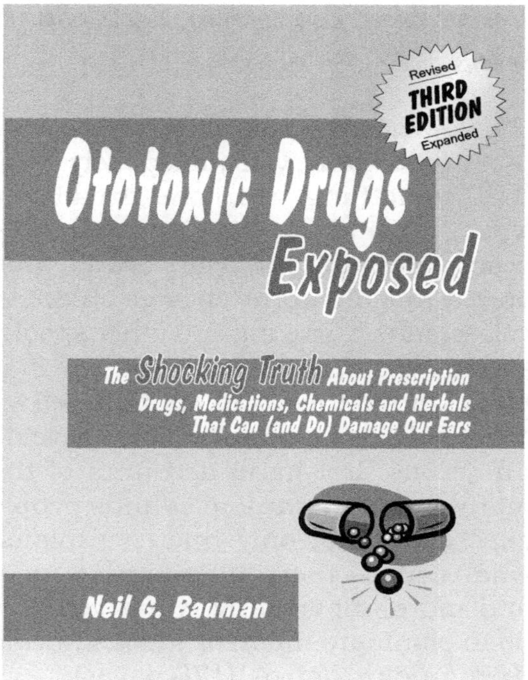


This book, now in its third edition, reveals the shocking truth that many prescription drugs can damage your ears. Some drugs slowly and insidiously rob you of your hearing, cause your ears to ring or destroy your balance. Other drugs can smash your ears in one fell swoop, leaving you with profound, permanent hearing loss and bringing traumatic change into your life. Learn how to protect your ears from the ravages of ototoxic drugs and chemicals. Describes the specific ototoxic effects of 877 drugs, 35 herbals and 148 chemicals. (798 pages)

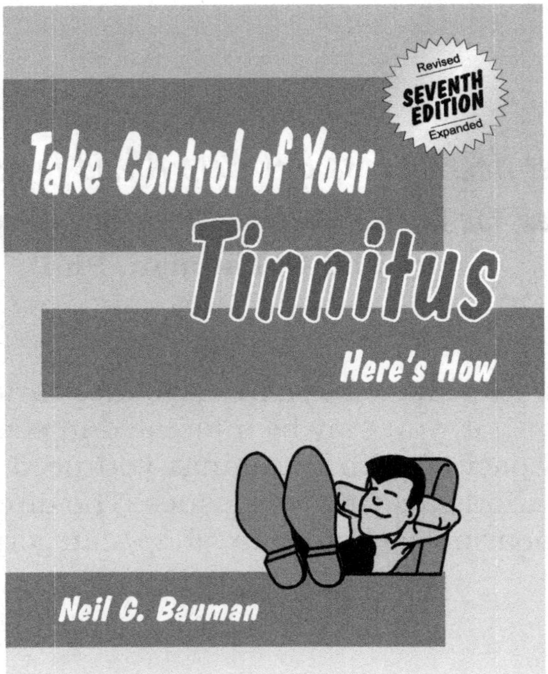


***Take Control of Your Tinnitus—Here's How*** ($29.95; eBook $22.99)

If your ears ring, buzz, chirp, hiss, click or roar, you know just how annoying tinnitus can be. The good news is that you do not have to put up with this racket for the rest of your life. You can take control of your tinnitus. Recent studies show that a lot of what we thought we knew about tinnitus is not true at all. Exciting new research reveals a number of things that you can do to eliminate or greatly reduce the severity of your tinnitus so that it no longer bothers you. This totally-revised, up-to-date and expanded 7th edition contains the very latest in tinnitus research and treatment. In this book you will learn what tinnitus is, what causes tinnitus and things you can do to take control of your tinnitus. (356 pages)

***Phantom Voices, Ethereal Music & Other Spooky Sounds*** ($22.49; eBook $16.99)

When you realize you are hearing phantom sounds, you immediately think that something has gone dreadfully wrong "upstairs"—that you are going crazy. Because of this, few people openly talk about the strange phantom voices, music, singing and other spooky sounds they hear. This book, the first of its kind in the world, lifts the veil on "Musical Ear syndrome" and reveals numerous first-hand accounts of the many strange phantom sounds people experience. Not only that, it explains what causes these phantom sounds, and more importantly, what you can do to eliminate them, or at least, bring them under control. (178 pages)

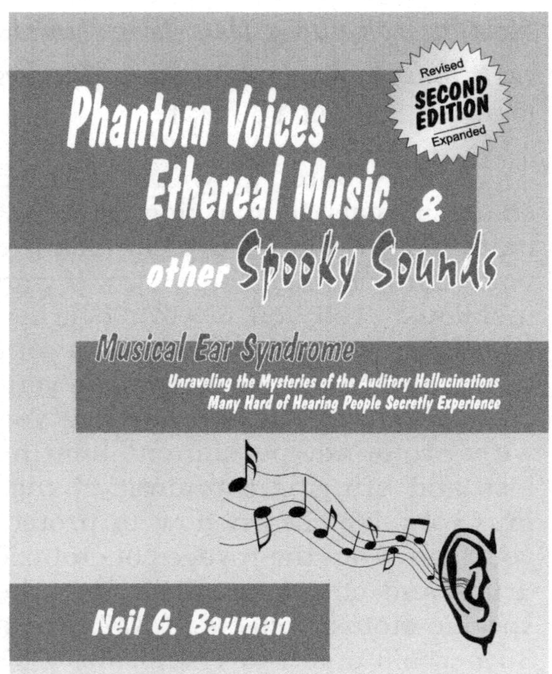

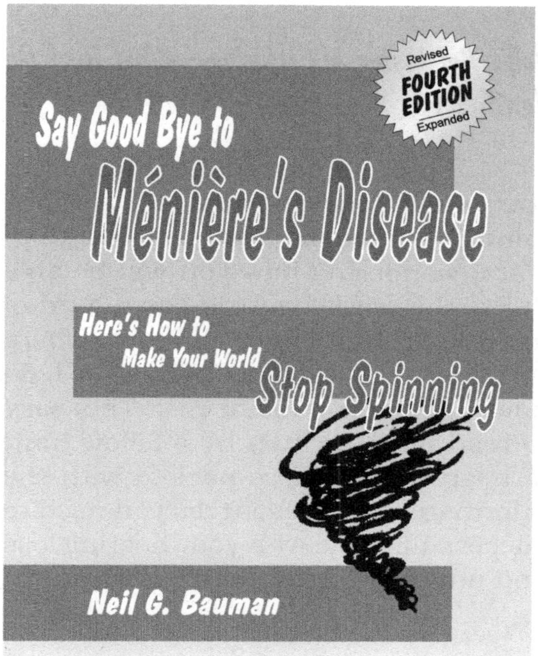


***Say Good Bye to Ménière's Disease—Here's How to Make Your World Stop Spinning*** ($21.95; eBook $16.49)

Ménière's disease is one of the more baffling and incapacitating conditions a person can experience. If you suffer from your world spinning, have a fluctuating hearing loss, tinnitus and a feeling of fullness in your ears, this book is for you. It details what Ménière's disease is like; explains the recent breakthrough into the underlying cause of Ménière's; and shows you how, at last, you can be free from the ravages of this debilitating condition. Each page is packed with practical information to help you successfully conquer your Meniere's disease. Join the hundreds and hundreds of people whose worlds have now stopped spinning (128 pages).

***Keys to Successfully Living with Your Hearing Loss*** ($19.97; eBook $15.49)

Do you know: a) the critical missing element to successfully living with your hearing loss? b) that the No. 1 coping strategy hard of hearing people instinctively use is wrong, wrong, wrong? c) what the single most effective hearing loss coping strategy is? d) how you can turn your hearing aids into awesome hearing devices? This book addresses the surprising answers to these and other critical questions. Applying them to your life will put you well on the road to successfully living with your hearing loss. (84 pages)

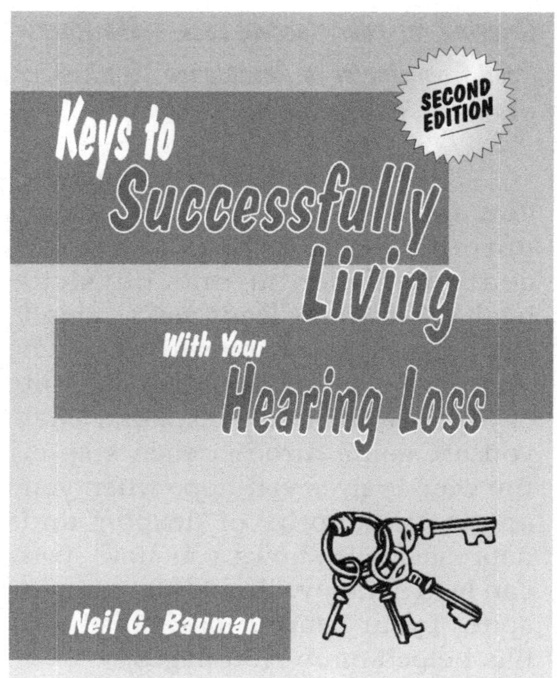

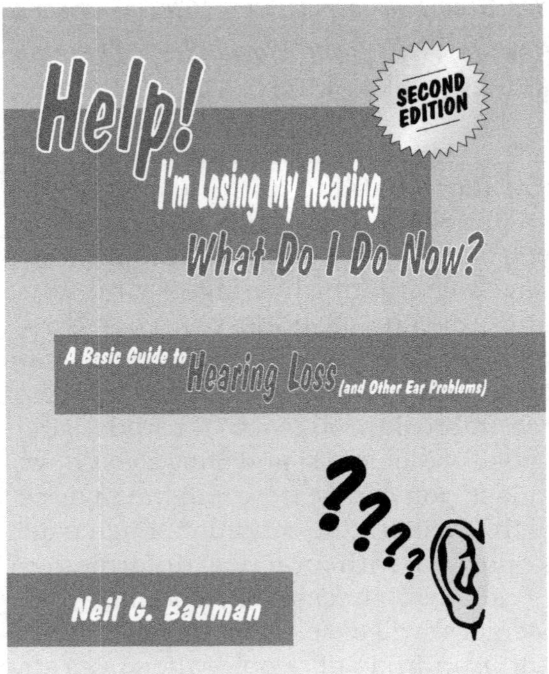


***Help! I'm Losing My Hearing—What Do I Do Now?*** ($18.95; eBook $14.49)

Losing your hearing can flip your world upside down and leave your mind in a turmoil. You may be full of fears, wondering how you will be able to live the rest of your life as a hard of hearing person. You don't know where to turn. You lament, "What do I do now?" Set your mind at rest. This easy to read book, written by a fellow hard of hearing person, is packed with the information and resources you need to successfully deal with your hearing loss and other ear conditions. (116 pages)

***Grieving for Your Hearing Loss—The Rocky Road from Denial to Acceptance*** ($12.95; eBook $9.95)

When you lose your hearing you need to grieve. This is not optional—but critical to your continued mental and physical health. This book leads you through the process of dealing with the grief and pain you experience as a result of your hearing loss. It explains what you are going through each step of the way. It gives you hope when you are in the depths of despair and depression. It shows you how you can lead a happy vibrant life again in spite of your hearing loss. This book has helped many. (56 pages)

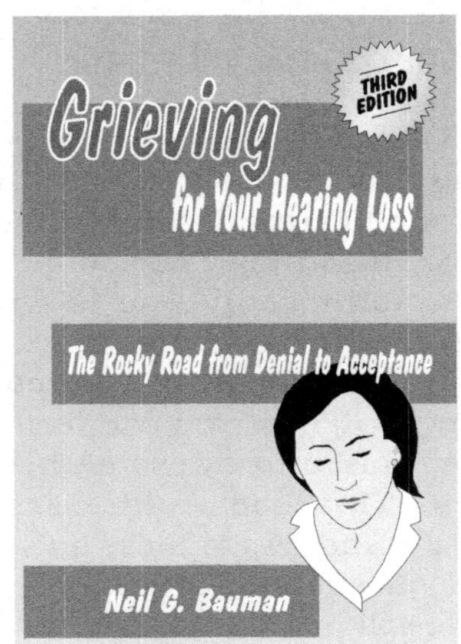

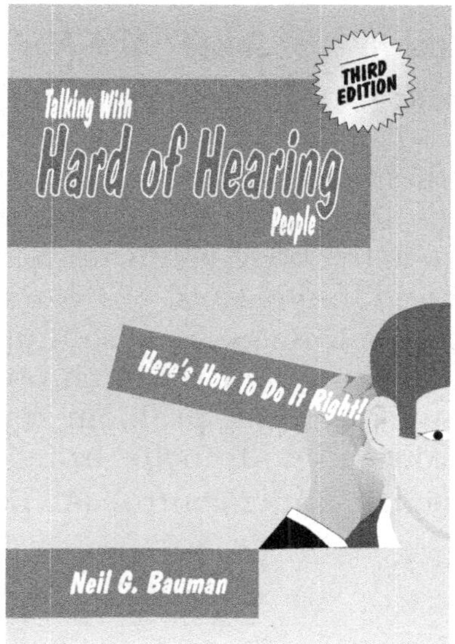


***Talking with Hard of Hearing People—Here's How to Do It Right!*** ($9.95; eBook $7.95)

Talking is important to all of us. When communication breaks down, we all suffer. For hard of hearing people this happens all the time. This book is for you—whether you are hearing or hard of hearing! It explains how to communicate with hard of hearing people in one-to-one situations, in groups and meetings, in emergency situations, and in hospitals and nursing homes. When you use the principles given in this book, good things will happen and you will finally be able to have a comfortable chat with a hard of hearing person. (38 pages)

***When Hearing Loss Ambushes Your Ears—Here's What Happens When Your Hearing Goes on the Fritz*** ($14.95; eBook $11.95)

Hearing loss often blind-sides you. As a result, your first step should be to learn as much as you can about your hearing loss; then you will be able to cope better. This most interesting book explains how your ears work, the causes of hearing loss, what you can expect to hear with different levels of hearing loss and why you often can't understand what you hear. Lots of audiograms and charts help make things clear. You will also discover a lot of fascinating things about how loud noises damage your ears. (88 pages)

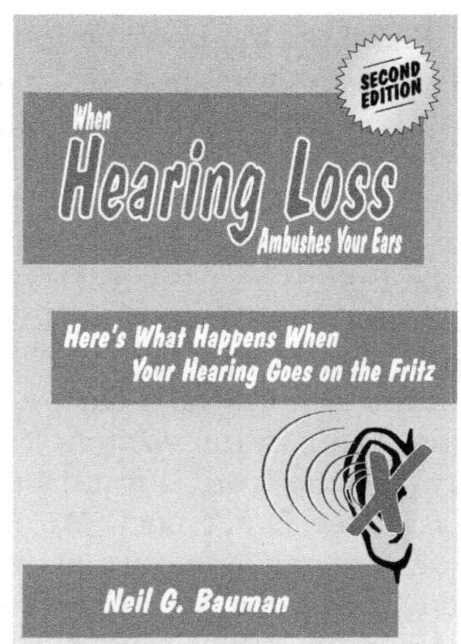

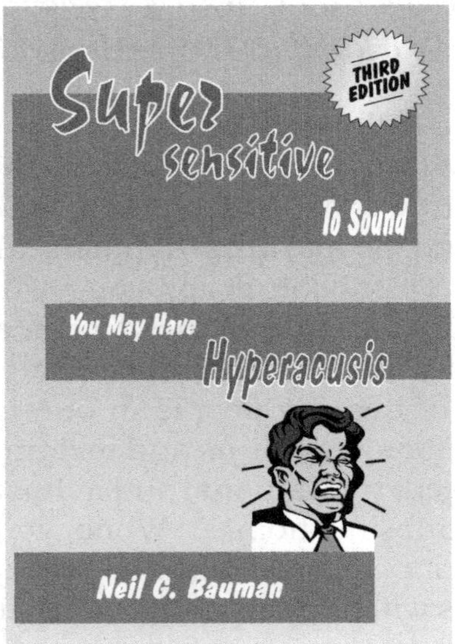


***Supersensitive to Sound? You May Have Hyperacusis*** ($9.95; eBook $7.95)

If some (or all) normal sounds seem so loud they blow your socks off, this is the book you want to read! You don't have to avoid noise or lock yourself away in a soundproof room. Exciting new research on this previously baffling problem reveals what you can do to help bring your hyperacusis under control. (42 pages)

***Here! Here! You and Your Hearing Loss/You and Your Hearing Aids*** ($12.95; eBook $10.95)

Part I of this book contains a series of my newspaper articles on hearing loss such as, "Hear Today. Gone Tomorrow?" "Hearing Loss Is Sneaky!" "The Wages of Din Is Deaf!" "When Your Ears Ring..." "Get In My Face Before You Speak!" "How's That Again?" "Being Hard of Hearing Is Hard" "I'm Deaf, Not Daft!" Part II contains articles on hearing aids such as, "You Better Watch Out..." "Before Buying Your First Hearing Aid..." "Please Don't Lock Me Away in Your Drawer" "Good-bye World of Silence!" "Becoming Friends with Your Hearing Aids" "Two's Better Than One!". (56 pages)

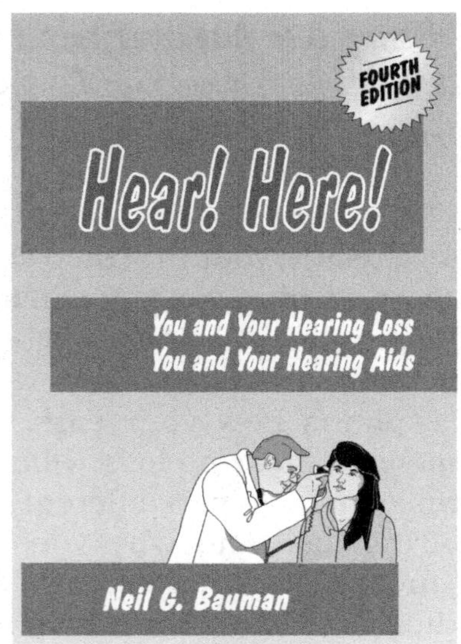

You can order any of the foregoing books/eBooks (plus you can read more than 1,000 other helpful articles about hearing loss and related issues) from the

**Center for Hearing Loss Help**

web site at

http://hearinglosshelp.com

or order them from the address below

Center for Hearing Loss Help

1013 Ridgeway Drive,
Lynden, WA 98264-1057
Phone: (360) 778-1266
FAX: (360) 389-5226
E-mail: info@hearinglosshelp.com
Web site: http://hearinglosshelp.com

26882055R00196

Made in the USA
Columbia, SC
23 September 2018